Addiction Psychiatric Medicine

Addiction Psychiatric Medicine

A COMPREHENSIVE BOARD REVIEW

HÉCTOR A. COLÓN-RIVERA, MD, CMRO

General, Addictions and Adolescent Psychiatrist,
Faculty and Attending Physician,
University of Pittsburgh Medical Center,
Psychiatry Department, Pittsburgh, Pennsylvania
Medical Director, APM, Philadelphia, Pennsylvania

ELIE G. AOUN, MD, MRO, FAPA

General, Addictions and Forensic Psychiatrist,
Assistant Professor of Clinical Psychiatry,
Columbia University College of Physicians and Surgeons - Division of Law,
Ethics, and Psychiatry, New York, New York

LEILA M. VAEZAZIZI, MD

Clinical Instructor and Addiction Psychiatrist,
Montefiore Medical Center/Albert Einstein College of Medicine, New York, New York
Faculty, New York University School of Medicine, New York, New York

ELSEVIER

Elsevier

1600 John F. Kennedy Blvd.
Ste 1800
Philadelphia, PA 19103-2899

ADDICTION PSYCHIATRIC MEDICINE: A COMPREHENSIVE BOARD REVIEW

ISBN: 978-0-323-75486-6

Notice

Practitioners and researchers must always rely on their own experience and knowledge in evaluating and using any information, methods, compounds or experiments described herein. Because of rapid advances in the medical sciences, in particular, independent verification of diagnoses and drug dosages should be made. To the fullest extent of the law, no responsibility is assumed by Elsevier, authors, editors or contributors for any injury and/or damage to persons or property as a matter of products liability, negligence or otherwise, or from any use or operation of any methods, products, instructions, or ideas contained in the material herein.

Senior Content Strategist: Melanie Tucker
Content Development Specialist: Laura Fisher
Senior Content Development Manager: Laura Schmidt
Publishing Services Manager: Deepthi Unni
Senior Project Manager: Manchu Mohan
Senior Book Designer: Margaret Reid

Printed in India.

Last digit is the print number: 9 8 7 6 5 4 3 2

Working together
to grow libraries in
developing countries

www.elsevier.com • www.bookaid.org

CONTENTS

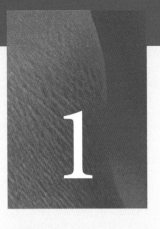

1

GENERAL PRINCIPLES OF SUBSTANCE USE DISORDERS

DEFINITIONS OF SUBSTANCE USE DISORDERS AND DIAGNOSTIC EVALUATIONS

Although persons with a substance use disorder (SUD) use drugs or alcohol, using these substances does not necessarily mean that a given person meets SUD diagnostic criteria. Indeed, in 2012, the *American Psychiatric Association's Diagnostic and Statistical Manual, 5th Edition* (DSM-5) set diagnostic phenomenological parameters for SUD diagnoses. These replace older diagnoses of substance abuse and substance dependence from the DSM's previous editions.

DSM-5 definition of SUD: A maladaptive substance use pattern leading to significant impairment or distress. This definition is met when a person meets at least two of the following 11 diagnostic criteria within a 12-month period:

Loss of Control
1. Substance taken in larger amount or for a longer period than intended
2. Persistent desire or unsuccessful efforts to control or stop substance use
3. Craving or a strong desire or urge to use the substance
4. Use continues despite knowledge of resultant physical or psychological problems
5. Continued use in situations in which it is physically hazardous

Adverse Consequences
6. Great deal of time spent to obtain, use, or recover from effects
7. Use resulting in a failure to fulfill major role obligations

8. Continued use despite recurrent social or interpersonal problems
9. Use resulting in important social, occupational, or recreational activities given up or reduced

Physiological Dependence
10. Tolerance
11. Withdrawal

Note that for individuals developing tolerance or withdrawal to a medically prescribed substance, tolerance and withdrawal do not count in diagnosing a SUD.

SUD severity is assessed by the number of diagnostic criteria (2–3: mild; 4–5: moderate; 6 or more: severe), not by the severity of substance use or the severity of any individual criteria.

A SUD diagnosis can be further qualified as:

- Early remission: When a person who previously met diagnostic criteria for SUD has not met any diagnostic criteria (except for craving) for longer than three months.
- Sustained remission: When a person who previously met SUD, diagnostic criteria has not met any diagnostic criteria (except for craving) for longer than 12 months.
- On maintenance therapy: When a person who previously met diagnostic criteria for SUD has not met any diagnostic criteria (except for tolerance or withdrawal) as a result of being prescribed maintenance medications (referring to full or partial agonists and antagonist medications such as naltrexone, buprenorphine, or methadone).

■ In a controlled environment: When a person who previously met diagnostic criteria for SUD is abstinent as a result of no longer having access to the substance when in an environment where access to the substance is restricted (such as correctional detention or residential rehabilitation programs).

Physiological dependence refers to the state resulting from repeated use of a substance marked by tolerance and/or withdrawal symptoms:

■ Tolerance to a given substance is a phenomenon marked by requiring a higher dose of the substance to achieve the same intoxicating effect (alternatively, it can be conceptualized as experiencing a reduced effect if the individual consumed their usual dose).
■ Withdrawal is a syndrome occurring following discontinuation or reduction of substance use marked by symptoms opposite to the expected effects of that substance. Resuming substance use would reverse the withdrawal and relieve these symptoms.

The 4 C's is another commonly used working description of the components of SUD.
Working Definitions of Addiction:

■ Compulsion
■ Loss of Control
■ Consequences
■ Craving

Know This:

1. Rebound symptoms and pseudo-withdrawal are two phenomena that are distinct from substance withdrawal. Rebound symptoms refer to situations in which symptoms preceding the drug use affected by the use worsen after discontinuation (e.g., persons with insomnia using benzodiazepines to sleep might experience worsening insomnia after benzodiazepines discontinuation). Pseudo-withdrawal refers to placebo-type symptoms experienced when a person using a substance considers or expects the substance's discontinuation. These symptoms resemble symptoms that would likely occur with drug discontinuation.
2. Conditioned (or learned) tolerance refers to a different phenomenon than the physiological tolerance described earlier. Conditioned tolerance refers to the presence of conditioned compensatory responses in response to using a substance in a novel environment, rather than their familiar place of use. Conditioned tolerance can be seen for example when a person with opioid use disorder experiences an opioid overdose when they use heroin in a new environment.
3. Incentive salience refers to yet another phenomenon. With incentive salience, specific environmental sensory or experiential cues become associated with using a given substance (such as smells, places of use, or persons with whom one uses). This leads to a physical state of expectation of substance use when encountering these cues. For example, someone using cocaine at a nightclub will experience a strong urge to use cocaine again every time they go to the nightclub.
4. Incentive salience is driven by operant conditioning (conditioning using positive or negative reinforcement) or classical conditioning (Pavlovian conditioning).

SUD SEVERITY AND PATIENT PLACEMENT CRITERIA

The American Society of Addiction Medicine (ASAM) patient placement criteria (PPC-2R) offer a standardized approach to connect a person's SUD severity and characteristics with the treatment level they require. Using the PPC-2R, persons with SUD are assessed for their treatment needs in six dimensions (each scored 0–4 based on the associated complication risks):

■ Dimension 1: Intoxication and withdrawal potential
■ Dimension 2: Biomedical conditions and complications
■ Dimension 3: Emotional, behavioral, or cognitive complications
■ Dimension 4: Readiness to change (trans-theoretical model of change or stages of change)
■ Dimension 5: Relapse or continued use potential
■ Dimension 6: Recovery environment (including social, legal, vocational, educational, financial, and housing factors)

Treatment type needs for every dimension are determined and classified by level:

- Level 0?
- Level 0.5: Early intervention
- Level I: Outpatient treatment
- Level II.1: Intensive outpatient
- Level II.5: Partial hospitalization
- Level III.1: Clinically managed low-intensity residential services
- Level III.3: Clinically managed medium-intensity residential treatment
- Level III.5: Clinically managed high-intensity residential treatment
- Level III.7: Medically monitored intensive inpatient treatment
- Level IV: Medically managed intensive inpatient treatment

When applicable, subspecifiers are used to denote treatment types further:

- D: Detoxification
- OMT: Opioid maintenance treatment
- BIO: Capable of managing complex medical comorbidity
- AOD: Alcohol or drug treatment only
- DDC: Dual diagnosis capable (the treatment facility can identify co-occurring psychiatric problems and refer to outside mental health treatment centers)
- DDE: Dual diagnosis enhanced, capable on-site of managing patients with co-occurring psychiatric problems

The PPC-2R model is presented as a matrix grid in which illness dimensions are listed on the Y-axis and treatment types on the X-axis.

For example, a patient with alcohol use disorder and depression seeking treatment might require initial care in a Level IV-D (inpatient detoxification) followed by a II.5-DDE (partial hospital program that is dual diagnosis enhanced)

Know This:

1. The role of coercion in treatment or the impact of one's experienced adverse consequences of substance use affects their motivation for treatment and is assessed in Dimension 4 (readiness to change).

2. Do not confuse **placement matching** and **modality matching**. **"Placement matching"** refers to the required intensity of treatment resources as identified in the PPC-2R, whereas **"modality matching"** refers to whichever clinical approach might be optimal in treating a patient's problems (such as using contingency management for stimulant use disorders, buprenorphine for opioid use disorder, or dialectical behavioral therapy [DBT] for borderline personality disorder).

Child and adolescent levels of care utilization services (CALOCUS) is a model similar to PPC-2R that is specific for identifying necessary levels of care for adolescent SUD. Basic services or prevention represent the least restrictive level of care in the CALOCUS model (Level 0), whereas a secure 24-hour medical management program is the most restrictive level (Level 6).

STATISTICS AND EPIDEMIOLOGICAL TIDBITS

It is not uncommon for the boards to ask a couple of basic statistical questions, most commonly addressing sensitivity, specificity, positive and negative predictive values, or the types of biases in scientific research.

	Test positive	**Test negative**
Condition present	True positive (TP)	False negative (FN)
Condition absent	False positive (FP)	True negative (TN)

Sensitivity and specificity present the means to assess how accurate a diagnostic test demonstrates the presence or absence of a condition. They address the likelihood of a given test outcome for persons who have or do not have the condition. A test with high specificity will help Rule-In the condition (Specificity – IN → SPIN), whereas a high sensitivity test will help Rule-Out the condition (Sensitivity – OUT → SNOUT). For example, gamma-glutamyl transferase is a highly specific but not very sensitive biomarker of alcohol use disorder.

In contrast, positive predictive value (PPV) and negative predictive value (NPV) address the likelihood of having a condition for persons who test positive or negative. As such, a test with high PPV will have a large number of TPs among all those who test positive, whereas a test with high NPV will have a large number of TNs among all those who test negative. Note that PPV and NPV are based on the assumption that the prevalence in the sample is representative of the prevalence in the general population.

Sensitivity = TP/(TP + FN)
Specificity = TN/(TN + FP)
PPV = TP/(TP + FP)
NPV = TN/(TN + FP)

Statistic and demographic data on SUD derives mainly from a few national surveys, including Monitoring the Future (MTF), the National Survey of Drug Use and Health (NSDUH), and the National Epidemiologic Survey on Alcohol and Related Conditions (NESARC).

MTF is conducted in schools and targets the youth with a sampling frame including only grades 8, 10, or 12. NSDUH, on the other hand, is a household survey.

Know This:

1. In general, remember that alcohol use disorders (AUD) are three to five times more common than illicit drug use disorders. The numbers below reflect an easy-to-memorize approximation. Alcohol use disorder in the United States:
   - Past year prevalence: 10%
   - Lifetime prevalence: 30% to 44%
   Illicit drug use disorders in the United States:
   - Past year prevalence: 2%
   - Lifetime prevalence: 10%
2. SUDs are roughly twice as prevalent in men than in women. Adolescents and the elderly are exceptions:
   - In adolescents, prevalence rates are comparable between genders.
   - In the elderly, the gender gap increases with age, for example, men over 65 are six times more likely than women to have AUD.
3. Caffeine is the most commonly used psychoactive substance, alcohol is the most commonly use addictive substance, marijuana is the most commonly used illicit substance, and opioid pain medications are the most commonly abused prescription drug (except in high school students who most commonly abuse prescribed amphetamines).

4. Cannabis use disorder is the most common SUD in adolescents (AUD is the second most common SUD in adolescents). In contrast, AUD is the most common SUD in adults.
5. Tobacco use and tobacco use disorder prevalence decreased over the past decade.
6. Telescoping refers to the phenomenon whereby SUD severity progresses faster for women than for men, with women more likely to seek SUD treatment and be in recovery faster than men.
7. PPV and NPV are conditional on the assumption that the sample prevalence reflects the prevalence in the general population.

Marijuana is the illicit drug with the highest new drug initiation rates, followed closely by prescription pain medications.

The board examinations often ask about SUD prevalence in different racial and ethnic groups. Overall, it is important to remember that racial and ethnic identity are not found to be risk factors for SUDs when adjusted for socioeconomic factors. With that in mind, Native Americans have the highest SUD rates in the United States (lifetime prevalence of AUD is 44% and illicit drug use disorders are 18%).

Racial and ethnic minorities are disproportionately affected by serious adverse health consequences of SUD, have less access to treatment, are less likely to achieve recovery, and more likely to engage in high-risk drug use behaviors, such as intravenous injecting.

Roughly half of high school students experiment with the illicit drug by the time of graduation, and a third of those develop a SUD later in life. Risk factors in children for future SUD:

- Poor school performance
- Poor social skills
- Aggressive behavior and lack of self-control
- Anxiety disorders

SUD rates in physicians are similar to those in the general population. However, recovery rates are significantly higher for physicians, likely due to the fear of losing one's license. AUD is the most common SUD in physicians, and marijuana is the most commonly used illicit drug. The age at which physicians present to physician health programs has decreased in recent years.

Tobacco is thought of as the substance with the highest addictive potential, followed by opioids, cocaine, alcohol, benzodiazepines, and marijuana consecutively. This is assessed by examining what percentage of those who used the substance once develop an SUD:

- 33% of those who use tobacco once develop tobacco use disorder
- 25% of those who use heroin once develop opioid use disorder
- 17% of those who use cocaine once develop cocaine use disorder
- 15% of those who use alcohol once develop AUD
- 10% of those who use benzodiazepine once develop a sedative use disorder
- 10% of those who use cannabis once develop cannabis use disorder

In contrast, cocaine use disorder is the SUD with the highest lifetime remission rates, with a median time for the remission of 5 years (in contrast with 14 years for alcohol and 26 years for nicotine).

PHARMACOKINETIC CONSIDERATIONS

The onset of drug effects depends on the form of administration, with smoked and injected drugs having a faster onset (seconds), snorted drugs (minutes), and orally ingested (up to hours) having a slower onset.

- Alcohol is metabolized by alcohol dehydrogenase (ADH) into acetaldehyde, which is further metabolized by aldehyde dehydrogenase (ALDH) into acetate, and finally to acetyl CoA.
- Benzodiazepines (except for lorazepam, oxazepam and temazepam – LOT) are metabolized by CYP 3A4.
- Cocaine is metabolized by cholinesterases into benzoylecgonine which is cleared renally.
- Methamphetamine is metabolized by CYP 2D6 and is cleared renally (hence, acidifying the urine can help with methamphetamine overdoses).
- Methadone is metabolized by CYP 3A4.
- CYP 2D6 metabolizes methylenedioxymethamphetamine (MDMA) into dihydroxymethamphetamine (HHMA).
- Nicotine is metabolized by CYP 2A6 into cotinine. Nicotine is also a CYP 1A2 inducer.

- Tetrahydrocannabinol (THC) is metabolized by CYP 2C9 and CYP 3A4 into 11-hydroxy-Δ9-THC, excreted in feces.

Know This:

1. Board examinations frequently ask questions about substance metabolism. We review here some important concepts:
    - Alcohol metabolism follows a zero-order kinetic model meaning that **a constant amount** of alcohol is cleared per unit time. As such, the drug dose (amount of alcohol consumed) is the most important factor for determining the time it takes to reach a steady state.
    - In contrast, cocaine follows a first-order kinetic model meaning that a **constant fraction (percent)** of the drug is cleared per unit time. As such, the drug's half-life is the most important factor for determining the time it takes to reach a steady state.
2. The concept of pharmacokinetic tolerance refers to the increased metabolism of a drug due to repeated administration. It is different from sensitization, which refers to decreased drug response after repeated administration.

ASSESSMENT SCALES

We review in the table some of the most commonly assessed standardized assessment scales used in patients with SUD:

Car, Relax, Alone, Forget, Friends, Trouble (CRAFFT)	Assesses SUD severity in adults
Drug Abuse Screening Test (DAST)	Screens for drug abuse
Diagnosis, Intractability, Risk, Efficacy (DIRE)	Assesses the risks of chronic opioid management
Prescription Drug Use Questionnairp-patient (PDUQp)	Screens for aberrant opioid behaviors in patients with chronic pain

Screener and Opioid Assessment for Patients with Pain (SOAPP-R)	Screens for aberrant opioid behaviors in patients with chronic pain	Short version of MAST-G (SMAST-G)	Screens for AUD in the elderly
Pain Medication Questionnaire (PMQ)	Screens for aberrant opioid behaviors in patients with chronic pain	NIAAA single-question alcohol screen	One question: "Do you sometimes drink alcohol? (in the past year)." Persons who screen positive should then receive an in-depth assessment to allow for the determination of the risk level. Brief intervention and providing advice follow (per the SBIRT – Screening, Brief Intervention and Referral to Treatment model)
Opioid Risk Tool (ORT)	Screens for aberrant opioid behaviors in patients with chronic pain		
Recovery Attitude and Treatment Evaluatory (RAATE)	Screens for resistance to treatment		
URICA	Screens for motivation level for treatment		
Alcohol Use Disorders Identification Test – Consumption (AUDIT-C)	Three questions: 1. How often do you have alcohol? 2. How many SDU do you drink in a typical day? 3. How often do you have six or more drinks on one occasion? A score of 4 or more for men or 3 or more for women is considered positive.	Tolerance, Annoyed, Cut down, Eye opener (T-ACE)	Screens for alcohol
		TWEAK	Screens for AUD in pregnant women
		Cut down, Annoyed, Guilty, Eye Opener (CAGE)	Screens for alcohol
		CAGE-AID	Screens for alcohol and drugs
Addiction Severity Index (ASI)	Assesses SUD severity in seven potential problem areas: medical status, employment and support, drug use, alcohol use, legal status, family and social status, and psychiatric status.	SAFE-T	Not SUD specific, assesses suicide risk factors
		PCL	Not SUD specific, assesses PTSD symptoms
Michigan Alcohol Screen-Geriatrics (MAST-G)	Screens for AUD in the elderly		

THE NATIONAL INSTITUTE ON ALCOHOL ABUSE AND ALCOHOLISM DRINKING GUIDELINES

- No-risk drinking: 4 or fewer drinks per day and 14 or fewer drinks per week for men; 3 or fewer drinks per day and 7 or fewer drinks per week for women.

- At-risk drinking: More than 4 drinks per day and more than 14 drinks per week for men; more than 3 drinks per day and more than 7 drinks per week for women.
- In men and women over age 65, NIAAA recommends no more than 7 drinks per week and no more than 3 drinks per day.

One standard alcoholic beverage or standard drinking unit contains 12 to 14 g of ethanol (0.6 oz of pure ethanol, or one 12 oz beer, one 5 oz glass of wine, one 1.5 oz of 80-proof liquor).

BEHAVIORAL ADDICTION

Beginning in the DSM-5, behavioral addictions were included in the same chapter as SUDs. Behavioral addictions are characterized by a recurrent pattern of behavior within a specific domain (gambling, eating, shopping, video gaming) that ultimately interferes with functioning in other domains (family, society, work). Unlike SUDs, there are no medically dangerous withdrawal states from behavioral addictions.

Gambling addiction is the only diagnosable behavioral addiction using the DSM-5 framework. Gambling disorder is the most studied behavioral addiction. Gambling was referred to as pathological gambling in the DSM-III under the impulse-control disorders category. It was then renamed to gambling disorder in the DSM-5 and moved to the new category of "Addictions and Related Disorders." Gambling disorder usually starts in the early stages of life, and males tend to start during childhood or adolescence years. Its lifetime prevalence is estimated to be between 0.1% and 7.6% of the adult population in the United States. The prevalence of adolescent gambling disorder is higher than that of adults. Twin studies have shown the role of a genetic etiology as a perpetuating factor for gambling activities. People with gambling disorders are at higher rates of comorbidity with alcohol, tobacco, and mood disorders.

A diagnosis of gambling disorder is made when persons meet at least four of the following diagnostic criteria:

- Needing to gamble with increasing amounts of money in order to achieve the desired excitement.
- Feeling restless or irritable when attempting to cut down or stop gambling.
- Making repeated unsuccessful efforts to control, cut back, or stop gambling.
- Being often preoccupied with gambling (e.g., having persistent thoughts of reliving past gambling experiences, handicapping or planning the next venture, thinking of ways to get money with which to gamble).
- Often gambling when feeling distressed (e.g., helpless, guilty, anxious, depressed).
- After losing money gambling, often returning another day to get even ("chasing" one's losses).
- Lying to conceal the extent of involvement with gambling.
- Having jeopardized or lost a significant relationship, job, or educational or career opportunity because of gambling.
- Relying on others to provide money to relieve desperate financial situations caused by gambling.

Not unlike other addictive disorders, the telescoping phenomenon has been studied in gambling disorders. This refers to the finding that gambling disorder in women has a later age of initiation and shorter times from the gambling initiation to having the disorder.

There are no U.S. Food and Drug Administration-approved pharmacotherapeutic treatments for gambling disorder. However, naltrexone has demonstrated efficacy in managing gambling urges and behavior compared to placebo in some studies. The mainstay of treatment for gambling disorder involves psychotherapies, cognitive-behavioral therapy utilizing the relapse prevention model, and motivational interviewing. Participation in 12-step based mutual support groups has also been found to support persons with behavioral addictions to maintain states of recovery effectively.

SUGGESTIONS FOR FURTHER READING

Calado, F., & Griffiths, M. D. (2016). Problem gambling worldwide: An update and systematic review of empirical research (2000–2015). *Journal of Behavioral Addictions, 5*(4), 592–613.

Diazgranados, N., & Goldman, D. (2020). The assessment and treatment of addiction: Best practices in a direct-to-consumer age. In B. A. Johnson (Ed.), *Addiction medicine: Science and practice,* (2nd ed., pp. 167–172). Elsevier.

Gowing, L. R., Ali, R. L., Allsop, S., Marsden, J., Turf, E. E., West, R., & Witton, J. (2015). Global statistics on addictive behaviours: 2014 status report. *Addiction, 110*(6), 904–919.

Grant, J. E., Odlaug, B. L., & Mooney, M. E. (2012). Telescoping phenomenon in pathological gambling: association with gender and comorbidities. *Journal of Nervous and Mental Disease, 200*(11), 996–998.

Mee-Lee, D., & Shulman, G. D (2018). The ASAM criteria and matching patients to treatment. In S. Miller, D. Fiellin, R. Rosenthal, & R. Saitz (Eds.), *The ASAM principles of addiction medicine* (6th ed., pp. 433–447). Wolters Kluwer.

American Psychiatric Association. (2013). Substance-related and addictive disorders. In *The diagnostic and statistical manual for mental disorders* (5th ed., pp. 481–590).

Teesson, M., & Mewton, L. (2015). Epidemiology of addiction. 2015. In M. Galanter, H. D. Kleber, & K. T. Brady (Eds.), *The American Psychiatric Publishing textbook of substance abuse treatment* (5th ed., pp. 47–58). American Psychiatric Publishing.

Zajicek, A., & Karan, L. D. (2018). Pharmacokinetic, pharmacodynamic and pharmacogenomic principles. In S. Miller, D. Fiellin, R. Rosenthal, & R. Saitz (Eds.), *The ASAM principles of addiction medicine* (6th ed., pp. 93–106). Wolters Kluwer.

REVIEW QUESTIONS

1. Which of the following are accurate risk factors for the development of alcohol use disorder?
   A. Male gender, younger, low socioeconomic status (SES), married
   B. Male gender, younger, low SES, single
   C. Male gender, older, high SES, married
   D. Female gender, younger, low SES, married
   E. Female gender, older, high SES, single

2. In understanding the ASAM patient placement criteria (PPC) dimensions, encouraging one's spouse to attend Al-Anon is an example of seeking to address problems in which dimension?
   A. Dimension 1
   B. Dimension 3
   C. Dimension 4
   D. Dimension 5
   E. Dimension 6

3. Which of the following best represents the telescoping effects seen in females with SUDs?
   A. Women get intoxicated with alcohol faster as a result of higher levels of gastric aldehyde dehydrogenase.
   B. Women get intoxicated with alcohol faster as a result of body water and fat distribution.
   C. The risk of developing alcohol use disorder is lower in women than it is in a man only when traditional gender roles are followed.
   D. Women with substance use disorders experience significantly more severe adverse medical and psychological consequences than men.

E. As a result of later onset of SUD in women compared to men, women use substances for fewer years than men.

4. Which of the following is true when thinking about treating SUD in females?
   A. Attending women only AA groups leads to better clinical outcomes than call and groups.
   B. Women respond better to medications for the treatment of SUD than men.
   C. Pregnancy and breastfeeding are contraindications for the use of medications for the treatment of SUD.
   D. Treating co-occurring psychiatric disorders leads to improved SUD outcomes.
   E. Women are treatment-resistant more often than men.

5. A 36-year-old married man who enjoyed day trading stocks since college started to move his money to an online casino phone application. Over the last 13 months, he has lost most of his family savings. His sleep has been affected, as he is always thinking about going back online to recover the money loss; he stopped going to the gym, his performance at work has decreased, and he stopped visiting his mother. What pharmacotherapies should be considered a first-line treatment for pathologic gambling?
   A. Naltrexone
   B. Lithium
   C. Buprenorphine
   D. Bupropion
   E. Topiramate

6. A 68-year-old female presents to your office with her son who is worried about his mother's late-night visits to the casino. His father suffered from gambling "issues," but his mother was never like that until a year ago. He describes that his mother has been increasing the time at the casinos, impairing her finances, and spending less time with the family. The behavior is affecting her sleep and mood. She has had two episodes of bankruptcy in 2 years. What phenomenon are we observing in this patient?

A. Rapid cycling
B. Interpersonal phenomenon
C. Telescoping phenomenon
D. Early initiation
E. Middle-life crisis

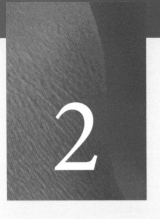

2 COMORBIDITIES OF SUBSTANCE USE DISORDERS

PSYCHIATRIC COMORBIDITIES OF SUBSTANCE USE DISORDERS

When thinking about the psychiatric manifestations of substance use disorder (SUD), one has to differentiate between:

1. The substance's effects: Drugs and alcohol intoxication or withdrawal cause psychiatric signs and symptoms that are part of a given substance's toxidrome. For example, feeling euphoric after using cocaine or anxious when going through alcohol withdrawal are expected effects of cocaine intoxication or alcohol withdrawal and should not be labeled as a manic or anxiety syndrome.

2. Substance-induced disorders: This category refers to the presence of psychiatric symptoms that:
   - Vastly exceed the expected effects of being intoxicated with or withdrawing from a substance.
   - Present with symptoms of an other psychiatric disorder (psychotic, bipolar, depressive, anxiety, obsessive-compulsive, sleep sexual or neurocognitive disorder), albeit there is no requirement to meet all the diagnostic criteria for the disorder.
   - Develop during or soon after substance intoxication or withdrawal.
   - The symptoms improve after a period of abstinence.

3. Co-occurring primary psychiatric disorders: This category refers to psychiatric disorders that either preceded or followed the onset of a SUD, but neither condition played a causative role in the other's onset. For example, tobacco use disorder and schizophrenia often co-occur. Still, schizophrenia does not cause the onset of a tobacco use disorder, and tobacco use disorder does not cause the onset of schizophrenia.

4. Secondary psychiatric disorders: This category refers to psychiatric disorders that follow the onset of a SUD, with the SUD playing a causative role in the onset of the co-occurring psychiatric disorder. Unlike substance-induced disorders, with secondary psychiatric disorders, the symptoms do not improve after a period of abstinence.

We review below some high-yield psychiatric comorbidities of SUD:

- Early-onset anxiety disorders are associated with an increased risk of developing a SUD in adolescents. In contrast, adolescents with SUD are at an increased risk of developing depressive disorders.
- In women with SUD, the most common comorbid psychiatric disorders are anxiety, depression, or posttraumatic stress disorder (PTSD). Other SUDs, attention deficit/hyperactivity disorder (ADHD), or antisocial personality disorder are more common in men.
- Overall, two-thirds of persons with cannabis or stimulant use disorders and one-third of those with nicotine or alcohol use disorder (AUD) will have a comorbid mood, anxiety, or personality disorder.

Know This:

- Panic attacks related to substance use are seen most commonly with marijuana and lysergic acid diethylamide (LSD) intoxication and alcohol withdrawal.
- Untreated substance-induced psychiatric disorders are associated with an increased risk of relapse.
- Substance use, substance use disorders, and withdrawal syndromes are associated with a significantly increased risk of suicidal behaviors including completed suicides.
- Drug use is associated with a significantly increased risk of violence perpetration. Alcohol use is associated with a significantly increased risk of violence perpetration and victimization.
- Forty percent of patients with schizophrenia have a SUD. The most commonly used substance by people with schizophrenia is nicotine (85%) followed by alcohol (35%), cocaine (30%), and cannabis (30%).
- Patients with bipolar disorder have the highest rates of co-occurring SUD.
- The prevalence of persistent psychosis among methamphetamine users is 11 times higher than the general population.
- ADHD treatment, including the use of stimulants, does not increase SUD risk. In fact, recent data suggest that it might reduce the risk.
- In patients with SUD, the most common comorbid personality disorder is an antisocial personality disorder.
- The misuse of prescription stimulants for treating ADHD is seen most commonly among friends of persons with ADHD rather than among individuals with the disorder themselves.
- Alcohol-related sleep impairments include decreased rapid eye movement (REM) sleep and slow-wave sleep, increased sleep latency, and decreased sleep efficiency and total sleep time.
- In patients with alcohol or sedative use disorders, insomnia is an independent risk factor for relapse on alcohol and benzodiazepines.
- The relationship between marijuana use and the onset of a psychotic disorder is not fully elucidated. It appears that although marijuana does not cause psychotic disorders, it might precipitate their onset, as such persons would have an earlier onset and a more severe course for their psychosis. Having the AKT1 mutation increases the lifetime risk of having a psychotic disorder in persons who use cannabis.
- The most common psychiatric disorders comorbids with cannabis use disorder are other SUDs followed by anxiety and depressive disorders.

NONPSYCHIATRIC, MEDICAL COMORBIDITIES OF SUBSTANCE USE

This section will review the impact of substance use on major bodily systems rather than list the medical conditions associated with every substance.

Know This:

1. Medical comorbidities of excessive alcohol use, including alcohol-related liver disease, cardiovascular complications, and neurologic problems, affect women more frequently and more severely than men. This is because women have lower levels of gastric alcohol dehydrogenase. As a result, less alcohol is metabolized at the gastric level resulting in higher circulating alcohol levels.
2. The impact of race on SUD rates is minimal. However, due to disparate access to care and medical services, serious adverse consequences of SUD disproportionately affect minority populations. For example, even though Black individuals have a later onset of heavy drinking and a lower prevalence of AUD, they are more likely to experience adverse medical consequences, including death, than White individuals. Similarly, liver cirrhosis-related mortality rates are higher in the Hispanic populations.

Cardiovascular Comorbidities of Substance Use

Excessive alcohol use can cause significant problems in cardiovascular function, including:

- Alcoholic cardiomyopathy (a dilated cardiomyopathy marked by hypercontractility, reduced cardiac output with increased systemic vascular resistance) caused by both the toxic effects of alcohol and acetaldehyde accumulation
- Portal venous diseases and portal hypertension are marked by a hyperdynamic cardiovascular function with increased cardiac output with decreased systemic vascular resistance
- Hypertension
- Arrhythmias including atrial fibrillation (holiday heart)

Excessive stimulant use can cause:

- Hypertension with increased cardiac workload, increased systemic vascular resistance, and vasoconstriction
- Left ventricular hypertrophy
- Coronary artery disease with vasculopathy and vasoconstriction
- Hyperthrombotic states
- Myocardial infarctions, angina, and strokes
- Aortic dissection and rupture
- Arrhythmias
- Mesenteric vasoconstriction and mesenteric ischemia

Know This:

Cocaine-related angina and myocardial infarction medical treatment should include benzodiazepines in addition to the standard protocols used for non–cocaine-related cardiac events. Benzodiazepines are necessary to manage hypertension and tachycardia and decrease the central stimulatory effects of cocaine.

Gastrointestinal Comorbidities of Substance Use

Excessive alcohol use can cause significant problems in gastrointestinal function, including:

- Alcoholic liver disease marked by moderately elevated transaminase levels, with aspartate aminotransferase (AST)/alanine aminotransferase (ALT) ratio 2:1. If ALT is more than AST, consider alternative causes of hepatocellular injury, such as acetaminophen toxicity or viral hepatitis, and severely elevated gamma-glutamyltransferase levels. Alcohol causes three types of liver syndromes including:

1. Alcoholic steatosis (fatty liver) manifesting with anorexia, nausea, vomiting, right upper-quadrant discomfort, hepatomegaly, and firm and tender liver on physical examination. Alcoholic steatosis does not require a long history of excessive alcohol use and may be seen in persons who drank heavily over a short time period. This condition is reversible with the discontinuation of alcohol use.
2. Alcoholic hepatitis manifesting with the signs and symptoms of steatosis in addition to liver function test abnormalities, hypercoagulable states and bruising, encephalopathy, and ascites. This condition is reversible with the discontinuation of alcohol use.
3. Alcoholic cirrhosis manifests with the signs and symptoms of hepatitis and portal venous disease, portal hypertension, ascites, bacterial peritonitis, hepatocellular carcinoma, varices, and hepatic failure. This condition is irreversible even with the discontinuation of alcohol use.

- Alcoholic esophagitis
- Esophageal varices
- Alcoholic gastritis
- Alcoholic pancreatitis (acute or chronic)
- Electrolyte abnormalities and nutrient deficiencies owing to malabsorption (thiamine, calcium, magnesium)

Know This:

1. Asterixis is seen with hepatic encephalopathy.
2. Alcoholic cirrhosis is associated with a 50% 2-year mortality rate and is the second most common cause of liver transplants. To be eligible for a transplant, one must abstain from alcohol use for at least 6 months. Transplants are indicated with ascites, encephalopathy, jaundice, or portal hypertension.
3. Untreated hypocalcemia and hypomagnesemia in AUD can cause arrhythmias.

4. Pentoxifylline is a steroid medication used as a part of the management of hepatitis. Its use is contraindicated in patients with gastrointestinal bleeding, renal insufficiency, or active infectious processes.

Other substances can also cause direct hepatotoxicity, including cocaine, heroin, 3-4 methylenedioxymethamphetamine (MDMA), phencyclidine (PCP), and androgenic steroids. Indirect substance-related hepatotoxicity can be caused by drug contaminants or viral hepatitis associated with drug and alcohol use discussed later.

Infectious Comorbidities of Substance Use

Injecting drugs (with contaminated needles, syringes, spoons, cotton swabs) or using intranasal instruments is associated with contracting HIV and hepatitis C virus (HCV). Toxic shock syndrome caused by group A beta-hemolytic *Streptococcus* is also seen as a result of injecting drugs and causes a generalized rash, hypotension, tachycardia, murmurs, abdominal pain, and diarrhea. Similarly, drug and alcohol use are associated with high-risk sexual behaviors, which are also associated with contracting HIV or hepatitis B virus (HBV). Finally, excessive alcohol use is associated with an increased risk of contracting various infectious processes, postoperative infections, along with impaired wound healing.

HIV-related immune suppression and AIDS cause opportunistic infections, including *Pneumocystis carinii* pneumonia (PCP), toxoplasmosis, or tuberculosis. Similarly, HIV infection and AIDS are associated with other complications, including Kaposi sarcoma and other neoplasms, HIV-associated nephropathy, cardiovascular disease, and neurocognitive decline. Highly active antiretroviral therapy (HAART) is recommended for all HIV-positive patients and slows or stops the progression of HIV infections, suppresses HIV viral loads, increases CD4 counts, and prevents the above-noted complications. Medications used in HAART have multiple interactions with commonly prescribed psychiatric medications and certain drugs.

HCV is the most common chronic bloodborne infectious agent, four times more prevalent than HIV. Up to 60% to 80% of injection drug users are HCV positive. Untreated HCV can lead to progressive hepatic disease, cirrhosis, and hepatocellular carcinoma. Risk factors for worse prognoses include alcohol use, HCV genotype 1, older age at the time of infection, male sex, co-occurring HBV, and higher viral load at the time of treatment initiation. The medical management of HCV includes ensuring that the person is vaccinated against hepatitis A virus/HBV and limiting alcohol consumption. Historically, HCV treatment consisted of interferon and ribavirin. Newer interferon-free HCV antivirals have been developed and are becoming more easily accessible. These include sofosbuvir, simeprevir, and ledipasvir.

Know This:

1. HIV patients should continue taking HAART during pregnancy, although the medication regimen should exclude efavirenz because of its teratogenicity (associated with renal tube defects).
2. Efavirenz is the antiretroviral medication most commonly associated with psychiatric adverse effects, including anxiety, depression, suicidal ideation, confusion, and hallucinations.

Renal Comorbidities of Substance Use

Acute renal failure can be caused by chronic hypertension (from alcohol or cocaine use) or rhabdomyolysis from seizures or volume depletion in persons using alcohol, cocaine, heroin, or bath salts. Contaminants found in heroin can cause nephropathy. Additionally, chronic and excessive alcohol use can cause hepatorenal syndrome (renal failure in patients with acute and severe liver failure from decompensated cirrhosis or acute fulminant hepatitis, causing jaundice, coagulopathy, and death from hepatic and renal failure or variceal bleeding). Finally, infectious processes seen in injection drug users, such as HBV or HCV or HIV, can cause nephrotic syndrome.

Know This:

1. Rhabdomyolysis symptoms include fever, muscle pain, and malaise. It is diagnosed by finding red blood cells in urine and myoglobin casts on sediment analysis (urine myoglobin analysis can take several days, so use urine blood and

sediment act as surrogate markers for hemo-globin and myoglobin). Treatment includes intravenous hydration, alkalization of the urine, and osmotic diuresis to decrease myoglobin toxicity and flush myoglobin casts.

2. Heroin and semisynthetic opioids but not synthetic opioids use is associated with rhabdomyolysis.

3. Ethylene glycol or methanol intoxication causes a metabolic acidosis with deposition of calcium oxalate crystals in renal tubules and brain tissue and pulmonary edema. They are treated with fomepizole, a potent alcohol dehydrogenase (ADH) inhibitor that prevents ethylene glycol or methanol's toxic metabolism. Severe cases may require dialysis.

Pulmonary Comorbidities of Substance Use

Tobacco use is associated with many pulmonary conditions, including chronic obstructive pulmonary disease, emphysema, airway reactivity, bronchospasm, bronchitis, pulmonary hypertension, pulmonary edema, and lung cancer. These conditions are 30 times more likely in heavy smokers compared with nonsmokers.

Excessive alcohol use is also associated with pulmonary pathology manifesting with obstructive sleep apnea, pulmonary hypertension, pulmonary edema, pneumonia due to alcohol-mediated impaired immune response, increased airway leakage and the accumulation of reactive oxygen species.

Inhalant use can cause pulmonary edema, bronchospasm, and alveolar hemorrhage. Cocaine and heroin use can also cause pulmonary edema.

Neuromuscular Comorbidities of Substance Use

Excessive alcohol use can cause significant neuromuscular function problems, including peripheral neuropathy, hepatic encephalopathy, Wernicke-Korsakoff disease, cerebellar dysfunction, myopathy, or subdural hematoma from falls. Additionally, alcohol withdrawal is associated with delirium, seizures, and epileptic activity.

Similarly, cocaine use can cause seizures, strokes, delirium, or other cognitive impairments.

Know This:

1. Alcohol myopathy presents with proximal symmetrical weakness, elevated creatine kinase levels, and sensory neuropathy.
2. Hypophosphatemia in patients with AUD caused by malabsorption presents with restlessness, agitation, and bilateral symmetrical motor weakness.

Hematologic Comorbidities of Substance Use

Excessive alcohol use can cause macrocytic anemia as a result of folic acid deficiency, pancytopenia as a result of direct bone marrow toxicity, and iron deficiency. Similarly, tobacco use is associated with prothrombotic hypercoagulable states.

Endocrine Comorbidities of Substance Use

Excessive alcohol use can cause type 2 diabetes and other glycemic control problems, hyperlipidemia, gout and hyperuricemia, hypercortisolemia, gynecomastia, alterations in gonadotropins, testicular atrophy, infertility, and erectile dysfunction. Similarly, chronic opioid use can be associated with osteopenia, amenorrhea, and abnormal sex hormones, including gonadotropins.

Know This:

Osteonecrosis of the hip is almost always due to excessive alcohol or steroid use. It presents with dull groin pain.

SUGGESTIONS FOR FURTHER READING

Addolorato, G., Mirijello, A., Vassallo, G. A., D'Angelo, C., Ferrulli, A., Antonelli, M., Caputo, F., Mosoni, C., Tarli, C., Rando, M. M., Sestito, L., Dioniso, T., Leggio, L., & Gabarrini, A. (2020). *Physical considerations for treatment complications of alcohol and drug use and misuse*. In B. A. Johnson (Ed.), *Addiction medicine: Science and practice* (2nd ed., pp. 811–832). Elsevier.

Batki, S. L., & Nathan, K. I. (2015). HIV/AIDS and hepatitis C. In M. Galanter, H. D. Kleber, & K. T. Brady (Eds.), *The American Psychiatric Association Publishing textbook of substance abuse treatment* (5th ed.). American Psychiatric Association Publishing.

Heit, H. A., & Gourlay, D. L. (2015). Psychiatric consultation in pain and addiction. In M. Galanter, H. D. Kleber, & K. T. Brady (Eds.), *The American Psychiatric Association Publishing textbook of substance abuse treatment* (5th ed.). American Psychiatric Association Publishing.

Saitz, R. (2018). Medical and surgical complications of addiction. In S. Miller, D. Fiellin, R. Rosenthal, & R. Saitz (Eds.), *The ASAM principles of addiction medicine* (6th ed.). Wolters Kluwer.

Youdelis-Flores, C., Goldsmith, R. J., & Ries, R. K. (2018). Substance-induced mental disorders. In S. Miller, D. Fiellin, R. Rosenthal, & R. Saitz (Eds.), *The ASAM principles of addiction medicine* (6th ed.). Wolters Kluwer.

REVIEW QUESTIONS

1. A 46-year-old woman with a long history of an AUD, hepatitis C, and cirrhosis is referred to your clinic for treatment. She expresses a desire to discontinue her alcohol consumption. In addition to psychotherapeutic interventions, which of the following pharmacologic agents is the medication of choice for treating this patient's condition?
   A. Disulfiram
   B. Gabapentin
   C. Ondansetron
   D. Acamprosate
   E. Naltrexone

2. A 59-year-old man with opioid and AUD is currently hospitalized for an abscess. He reports depression and sleep disturbances. Which of the following would be the best time to perform psychiatric evaluation to determine whether he would benefit from treatment for an underlying depressive pathology?
   A. His treatment should be started in the emergency room, as soon as he arrives at the hospital.
   B. His treatment should be started after completing medically assisted detoxification but before starting maintenance treatment.
   C. He should be screened for depression on admission and reassessed frequently thereafter.
   D. He benefits only after being sober from all drugs and alcohol for at least 1 month.
   E. Never, this man's depression results from his heroin and alcohol use.

3. A 34-year-old man with severe AUD, cocaine and ketamine use is referred to you for chronic and severe anxiety and frequent panic attacks. The panic attacks are associated with significant avoidance behaviors leading to him to skip work often. The panic attacks often happen in the morning. When meeting with him, he tells you that he drinks alcohol to "self-medicate his anxiety and panic attacks." Which of the following is the most likely explanation for this patient's anxiety and panic attacks?
   A. Cocaine intoxication
   B. Alcohol intoxication
   C. Alcohol withdrawal
   D. Generalized anxiety disorder
   E. Panic disorder without agoraphobia

4. In patients with comorbid SUDs and depression, which of the following factors is most strongly associated with improved response to antidepressant treatments?
   A. Using selective serotonin reuptake inhibitors (SSRI) antidepressants
   B. Diagnosis of depression made while patient is actively drinking
   C. Diagnosis of depression made at least 1 week after patient discontinues drinking
   D. Using antidepressant medications without psychosocial interventions to treat depressive symptoms
   E. Greater initial severity of the depressive symptoms

5. A 42-year-old man with severe AUD is admitted into a combined program, including medically supervised alcohol detoxification followed by a long-term residential rehabilitation program. He reports that he has been drinking 8 to 10 alcoholic drinks daily for the past 6 years. Also, he describes symptoms of major depressive disorder for the past 7 months. Which of the following would be the most appropriate strategy to treat his depressive symptoms?
   A. His alcohol use causes this person's depression. Abstinence during the residential rehabilitation program will be curative for his depression.

B. Because of the comorbid AUD, antidepressant medications are not indicated. This patient's depression should be treated using intensive cognitive behavioral therapy alone.

C. This patient's depression has lasted more than 6 months. This is consistent with a diagnosis of major depressive disorder, and he should be prescribed antidepressant medication immediately.

D. Start an antidepressant medication after this patient completes the residential rehabilitation program if he remains symptomatic.

E. Start an antidepressant medication after this patient completes a medically supervised alcohol detoxification if he remains symptomatic.

6. A 42-year-old woman is brought to the emergency room by emergency medical services for chest pain and dyspnea. ST depressions are seen on electrocardiogram. The patient admits to using cocaine regularly, including snorting 1 g of cocaine on the day of admission. Assuming that her drug use played a causal role in her current presentation, what is cocaine-induced ischemia's physiological mechanism?

A. Increased cardiac workload and systemic vascular resistance

B. Dilated cardiomyopathy

C. Superficial venous thrombosis

D. Severe hypotension following a vasovagal episode

E. Coronary thromboembolism

7. A 34-year-old man with severe opioid use disorder and comorbid major depressive disorder comes into the clinic to evaluate and consider treatment with buprenorphine. The patient tells you that he has been injecting heroin at least four times daily on and off for the past 15 years. He also acknowledges using illicitly obtained buprenorphine on multiple occasions in the past in an attempt to treat his opioid use disorder on his own. During your evaluation, the patient admits that his father died of an opioid overdose a month ago, and as a result, he has been feeling very depressed. He adds that 1 month ago, he attempted suicide by intentionally overdosing on heroin. Which of the following is the most appropriate next step of this evaluation?

A. Order stat laboratory testing for HIV and HCV.

B. Assess the severity of the patient's depression and current suicidal thoughts.

C. Inform the patient that he is not eligible for treatment with buprenorphine because he has a history of obtaining it from illicit sources.

D. Inform the patient that he is not eligible for treatment with buprenorphine because of his recent suicide attempt.

E. Prescribe fluoxetine.

8. A patient with severe opioid use disorder who injects heroin is referred to your office for an evaluation. The patient tells you that he is interested in being prescribed medication to treat opioid use disorder. The patient tells you that his opioid use began 10 years ago when he was prescribed opioid pain medications for chronic and severe back pain. He continued using illicitly obtained opioid pain medication after his physician "cut him off" and ultimately transitioned to heroin use. The patient reports more than seven suicide attempts by intentional opioid overdose but denies any current suicidal thoughts or depression. The patient is hopeful that treatment will improve his condition. During your evaluation, the patient appeared to be in insignificant distress as a result of opioid use disorder. What is the most appropriate next step?

A. The patient should be assessed for suicide risk and consideration for inpatient hospitalization given prior suicide history.

B. Prescribe clonidine, ibuprofen, and loperamide for his withdrawal symptoms and schedule him for a follow-up appointment in 1 week.

C. Perform a naloxone challenge test. If no evidence of withdrawal is seen, prescribe oral naltrexone in preparation for starting long-acting injectable naltrexone.

D. Send the patient to the emergency room to be admitted for a medically supervised detoxification.

E. Assess the severity of his opioid withdrawal and begin initiation with buprenorphine.

9. A 17-year-old boy presents for an intake evaluation. He tells you that he has been using heroin and cocaine together by injection for 6 months and admits to sharing needles. He mentions that he has been experiencing chest discomfort, low energy, and generalized fatigue during the examination. You find him febrile, tachycardic, and normotensive on physical examination. What is the most appropriate next step?

A. Refer him to a methadone clinic.

B. Send him to the emergency room.

C. Obtain laboratory testing for HIV and HCV.

D. Refer him to a medically supervised inpatient detoxification program.

E. Initiate treatment with buprenorphine as soon as he presents with moderate symptoms of opioid withdrawal.

10. A 27-year-old woman with AUD and a history of cocaine and heroin use by injection is referred to your methadone clinic. On methadone initiation, she discontinues all illicit opioid use but continues to drink alcohol excessively and inject cocaine. Laboratory testing reveals that she is HIV positive. When is the most appropriate time for her to begin treatment for HIV using highly active antiretroviral treatment (HAART)?

A. Only if she develops Kaposi sarcoma

B. Only if she just continues all injection drug use

C. Only if she discontinues all alcohol use

D. When her CD4 count is less than 200

E. Immediately

11. Which of the following is accurate regarding the effects of chronic excessive alcohol use?

A. Brain imaging studies reveal frontal lobe hypertrophy, and neuropsychological testing reveals cognitive deficits.

B. Neuropsychological testing of cognitive function does not reveal any impairments.

C. No changes are noted on brain imaging, and neuropsychological testing reveals cognitive deficits.

D. Brain imaging studies reveal a loss of brain tissue, and cognitive impairments are noted on neuropsychological testing.

E. Elevated concentration of serotonin is found in the cerebrospinal fluid.

12. Which of the following personality disorders has the highest comorbid SUD rates?

A. Borderline personality disorder

B. Obsessive-compulsive personality disorder

C. Dependent personality disorder

D. Schizoid personality disorder

E. Antisocial personality disorder

13. The FDA approves several medications for the treatment of opioid use disorder. Which of the following is an FDA-approved medication for treating co-occurring PTSD and opioid use disorder?

A. Buprenorphine

B. Naltrexone

C. Methadone

D. Baclofen

E. None of the above

3 NEUROBIOLOGY OF ADDICTION

GENERAL TERMS AND CONCEPTS

Following initiation of substance use, using is typically impulsive and a positively reinforcing experience. The chronic and repeated use of it leads to possible tolerance accompanied by diminishing returns on the substance's positively reinforcing effects. In parallel, there is an increase in the negative reinforcing effects, such as using the substance to avoid withdrawal symptoms. Over time, substance use becomes less impulsive and rewarding and more compulsive and habitual. There is strong evidence of how the brain changes in substance use that explains long-term changes in behavior and motivation, the key points of which will be reviewed in this chapter.

Know This:

The following general terms and definitions are fundamental to know for the board examination.

- **Impulsivity:** Tendency to perform actions without forethought or consideration of consequences. Impulsive actions are typically preceded by arousal, followed by gratification with the act's performance, and then regret or guilt afterward. Impulsivity can be measured experimentally by tasks of delay-to-gratification (Go/No-Go Tasks and delayed discounting).
- **Compulsivity:** Actions that persist despite not being pleasurable, not being related to an overall goal, often resulting in negative consequences. Compulsive actions are typically preceded by thoughts (obsessions) causing anxiety and stress. Following the performance of the compulsive act, one experiences relief. Compulsivity can be measured experimentally

in animal models by pairing substance use with an adverse consequence or progressive-ratio reinforcement schedule.

- **Delayed discounting**: It is the tendency to choose immediate, smaller rewards over larger, delayed rewards. Higher rates of discounting are associated with substance use disorders (SUDs) and many negative life outcomes.
- **Positive reinforcement:** A reward or punishment is paired with behavior in an additive fashion, making it more likely that the behavior will be repeated or extinguished. Example: Experiencing euphoria following heroin use, or withdrawal symptoms after substance use discontinuation.
- **Negative reinforcement:** A stimulus is removed with a behavior, making it more likely that the behavior will be repeated or extinguished. Example: Removal of opioid withdrawal symptoms following resumption of heroin use or revoking social privileges following substance use.
- **Operant conditioning:** Behavior modification (e.g., decrease or increase in frequency) through positive and negative reinforcement by using punishing and rewarding consequences. Example: Contingency management (CM) treatment for SUDs.
- **Classical conditioning:** A previously neutral (unconditioned) stimulus elicits a response after being paired with a biologically potent (conditioned) stimulus. Example: If someone always drinks alcohol while going to the bar, then that setting becomes the conditioned stimulus and can produce cravings.

THE ADDICTION CYCLE AND RELATION TO ANIMAL MODELS

The current body of human and animal research provides robust support for a conceptual model of addiction, first described by Dr. George Koob that involves three recurring stages: (1) binge/intoxication, (2) withdrawal/negative affect, and (3) preoccupation/anticipation. The addiction cycle is an organizing principle to understand the neurochemical and neurobiological changes that a person undergoes as their SUD intensifies, for example, as they move from impulsive to compulsive substance use. Definitions of these stages are as follows:

1. **Binge/intoxication:** The stage in which a person uses an intoxicant and experiences pleasure and reward (positively reinforcing effect). For example, a person experiences a pleasurable high from heroin or cocaine.
2. **Withdrawal/negative affect:** The stage in which a person experiences the negative emotional and physiological effects in the absence of the intoxicant and removes these negative effects on resumption of substance use (negatively reinforcing effect). For example, opioid or alcohol withdrawal.
3. **Preoccupation/anticipation:** The stage in which a person seeks out an intoxicant after a period of abstinence (stress-, cue-, or drug-induced reinstatement). For example, a relapse of alcohol after decades of abstinence following a stressful life event.

In the subsequent sections, we will describe each stage in more detail and the relevant animal models, neuroanatomy, neurocircuitry, and neurotransmitter systems that are frequently tested on in board examinations.

Stage I: Binge/Intoxication

In this stage, an individual consumes a substance that is acutely experienced as rewarding and positively reinforcing. This stage's neurobiological processes involve the acute effects of substances, activation of reward circuitry, development of incentive salience circuits, and drug-seeking habits. Key points to remember regarding this stage:

- The "reward pathway" refers to the mesolimbic dopamine pathway, which includes dopaminergic cell bodies in the ventral tegmental area (VTA; midbrain) that project to the nucleus accumbens (NAc) in the ventral striatum (part of the basal ganglia).
- The acute effects of drugs are generally mediated through one of several mechanisms: they can directly increase extracellular dopamine release in the reward pathway (e.g., amphetamines, cocaine), activate or inhibit channels (e.g., phencyclidine, ketamine, or ethanol), or mimic neurotransmitters by activating receptors (opioids, cannabis, nicotine). Table 3.1 summarizes substances of abuse and affected neurotransmitter systems.

TABLE 3.1

Common Drugs of Abuse and Primary Receptor Signaling Mechanism

Drug	Molecular Target and Action	Receptor Signaling Mechanism
Nicotine	Nicotinic acetylcholine receptor agonist	Ligand-gated channel
Alcohol	GABA-A receptor agonist, NMDA receptor antagonist	Ligand-gated channel
Cannabinoids	CB1 and CB2 receptor agonist	G_i[a]
Opioids	Mu-, delta- and kappa-opioid receptor agonist	G_i
Cocaine	Inhibits dopamine transporter, increasing extrasynaptic DA	G_i and G_s
Amphetamine	Stimulates dopamine release, increasing extrasynaptic DA	G_i and G_s
Phencyclidine	NMDA glutamate receptor antagonist	Ligand-gated channels
Ketamine	NMDA glutamate receptor antagonist	Ligand-gated channels
Hallucinogens	5-HT2A agonist	Ga_q

[a]G_i receptors couple D_2-like receptors and G_s receptors couple D_1-like receptors, both of which are important for their reinforcing effects.
5-HT2A, 5-Hydroxytryptamine 2A; DA, dopamine; GABA, γ-aminobutyric acid; NMDA, N-methyl-D-aspartate.

- "Incentive salience" refers to the phenomenon of cue learning, in which associated stimuli become conditioned with a substance's rewarding effect to the point in which the associated stimuli alone can induce motivation to drug-seek and dopamine release. Incentive salience is regulated by glutamatergic projections from the prefrontal cortex (PFC) to dopamine neurons in the VTA, leading to dopaminergic cell excitation and dopamine release. Incentive salience is the principle behind the Alcoholics Anonymous aphorism of "people, places, and things," referring to the environmental cues that can lead to urges and drug-like effects.
- The dorsal striatum (part of the basal ganglia) is key for habit strengthening and development of compulsive substance use.

Know This:

Stimulants are the main drugs of abuse that directly increase dopaminergic neurotransmission in the NAc; other drugs of abuse increase dopaminergic neurotransmission indirectly. Fig. 3.1 summarizes the acute effects of substances on the reward pathway. These are some key features to remember regarding the specific biological effects of substances on the reward pathway:

- Opioids inhibit γ-aminobutyric acid (GABA)-ergic interneurons in the VTA, which disinhibit VTA dopaminergic neurons, thus increasing dopaminergic neurotransmission. They also act on opioid receptors directly in the NAc.
- Nicotine activates VTA dopamine neurons through stimulation of nicotinic acetylcholine receptors, stimulates glutamatergic nerve terminals that innervate VTA dopamine neurons and may also activate endogenous opioid pathways.
- Alcohol increases GABA-A function, and is also believed to inhibit GABA-ergic nerve terminals in the VTA, thus disinhibiting VTA dopamine neurons and increasing dopaminergic neurotransmission. Alcohol also activates endogenous opioid pathways.
- PCP and ketamine act by inhibiting postsynaptic N-methyl-D-aspartate (NMDA) glutamate receptors in the NAc.
- Cannabis activates CB1 receptors on NAc cell bodies, as well as on glutamatergic and GABAergic nerve terminals in the NAc.

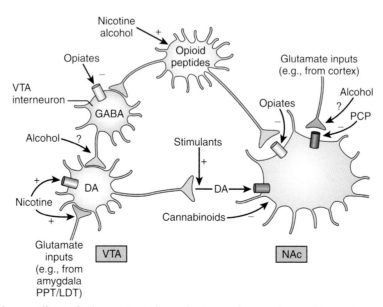

Fig. 3.1 ■ Scheme of acute effects of substances on the nucleus accumbens and ventral tegmental area. (From Nestler, E. J. (2005). Is there a common molecular pathway for addiction? *Nature Neuroscience*, 8(11), 1445–1449. https://doi.org/10.1038/nn1578).

Binge/Intoxication: Animal Models

A summary of all animal models and their relation to specific stages of addiction is presented in Table 3.2. The most important animal models related to the binge/intoxication stage are intracranial self-stimulation (ICSS), self-administration, and conditioned place preference.

- ICSS: The landmark Olds and Milner (1954) study was an ICSS animal study showing that animals would perform a response (lever pressing) to self-administer a stimulus delivered via implanted brain electrodes to brain reward circuits. ICSS provides a way to study substances' effects on brain reward thresholds. Drugs and alcohol generally decrease ICSS threshold; the addictiveness of substance is correlated with its ability to lower ICSS threshold.

- Self-administration: These studies differ from ICSS in that experimental animals will perform a response to self-administer a substance. Self-administration provides a reliable measure of the animal's motivation to use a substance by measuring the amount of work an animal is willing to exert for the reward.

- Conditioned place preference: This model provides a measure of the reinforcing effect of a substance. Administration of a drug is paired with a specific environment, whereas placebo is paired with another. Substances that are positive reinforcers will cause animals to prefer a drug-paired

TABLE 3.2		
Summary of the Most Important Animal Models Used to Study Addiction, Categorized by Relevant Stage of the Addiction Cycle		
Stage of Addiction	**Animal Models**	**Description**
I. Binge/intoxication	Self-administration	The animal receives a drug dose by performing a discrete response, such as pushing a lever. The pattern of response required for a dose depends on the reinforcement schedule (e.g., fixed or variable-interval schedule).
	Conditioned place preference	A drug is paired with one specific environment, whereas placebo is paired with another. The choice of the animal to spend time in one environment or another is a measure of conditioned place preference.
	Brain stimulation reward	ICSS, e.g., the classic Olds and Milner (1954) study in which animals pressed a lever to self-administer a stimulus delivered via brain-implanted electrode.
II. Withdrawal/negative affect	Conditioned place aversion	Animals are exposed to the effects of drug withdrawal in one environment and are not in withdrawal in another. The choice of the animal to spend time in one environment or another is a measure of conditioned place aversion.
	Brain stimulation reward	ICSS as described above; animals in withdrawal show increased ICSS thresholds (e.g., decreased ICSS reward).
	Elevated maze test (anxiety)	A maze is placed approximately 2 feet above ground and an animal is placed at the intersection of a cross, where two arms are dark and walled off, and the other two are open and well lit. An anxious animal will generally spend more time in the "safer" region (the dark, walled off arms), and an animal's behavior in this paradigm is very sensitive to drug withdrawal.
	Defensive burying (anxiety)	An animal is placed in a box filled with woodchip bedding and an electrified probe protruding into the box. After touching the probe and receiving a mild shock, the active response is generally to bury the probe with the woodchips; observers will then measure the time to burying (latency), the height of the woodchip mound, total time spent burying, and number of burying acts.
III. Preoccupation/anticipation	Drug-induced reinstatement	Exposure to a reinforcing drug can reinstate drug use after the behavior has been extinguished.
	Cue-induced reinstatement	Cues previously paired to drug use act as a conditioned stimuli and lead to reinstatement of drug self-administration after the behavior has been extinguished.
	Stress-induced reinstatement	Reinstatement of drug self-administration provoked by stress; first shown with intermittent foot shock stressor in rats leading to reinstatement of substance use.

ICCC, Intracranial self-stimulation.

environment, whereas substances that have aversive effects will cause animals to prefer the placebo-paired environment.

Know This:

In the ICSS paradigm, rewarding drugs lower ICSS threshold, whereas substance withdrawal increases ICSS threshold.

Stage II: Withdrawal/Negative Affect

Using substances repeatedly over extended periods can lead to the *withdrawal/negative affect* stage. Key alterations in the withdrawal/negative affect stage include the (1) blunting of one's neurobiological responsiveness to rewards, (2) development of withdrawal syndromes, and (3) dysregulation of brain stress response systems, with perturbations in the hypothalamic-pituitary-adrenal (HPA) axis, corticotropin-releasing factor (CRF), dynorphin, norepinephrine, and neuropeptide Y (NPY).

- Loss of reward responsiveness has been demonstrated in both animal and human subjects following chronic substance use. Among individuals who have a SUD, imaging studies have found decreased dopamine D2 receptors in the striatum compared to controls and lower dopaminergic cellular activity in response to a stimulant drug challenge. These findings point to the development of diminished reward responsiveness that may reduce interest in natural stimuli such as food or sex and increased interest in substances that more robustly activate reward pathways.
- Although substance withdrawal syndromes have unique physiological signs and symptoms, there are general negative emotional and motivational changes in substance withdrawal common to all substances of abuse. These symptoms include irritability, anxiety, dysphoric affect, alexithymia (difficulty describing one's emotional state), and hyperkatifeia (hypersensitivity to emotional distress).
- Dysregulation in the brain's stress response system in the habenula and extended amygdala is hypothesized to cause the emotional perturbations in withdrawal. Implicated in this are perturbations in the HPA axis, CRF, dynorphin, norepinephrine, and NPY.
  - Withdrawal from all substances leads to activation of the **HPA axis** with an elevation of adrenocorticotropic hormone (ACTH), glucocorticoids, and extrahypothalamic **CRF** in the amygdala. With repeated cycles of withdrawal, HPA responsiveness diminishes, whereas extrahypothalamic CRF sensitization develops in the amygdala.
  - **NPY** is a neuromodulator shown to have anxiolytic effects and is part of the brain's putative "antistress" system that functionally opposes CRF. In withdrawal, NPY levels in the amygdala are diminished, thereby increasing vulnerability to negative emotional states.
  - **Dynorphin** and **norepinephrine** are also implicated in stress response; upregulation of dynorphin in the withdrawal/negative affect stage leads to increased dysphoria, whereas central noradrenergic systems activated during withdrawal lead to anxiety and agitation.

Know This:

The "reward deficiency syndrome" theory posits that those who are vulnerable to SUDs have hypodopaminergic functioning in the midbrain. This, in turn, predisposes vulnerable individuals to seek out substances to overcome dopamine deficits. It is thought to be regulated by specific polymorphisms of the DRD2 gene coding for the D2 receptor.

Withdrawal/Negative Affect: Animal Models

The key animal models in the withdrawal/negative affect stage of addiction include ICSS, conditioned place aversion, and models examining anxiety-like responses in animals, including the defensive burying and the elevated maze test.

- Conditioned place aversion: This paradigm is analogous to the conditioned place preference experiment described previously. Animals are exposed to the effects of drug withdrawal in one environment and are not in withdrawal when exposed to the other. This paradigm demonstrates that withdrawal is an aversive stimulus for animals and that they will avoid cues associated with it.

- Elevated maze test: A maze is elevated and an animal is placed at the intersection of a cross where two arms are dark and walled off, and the other two are open and well lit. An anxious animal will generally spend more time in the "safer" (dark and walled off) arms. An animal's behavior in this paradigm is very sensitive to drug withdrawal.

- Defensive burying test: The animal is placed in a box filled with woodchip bedding and a protruding electrified probe. After receiving a shock from the probe, the animal generally buries the probe with woodchips; observers will measure variables related to burying including the time to burying, the height of the woodchip mound, and time spent burying.

Know This:

Withdrawal from substances produces higher anxiety-like responses in the elevated maze and defensive burying test, and both of these responses can be reversed by administration of CRF antagonists.

Stage III: Preoccupation/Anticipation

The *preoccupation/anticipation* stage of addiction best captures the concept of addiction as a chronic, relapsing, and remitting disease. It describes the stage of addiction in which one seeks a substance following a period of abstinence. The construct of drug "craving" is generally linked to this stage as well, although it has proven difficult to study in humans and does not always correlate with relapse. Key alterations relevant to the *preoccupation/anticipation* stage include (1) deficits in PFC functioning leading to loss of executive control, (2) excessive incentive salience for a substance when relevant cues are presented to the individual, and (3) the development of drug cravings.

- The PFC is the key brain region implicated in the loss of control over substance use that characterizes this stage of addiction. The PFC regulates the limbic reward region and is critical for higher-order executive functioning, for example, self-control, emotional regulation, inhibitory control, self-awareness, attention, interoception, and salience attribution. Deficits in PFC functioning are associated with more negative outcomes, and chronic substance use can damage the PFC's selective regions.

- The anterior cingulate cortex and orbitofrontal cortex also modulate activity in the VTA-NAc through glutamatergic projections. Reduced cortical activity in these areas has also been linked to increased impulsive and compulsive substance use.

- In the presence of frontal lobe deficits, excessive incentive salience to drug-associated cues can lead to relapse and uncontrolled substance use.

- During abstinence, an important risk factor for relapse is cue-induced drug cravings. Cravings' development involves multiple cellular processes, but a key pathway involves AMPA-mediated synaptic remodeling of the medium spiny neurons of the NAc.

Know This:

In the *preoccupation/anticipation stage*, hypofrontality in the PFC, orbitofrontal cortex, and anterior cingulate cortex contributes to the inability to modulate the drive to use drugs despite the presence of negative consequences.

Preoccupation/Anticipation: Animal Models

Animal models of "craving" are divided into *reward cravings* and *relief cravings*. Reward cravings are provoked by stimuli previously coupled with drug self-administration, and stressful situations provoke relief cravings. Animal models of reward craving include *drug-induced reinstatement* and *cue-induced reinstatement*; the animal model most relevant to relief cravings is *stress-induced reinstatement*. Among animals for whom drug self-administration was established and subsequently extinguished, reinstatement of drug-seeking behavior can occur following exposure to a reinforcing drug (drug-induced reinstatement) or a cue previously paired to drug use (cue-induced reinstatement). On the other hand, relief cravings are induced by stressful stimuli, for example, foot shocks or social defeat experiments. Animal models of stress-induced reinstatement demonstrate that stress can lead to reinstatement among animals where drug self-administration was previously extinguished.

Know This:

The board examination may test you on the brain regions involved in drug, cue, and stressed-induced reinstatement. In summary:

- Drug-induced reinstatement is localized to the glutamatergic circuit involving the medial prefrontal cortex and ventral striatum.
- Cue-induced reinstatement involves the basolateral amygdala with hypothesized feed-forward inhibition of the prelimbic prefrontal cortex.
- Stress-induced reinstatement depends on activation of CRF and norepinephrine in the amygdala and VTA.

The three stages of addiction and their key features are summarized in Table 3.3.

GENETICS OF ADDICTION

SUDs are heritable conditions comparable to other highly heritable psychiatric disorders, such as schizophrenia and autism. With the development of rapidly improving genetic techniques and research studies with unprecedented sample sizes, we are approaching an era in which knowing individual genotypes will have substantive diagnostic value and treatment implications for SUDs. In this section, we review:

1. Heritability of SUDs and current estimates.
2. Contribution of genetic linkage and association studies.
3. Key candidate genes.
4. Epigenetic contributions.
5. Genetic overlap with psychiatric conditions.

The *heritability* of a trait or disorder refers to the proportion of the variability attributed to genetic factors and is typically estimated through family, adoption, and twin studies. Based on national surveys of adult twins, heritability is lowest for hallucinogen abuse (0.39) and highest for cocaine abuse (0.72), placing SUDs among the most highly heritable of psychiatric disorders (Fig. 3.2).

The finding of moderate to high heritability for SUDs is a precondition for searching for relevant genetic polymorphisms using molecular genetic approaches. Two approaches used to identify genetic causes of variability in SUDs are (1) genetic linkage and (2) genetic association studies.

- Genetic linkage studies search for chromosomal regions co-inherited with the phenotype of interest. The major aim is to identify risk genes within these regions on follow-up studies. Genetic linkage studies have identified important susceptibility loci for a number of SUDs, such as

---

TABLE 3.3
Summary of the Three Stages of Addiction

Stage of Addiction	Definition	Key Brain Regions	Key Neurotransmitters
Binge/intoxication	Stage of addiction in which the person uses an intoxicant and experiences the rewarding and reinforcing effects.	Nucleus accumbens Ventral tegmental area Dorsal striatum	Dopamine (directly or indirectly for all drugs) Opioid system (opioids, alcohol, cannabis) Serotonin (alcohol, stimulants) Endogenous cannabinoid system GABA (alcohol)
Withdrawal/negative affect	Stage of addiction in which the person experiences the negative physiological and emotional state in the absence of the substance.	Extended amygdala Habenula	Corticotrophin-releasing factor Dynorphin Neuropeptide Y Norepinephrine
Preoccupation/anticipation	Stage of addiction in which one seeks the substance after a period of abstinence.	Prefrontal cortex Orbitofrontal cortex Anterior cingulate cortex	Glutamate Dopamine

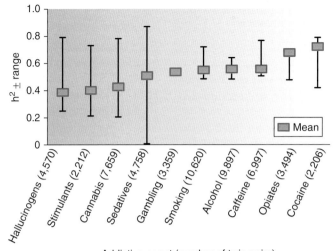

Fig. 3.2 ■ Heritability of common substance use disorders and behavioral addictions. (From Ducci, F., & Goldman, D. (2012). The genetic basis of addictive disorders. *Psychiatric Clinics of North America, 35*(2), 495–519. https://doi.org/10.1016/j.psc.2012.03.010)

the ADH and GABRA2 gene cluster, which are relevant for risk of alcohol use disorder.

■ Genome-wide association studies (GWAS) have largely replaced genetic linkage studies in the search for candidate genes. GWAS is typically performed by querying the genome with microarrays of thousands to millions of genetic markers to examine whether particular alleles are common among individuals with the disease versus controls. GWAS for SUDs have largely replicated prior candidate gene findings, and have identified novel genes such as CHRNA5/A3/B4 on chromosome 15 (encoding neuronal nicotinic acetylcholine receptor subunits) that are associated with tobacco, alcohol, and cocaine use disorders.

Notable genes that may be tested are presented in Table 3.4.

Epigenetic modification is another mechanism by which substance use is believed to alter gene expression and result in longer-term changes in neuralplasticity and behavior. Epigenetics refers to DNA modification that does not involve changes in DNA base pair sequence, but rather involves changes in gene expression through transcription factors and histone modification. The best-known transcription factors relevant for drug-induced neuroplasticity are ΔFosB and cAMP response element-binding (CREB)

protein. CREB and ΔFosB are the two main transcription factors relevant for drug-induced neuroplasticity and long-term changes in addictive behavior caused via epigenetic modification. The actions of CREB and ΔFosB can be summarized as follows:

■ CREB rapidly increases in the NAc with opioids, cocaine, and alcohol and leads to upregulation of dynorphin.
■ CREB rapidly decreases in the central nucleus of the amygdala with alcohol and nicotine and leads to reductions in levels of NPY.
■ ΔFosB accumulates slowly with substance use and remains stably high for months following abstinence. It increases the positive rewarding effects of substances and susceptibility to addiction.

Other important discoveries include the prominent genetic overlap between substance use disorders and several psychiatric illnesses. Epidemiological studies have established the significant comorbidity between substance use disorders and most psychiatric illnesses, and this overlap has been supported by genetic studies that have identified overlapping risk alleles. Examples of this are ADHD and tobacco use disorders. Both have been associated with monoamine regulating genes, including the dopamine D4 and D5 receptor genes (DRD4 and DRD5), the dopamine transporter (DAT1)

TABLE 3.4		
Identified Genetic Variants Relative to Specific Substance Use Disorders		
Substance	Gene	Relevance
Nicotine		
	CYP2A61B	Involved in metabolism of nicotine; if homozygous, more likely to be a heavier smoker
	GABRA2	Impulsivity and external behavior problems in nicotine and alcohol use disorder
	GABRA6	Implicated in flushing reaction, as well as impulsivity
	CHRNA5	Increased risk of nicotine use disorder
	DRD2	Associated with increased risk of smoking and reward deficiency syndrome
Alcohol		
	AUTS2	Prefrontal cortex
	SLC6A4	Implicated in activation of amygdala and linked to psychiatric issues in alcohol use
	OPRM1	Moderates naltrexone response; mediates greater reduction of heavy drinking in alcohol users prescribed naltrexone
	ALDH1A1	Linked to epigenetic changes that occur in patients who suffer childhood adversity leading to later alcohol abuse
	ADH1B	Associated with upper GI cancers and alcohol consumption
	ADH2	Increases risk for alcohol use disorder
Opioids		
	ALDH5A1	Associated with nonresponsiveness in patients who receive maintenance therapy for opioid use disorder
	ORPD1	Associated with treatment efficacy with long-term use of methadone
	CYP2D6	Associated with risk of respiratory depression particularly among European Whites who abuse codeine
	OPRM1	Variants A118G and C17T SNPs are most important: A118G variant associated with increased risk of heroin addiction and alcohol abuse
Cocaine		
	CAMK4	Associated with higher susceptibility to cocaine addiction
	PER1	Associated with changes in circadian rhythm and cocaine addiction
	VNTR	Associated with cocaine-induced paranoia
	H3K9E3	Associated with cocaine use
Marijuana		
	FAAH	Associated with striatal activation to marijuana cues and linked to withdrawal and cravings in patients who use marijuana
	CRN1	Encodes CB1 receptor
	AKT1	Associated with psychosis in cannabis users
	COMT	Associated with schizophrenia in cannabis users

GI, Gastrointestinal; *SNPs*, single nucleotide polymorphisms.

gene, and the dopamine beta-hydroxylase (DBH) gene. Co-morbidities of substance use disorder with psychiatric illnesses were reviewed in more details in Chapter 2.

Know This:

GWAS is the method of choice for confirming previously identified candidate genes and novel genes associated with substance use disorders.

PHARMACOTHERAPEUTIC APPROACHES FOR SUDs

Research into medication treatments for substance use disorders primarily focuses on treatments that act by one of several approaches:

1. Blocking drug targets in the brain
2. Simulating the actions of drugs
3. Modifying relevant biological elements of addiction

Here we provide examples of medications used for SUDs that follow each of these principles and are frequently asked about on board examinations. Subsequent chapters on individual substances of abuse will review treatment approaches in greater depth.

Examples of medications that block drug targets include receptor antagonists, for example, **naltrexone** (an opioid receptor antagonist used for opioid and alcohol use disorder) and **rimonabant** (an inverse agonist that acts as an antagonist at the cannabinoid 1 receptor; researched but not approved for cannabis use disorder). Other research efforts are focused on developing vaccines for addiction. The therapeutic cocaine vaccine (i.e., **TA-CD**) has been shown to produce antibodies against cocaine and reduce self-administration of cocaine in animals; however, phase III trials in humans with cocaine use disorder showed no significant treatment effect.

Another common approach involves simulating the actions of drugs of abuse in the brain; some treatments following this paradigm include **methadone** (a full mu-opioid receptor agonist), **stimulant medications** and other dopamine agonists for stimulant use disorders (e.g., mixed amphetamine salts), and **nicotine replacement therapy** for tobacco use disorder. Partial agonists both simulate drugs' actions while also blocking drug targets in the brain; these include **buprenorphine** for opioid use disorder and **varenicline** for tobacco use disorder.

Although many treatments act directly on a drug's direct molecular target or modulating the dopamine system, many other neurotransmitters are important in addiction, which are potential treatment targets. These include glutamate, GABA, NPY, CRF, serotonin, norepinephrine, and brain-derived neurotrophic factor. Glutamatergic input from the prefrontal cortex, hippocampus, and amygdala is essential in modulating dopamine release in the NAc and VTA. Medications with glutamatergic actions are of interest in addiction treatment; some examples of medications with glutamatergic actions include **acamprosate**, **topiramate**, and **N-acetylcysteine**.

REFERENCE

Olds, J., & Milner, P. (1954). Positive reinforcement produced by electrical stimulation of septal area and other regions of rat brain. *Journal of Comparative and Physiological Psychology, 47*(6), 419–427. https://doi.org/10.1037/h0058775.

SUGGESTIONS FOR FURTHER READING

Koob, G. F. Volkow N.D. (2005). Neurocircuits of Addiction. In M. Galanter, H. D. Kleber, & K. Brady (Eds.), *The American Psychiatric Association Publishing textbook of substance abuse treatment* (5th ed., pp. 3–18). American Psychiatric Association Publishing.

Koob, G. F., & Volkow, N. D. (2016). Neurobiology of addiction: A neurocircuitry analysis. *The Lancet. Psychiatry, 3*(8), 760–773. https://doi.org/10.1016/S2215-0366(16)00104-8.

Li, M. D., & Burmeister, M. (2009). New insights into the genetics of addiction. *Nature Reviews Genetics, 10*(4), 225–231. https://doi.org/10.1038/nrg2536.

Nestler, E. J. (2005). Is there a common molecular pathway for addiction? *Nature Neuroscience, 8*(11), 1445–1449. https://doi.org/10.1038/nn1578.

Olds, J., & Milner, P. (1954). Positive reinforcement produced by electrical stimulation of septal area and other regions of rat brain. *Journal of Comparative and Physiological Psychology, 47*(6), 419–427.

REVIEW QUESTIONS

1. Which of the following animal models would be most appropriate in studying the aversiveness (i.e., negative reinforcing effects) of opioid withdrawal?
   A. Conditioned place preference
   B. Conditioned place aversion
   C. Self-administration
   D. Drug-induced reinstatement
   E. Cue-induced reinstatement

2. Which of the following is believed to be a key neuromodulator for reducing stress and counteracting the effects of corticotropin-releasing factor (CRF)
   A. Dynorphin
   B. Neuropeptide Y
   C. Norepinephrine
   D. Adrenocorticotropic hormone
   E. Glutamate

3. Which neurotransmitter system is least important in mediating the rewarding effects of substances in the binge/intoxication stage?
   A. Norepinephrine
   B. Serotonin
   C. GABA
   D. Opioid
   E. Dopamine

4. Which of the following statements accurately represents the findings of Olds and Milner's classic brain stimulation reward animal experiment?
   A. Animals that are exposed to aversive effects of a substance will spend less time in the area of the cage where they experienced those symptoms.
   B. Animals that are exposed to the rewarding effects of a substance will spend more time in the area of the cage where they experienced those symptoms.
   C. Reinforcing drugs will lower the threshold for ICSS.
   D. Reinforcing drugs will increase the threshold for ICSS.
   E. Reinforcing drugs will not change the threshold for ICSS.

5. Which of the following experimental models would best measure the anxiety-like responses of an animal in opioid withdrawal?
   A. Defensive burying
   B. Conditioned place aversion
   C. Conditioned place preference
   D. Drug self-administration
   E. Intracranial self-stimulation

6. You are seeing a 23-year-old man with a history of heroin use. He tells you that he experiences severe withdrawal symptoms such as anxiety, irritability, body aches, and tremor, but that he experiences quick relief of symptoms once he resumes heroin use. This phenomenon is an example of:
   A. Positive reinforcement
   B. Negative reinforcement
   C. Classical conditioning
   D. Operant conditioning
   E. Incentive salience

7. *Contingency management* is a behavioral treatment that seeks to shape behavior by using punishing and rewarding reinforcements. This treatment modality is an example of:
   A. Positive reinforcement
   B. Negative reinforcement
   C. Classical conditioning
   D. Operant conditioning
   E. Incentive salience

8. Incentive salience is regulated through which of the following biological processes?
   A. Glutamatergic projections from the PFC to dopamine neurons in the VTA
   B. Dysregulation in the brain's stress response systems in the extended amygdala and the habenula
   C. Activation of CRF and norepinephrine in the amygdala and VTA
   D. AMPA-mediated synaptic remodeling of the medium spiny neurons in the NAc
   E. Inhibition of GABA-ergic nerve terminals in the VTA, which then disinhibit VTA dopamine neurons and increase dopaminergic neurotransmission

9. Which of the following substances has the lowest heritability in terms of the risk of developing a SUD?
   A. Alcohol
   B. Hallucinogens
   C. Nicotine
   D. Opioids
   E. Cocaine

10. Which of the following genetic methods is most commonly used to identify novel genes associated with SUDs?
    A. GWAS
    B. Genetic linkage studies
    C. Twin studies
    D. Adoption studies
    E. Epigenetic studies

ALCOHOL USE DISORDER

GENERAL CHARACTERISTICS AND HISTORY

Evidence of alcohol consumption has been noted as far back as 9,000 years ago by Neolithic farmers in Northern China, and recipes for producing alcohol have been discovered worldwide for thousands of years. Dr. Benjamin Rush is believed to have been the first person to characterize excessive alcohol use as a disorder in 1784. By the late 1800s, temperance movements sprung up across the United States, inspired mainly by religious groups who considered drunkenness a national threat. In 1920, Prohibition was enacted in the form of the 18th Amendment, which prohibited the manufacture and sale of alcohol. This was later repealed in 1933 because of its unpopularity. In 1935, Alcoholics Anonymous (AA) was founded by Bill Wilson and Dr. Robert Smith as a peer-based fellowship to provide group support to other recovering alcoholics when no other treatment options were available. Since then, enormous advances have been made in understanding alcohol use disorder (AUD), including the biological effects of alcohol, treatment approaches for alcohol intoxication and withdrawal, development of medications, and establishment of evidence-based therapies for AUD of which will be reviewed in this chapter.

PHARMACOLOGY OF ALCOHOL

Chemical Structure and Metabolism

Fig. 4.1 shows the chemical structure and metabolism of ethanol and several other alcohols that are clinically relevant to know about and which you may be asked about on the board examination.

Here are some key points to remember about alcohol's pharmacokinetics and pharmacodynamics:

- Alcohol undergoes first-pass metabolism in the stomach due to alcohol dehydrogenase (ADH) in the gastric mucosa.
- Alcohol is metabolized by ADH to acetaldehyde, which is toxic and a known carcinogen. Acetaldehyde is then metabolized by aldehyde dehydrogenase (ALDH) to acetate, which is converted to water and carbon dioxide for easy elimination (Fig. 4.1). CYP2E1 also metabolizes alcohol at higher blood concentrations and produces reactive oxygen species as a byproduct.
- ADH and ALDH are responsible for metabolizing a range of alcohols encountered in the body, including ethanol, methanol, ethylene glycol, and isopropyl alcohol (Fig. 4.1).
- Alcohol metabolism follows zero-order kinetics because ADH saturates at very low serum levels of ethanol, leading to constant levels of elimination.
- Alcohol is metabolized at roughly 0.015 g/dL per hour. The rate of alcohol metabolism is dependent on factors including age, sex, body weight, and differences in expression and enzyme isotypes of ADH and ALDH. Women have a higher blood alcohol concentration than men for an equivalent amount of alcohol use because of lower levels of gastric ADH and first-pass metabolism and lower total body water. Lower body weight and increased age are both associated with a slower metabolism. Gastric ADH levels decline with age.
- The peak effect of ethanol occurs 30 minutes after consumption.

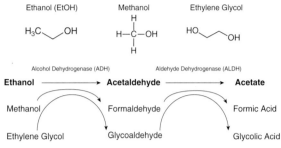

Fig. 4.1 ■ Chemical structure and metabolism of alcohols.

Nonethanol alcohols that you may be asked about are methanol, ethylene glycol, and isopropyl alcohol.

- **Methanol** is found in windshield wiper fluid and is a common impurity in home-distilled spirits (a.k.a. "moonshine"). It is metabolized to formaldehyde and formic acid, which is highly toxic and can lead to blindness by damaging the optic nerve.
- **Ethylene glycol** is a common odorless antifreeze component and is metabolized to glycolic acid and other byproducts. Its most toxic byproduct is calcium oxalate, which can accumulate in the body and lead to kidney damage.
- **Isopropyl alcohol** is a flammable component of hand sanitizers, rubbing alcohol, disinfectants, and detergents and has a strong odor. ADH metabolizes it to acetone, which is nontoxic and nonacidic.

Neurobiology of Alcohol

Unlike other drugs of abuse that have more targeted pharmacologic effects (e.g., cocaine), alcohol affects many neurotransmitter systems. Here we summarize the key neurotransmitter and receptor systems affected by alcohol and are essential to know for the board examination.

- **γ-aminobutyric acid (GABA):** GABA-A and GABA-B receptors are the two main GABA receptor types and are the primary inhibitory receptor system in the central nervous system (CNS); GABA-A is ionotropic and GABA-B is metabotropic. Alcohol's CNS depressant effects are primarily mediated through enhancement of GABA-A receptor function.
- **Glutamate:** Glutamate is the primary excitatory neurotransmitter in the CNS. The three main glutamate receptors are N-methyl-D-aspartate receptor (NMDA), α-amino-3-hydroxy-5-methyl-4-isoxazolepropionic acid (AMPA), and kainate. Alcohol inhibits glutamatergic NMDA receptors, and alcohol withdrawal leads to glutamatergic overactivity owning to loss of NMDA receptor inhibition.
- **Dopamine:** The rewarding effects of alcohol are indirectly mediated through the same common pathway as other drugs of abuse, that is, via dopamine release in the ventral tegmental area. Alcohol indirectly increases dopamine levels in the mesocorticolimbic system.
- **Serotonin:** Alcohol potentiates 5-hydroxytryptamine 3 (5-HT3) receptor activity; lower overall serotonin neurotransmission is believed to be implicated in AUD. In individuals who abuse alcohol, levels of 5-HT and 5-HT metabolites have been found to be lower in the cerebrospinal fluid.
- **Opioids:** Alcohol leads to the release of endogenous endorphins in the ventral tegmentum and nucleus accumbens, which leads to increases in dopaminergic neurotransmission. The use of naltrexone reduces alcohol consumption by blocking opioid receptors.
- **Endocannabinoids:** The endocannabinoid system is an important modulator of alcohol's reinforcing properties.

TOXICOLOGY

Testing for alcohol and other substances is covered at length in Chapter 12 (Drug Testing, Forensic Addictions, and Ethics). Biomarkers for alcohol intoxication or very recent ingestion (typically on the order of hours) include:

- **Blood alcohol concentration (BAC):** Tests for alcohol concentration in whole blood samples.
- **Breath alcohol testing, a.k.a. breathalyzer:** Tests for alcohol in exhaled air; used by law enforcement agencies and the Department of Transportation.
- **Ethyl glucuronide (EtG):** A direct biomarker of alcohol use and a metabolite of ethanol. It can be detected in urine from 1 hour after alcohol intake and up to 3 to 5 days, and then in hair for up to 3 months.
- **Ethyl sulfate (EtS):** A direct biomarker of alcohol use and a metabolite of ethanol. It can be detected in urine from 1 hour after alcohol intake and up to 3 to 5 days, and then in hair for up to 3 months.

Know This:

The Widmark Equation is commonly used in legal settings to estimate BAC. BAC = A/(Wr), where A = weight of alcohol absorbed (in oz), W = weight of subject (in oz), and r = Widmark factor, a constant ratio of total body water compared with water in blood.

ALCOHOL INTOXICATION

Alcohol intoxication is associated with a number of complications, including accidents, trauma, homicide, and suicide and accounts for over 600,000 (0.6%) emergency department visits in the United States per year. The following symptoms can be observed at these approximate BACs in nontolerant individuals:

- 50 to 100 mg/dL: Euphoria, disinhibition, slower reaction times
- 100 to 200 mg/dL: Ataxia, slurred speech, deficits in psychomotor skills, impaired judgment
- 200 to 300 mg/dL: Nausea, vomiting, confusion, stupor
- 300 to 400 mg/dL: Hypothermia, amnesia, dysarthria
- >400 mg/dL: Obtundation, coma, respiratory depression, seizures, arrhythmias, death

In general, uncomplicated alcohol intoxication is not life-threatening, except for alcohol poisoning, which can be fatal. Patients presenting with a BAC greater than 300 mg/dL are at risk for coma, respiratory depression, and death. Keep in mind that an elevated BAC may not be accompanied by any notable signs of intoxication among individuals who use large amounts of alcohol chronically.

Other common sequelae of alcohol intoxication include:

- Anterograde amnesia (a.k.a. "blackouts"): A common consequence of heavy alcohol use and frequently seen in college-age adults. Some risk factors include a rapid rise in BAC, fatigue, drinking on an empty stomach, and drinking quickly (a.k.a. chugging).
- Hangovers: They are not well understood but are believed to be caused by a build-up of the intermediate metabolite, acetaldehyde, in addition to dehydration, electrolyte imbalance, and poor sleep. Alcohols with congeners (e.g., red wine and other dark liquors such as rum and brandy) are more likely to cause hangovers than clear alcohols.

Know This:

Alcohol poisoning deaths are most common among middle-aged non-Hispanic White men.

Treatment of Alcohol Intoxication

- Management is typically supportive to prevent harm from agitation, respiratory depression, or loss of airway protection. Most patients will only require observation and serial examinations until they reach clinical sobriety.
- Patients presenting with alcohol intoxication should be asked about co-ingestion of other substances, have a rapid glucose test, and be assessed for dehydration and traumatic or occult injuries.
- If patients require dextrose because of hypoglycemia, high-dose thiamine should be co-administered to prevent Wernicke encephalopathy.
- The evaluation and referral for substance use treatment should be encouraged following the resolution of intoxication.

Know This:

Other types of alcohol can present with different signs, symptoms of intoxication. Please review the types of alcohol and the treatments (Table 4.1) for your board exams.

Intoxication with methanol or ethylene glycol should always be considered if a patient presents with a profound metabolic acidosis (serum bicarbonate <8 mEq/L) and a high unexplained osmolal gap. All alcohol intoxication syndromes will present with an elevated serum osmolality. Early treatment of methanol and ethylene glycol ingestion includes administration of fomepizole, which competitively inhibits ADH and prevents build-up of their toxic byproducts. Because ethanol has a higher affinity for ADH than methanol, ethanol can also be used to treat methanol ingestion.

	TABLE 4.1			
Methanol, Ethylene Glycol, and Isopropyl Alcohol				
Alcohol	Byproducts	Clinical Findings	Unique Laboratory Findings	Treatment
Methanol	Formic acid (toxic)	Blindness, visual blurring, and central scotomata	Anion gap metabolic acidosis, elevated lactate	Fomepizole +/– dialysis, Ethanol
Ethylene glycol	Glycolic acid (toxic)	Hematuria, oliguria, flank pain, fluorescent urine	Anion gap metabolic acidosis, elevated lactate, urine calcium oxalate crystals	Fomepizole +/– dialysis,
Isopropyl alcohol	Acetone (nontoxic)	Fruity breath, intoxication syndrome similar to ethanol	No anion gap, ketosis without metabolic acidosis	Supportive

ALCOHOL WITHDRAWAL

Following an abrupt reduction or cessation of alcohol use, alcohol withdrawal symptoms can emerge within 6 to 8 hours and may last for up to 7 days. Alcohol enhances inhibitory GABA-A receptor function and inhibits excitatory glutamatergic NMDA receptors; therefore cessation of alcohol in an individual who is physiologically dependent results in alcohol withdrawal pathophysiology: loss of GABAergic inhibition, glutamatergic overactivity, and a severe hyperadrenergic state. Predictors of more severe alcohol withdrawal include longer duration of alcohol use, medical comorbidities, history of prior alcohol withdrawal, seizures or delirium tremens (DTs; due to kindling effects), presence of medical illness (notably electrolyte abnormalities and elevated liver function tests), presentation with BAC greater than 300 mg/dL, and elevated blood pressure and heart rate. There is high individual variation in the severity and duration of alcohol withdrawal symptoms. Keep in mind that patients can experience alcohol withdrawal symptoms before the BAC returns to zero.

Symptoms of mild alcohol withdrawal include anxiety, sweating, irritability, tremor, agitation, nausea, and vomiting, with normal mental status. More severe sequelae of alcohol withdrawal include the following:

- Alcoholic hallucinosis: Hallucinations are predominantly auditory but can include visual and tactile hallucinations as well. Hallucinosis can occur without the presence of other withdrawal symptoms and the patient's mental status is otherwise clear. Hallucinosis is not synonymous with DTs.
- Alcohol withdrawal seizures: Typically tonic-clonic seizures; status epilepticus is uncommon.

- DTs: This is the most serious complication of alcohol withdrawal with high mortality rates if left untreated. Symptoms include fluctuating levels of consciousness, visual and auditory hallucinations, autonomy instability, and hyperpyrexia.

The general timeline of alcohol withdrawal symptoms is presented here.

Symptoms	**Time of Onset After Last Drink**	Duration
Mild alcohol withdrawal symptoms	6–8 hours	36 hours
Alcoholic hallucinosis	12–24 hours	48 hours
Alcohol withdrawal seizures	8–24 hours	5 days
DTs	2–4 days	7 days

After resolution of acute alcohol withdrawal and establishment of abstinence, patients can continue to experience protracted withdrawal symptoms that resemble some of the symptoms of acute withdrawal. These include sleep disruption, depression, mood swings, anxiety, and agitation, and they can render the patient vulnerable to relapse during early abstinence.

Evaluation of Withdrawal

A broadly used and well-validated rating scale measuring the severity of alcohol withdrawal is the **Clinical Institute Withdrawal Assessment for Alcohol—Revised (CIWA-Ar)** (Sullivan et al., 1989). It is a 10-item, clinician-rated scale that ranges from 0 to 67; the 10 items include nausea and vomiting, tremor, sweating, anxiety, agitation, tactile disturbance, auditory disturbances, visual disturbances, headache, and clouding of sensorium. Scores greater than 15 indicates severe withdrawal. CIWA scores are also used to guide the need for medication dosing. Individuals with a CIWA score less than or equal to 8 generally do not require medications to manage alcohol withdrawal symptoms.

Administration of the CIWA-Ar relies on patient's ability to communicate and should only be used if other etiologies of the patient's condition have been excluded (e.g., delirium, dementia, acute psychosis, opioid withdrawal). If the patient is unable to communicate, the CIWA-Ar is not an appropriate assessment tool. Other assessment tools such as the Richmond Agitation-Sedation Scale (RASS) can be used to manage withdrawal in patients who are intubated or in the intensive care setting.

Know This:

The CIWA does not include scored items for vital signs. The decision not to include vital signs was based on data showing that pulse and blood pressure did not correlate with the severity of alcohol withdrawal than the other signs and symptoms included in the CIWA-Ar.

Treatment of Withdrawal

The mainstay of pharmacological treatment for alcohol withdrawal are benzodiazepines; commonly used benzodiazepines are those with longer half-lives, including diazepam, chlordiazepoxide, or clonazepam. Some key points regarding the treatment of alcohol withdrawal include the following:

- Benzodiazepines are cross-tolerant with alcohol and are considered the first line for the treatment of alcohol withdrawal.
- Benzodiazepines are typically metabolized by hepatic oxidation followed by hepatic glucuronidation. For patients with liver damage, alternative benzodiazepines that do not undergo hepatic oxidation include lorazepam (L), oxazepam (O), and temazepam (T); use the LOT mnemonic to remember safer benzodiazepines in patients with liver damage.

- Barbiturates such as phenobarbital can be used to treat alcohol withdrawal but are far less commonly employed than benzodiazepines because of their narrow therapeutic index.
- Other medications that can be used for treating alcohol withdrawal include anticonvulsants (such as carbamazepine, gabapentin, levetiracetam and valproic acid) and adrenergic agents (such as clonidine and dexmedetomidine).
- Benzodiazepines-sparing protocols for the treatment of alcohol withdrawal (such as protocols using anticonvulsant medications) are particularly useful for treating alcohol withdrawal in outpatient settings.
- For patients with refractory DTs, treatment options include phenobarbital or propofol. Propofol is a sedative-hypnotic that acts as a GABA-A receptor agonist and NMDA receptor antagonist. Intubation is frequently necessary if phenobarbital or propofol are given.

Two commonly employed strategies are *fixed multiple daily dosing* and *symptom-triggered treatment* for individuals requiring medications to manage alcohol withdrawal. In fixed multiple daily dosing schedules, patients are typically placed on a gradual, tapering benzodiazepine schedule once their withdrawal symptoms are stabilized. In symptom-triggered treatment, benzodiazepines are only administered if patients are showing sufficient symptoms of alcohol withdrawal. The current evidence favors symptom-triggered treatment, as it reduces the average length of stay, the total dosage of administered benzodiazepines, and the level of patient sedation. Despite this, the fixed-dose schedule is still widely used. CIWA-Ar can be used to guide the need for symptom-triggered medication and ancillary rescue medication if a patient is on a fixed-dose schedule.

Know This:

For the board examination, you may be asked whether a patient in alcohol withdrawal can be safely treated in the inpatient versus outpatient setting. The American Society of Addiction Medicine (ASAM) patient placement criteria provide a guide to help you determine which patients are appropriate for outpatient care (see Chapter 1). In general, inpatient treatment is preferred for patients who:

Present in more severe withdrawal (CIWA >15)

A history of severe or complicated withdrawal (history of seizures or delirium tremens)

Have high levels of recent alcohol consumption

Have severe co-occurring medical or psychiatric illness that may complicate treatment

Lack an adequate support network

Patients who have only mild or moderate withdrawal, no significant medical or psychiatric illness, can come to the clinic daily, and have social support to assist through the detoxification process are good candidates for outpatient detoxification.

AT-RISK DRINKING AND AUD

Screening for At-Risk Alcohol Use

There are a number of screening tests designed to identify unhealthy alcohol use or AUD. When patients are identified as having harmful or unhealthy alcohol use, they should be assessed for an AUD and referred to treatment if warranted.

Some important terminology:

- **Standard drink:** Definition varies by country; in the United States, one standard drink contains approximately 12 to 14 g of ethanol and is equivalent to 12 oz beer, 5 oz wine, and 1.5 oz 80-proof liquor.
- **At-risk drinking (unhealthy alcohol use):** According to the National Institute on Alcohol Abuse and Alcoholism (NIAAA), unhealthy alcohol use is defined for women as more than seven standard drinks per week and more than three standard drinks per day. For men, it is defined as more than 14 standard drinks per week and more than 4 standard drinks per day. Drinking above these levels increases the likelihood of social and health consequences.
- **Binge drinking:** Pattern of drinking that brings BAC to 0.08 mg/dL; this is approximately five or more drinks for men and four or more drinks for women consumed on one occasion.
- **Heavy alcohol use:** Defined as binge drinking on 5 or more days during the past 30 days.

Important screening instruments for alcohol use include the National Institute on Alcohol Abuse and Alcoholism (NIAAA) single-question alcohol screen Alcohol Use Disorders Identification Test (AUDIT), The Alcohol Use Disorders Identification Test-Concise (AUDIT-C), (CAGE) stand for Cut, Annoyed, Guilty, and Eye questionnaire, Michigan Alcohol Screening Test (MAST), Michigan Alcoholism Screening Test- Geriatric Version (MAST-G), TWEAK is an acronym for Tolerance (T1 number of drinks to feel high; T2, number of drinks one can hold), Worry about drinking, Eye-opener (morning drinking), Amnesia (blackouts), and Cut down on drinking (K/C) and Screening, Brief Intervention, and Referral to Treatment (SBIRT), all of which have been covered in Chapters 1 and 2.

You will frequently encounter the DSM-IV definitions of alcohol dependence and alcohol abuse. In the DSM-5, these distinct diagnoses were replaced by the single diagnosis of AUD. The DSM-5 also removed the DSM-IV criterion of "legal problems" and added the criterion of "cravings." According to the DSM-5, the diagnosis of AUD is established based on the diagnostic criteria listed in Chapter 1.

AUD Typologies

A number of early research studies have led to the idea that there are typologies of individuals with alcohol dependence, and these typologies are frequently referenced in clinical practice. The most well-known of these are the Cloninger type I vs. II and Babor type A vs. B. These typologies are summarized in Table 4.2.

EPIDEMIOLOGY OF ALCOHOL USE

In terms of the overall epidemiology of alcohol use, some key facts to remember are:

- Alcohol use, heavy alcohol consumption, and lifetime AUD among adults 18 and older have increased in the United States over the past 2 decades.
- Alcohol-related deaths in the United States have doubled from 1999 to 2017; in 2017, alcohol-related mortalities accounted for nearly 3% of all mortalities predominantly from liver disease (31%) and followed by overdoses (18%).

TABLE 4.2
Typologies of Alcohol Dependence

Cloninger Typologies of Alcohol Dependence

Type I	Type II
Genetics and environment both contribute to risk	Predominantly genetic; environment has limited contribution
Late onset (after age 25 years)	Early onset (before age 25 years)
Affect men and women equally	Predominantly men
Ability to abstain temporarily	Inability to abstain temporarily
Harm avoidance high	Harm avoidance low
Drinking to self-medicate (e.g., to relieve anxiety)	History of antisocial behaviors (e.g., drinking followed by aggressive behaviors)
Typically respond better to treatment	Drinking to induce euphoria

Babor Typologies of Alcohol Dependence

Type A	Type B
Late onset	Early onset
Fewer childhood risk factors	Greater childhood risk factors
Less severe dependence	Family history of alcohol use
Fewer problems associated with alcohol	More severe dependence
Less psychopathology	More serious consequences of alcohol use
	Greater psychopathology
	More frequent polysubstance use
	More chronic treatment history

- Prevalence of lifetime DSM-IV alcohol abuse and/or dependence among those 18 and older was 30% between 2001 and 2002 and 44% between 2012 and 2013.
- In 2018, 25% of individuals aged 12 years and over were current binge alcohol users, and 6.1% were heavy alcohol users. However, among adolescents aged 12 to 17 years, binge alcohol use has been declining over the past 2 decades.
- The financial burden of excessive alcohol use in the United States (nearly $250 billion in 2010) is predominantly from drinking-related crimes and *binge drinking.*
- Keep in mind that more than 50% of individuals will remit from AUD without any treatment, depending on the severity of the problem.

In terms of other demographic risk factors:

- Age: Adults aged 18 to 25 years old have the highest prevalence of past year and lifetime AUD than other age groups (National Epidemiologic Survey on Alcohol and Related Conditions-III [NESARC-III] 2012–2013).
- Sex: Males are approximately twice as likely to have an AUD compared with females. During pregnancy, AUD is less prevalent than in nonpregnant females, and alcohol use has been declining in pregnant adult females over the past 2 decades.
- Race: Lifetime prevalence of AUD varies by race/ethnicity. From highest to lowest: Native American (43%), White (33%), Hispanic (23%), Black (22%), and Asian/Pacific Islander (15%) according to data collected between 2012 and 2013.
- Low income is also a risk factor for having an AUD.

RISK FACTORS FOR AUD

This section will cover the key genetic, psychopathological, and personality factors that increase the risk for developing an AUD.

Genetics of AUD

The heritability of AUD is estimated to be approximately 50% based on twin and adoption studies, indicating that positive family history is a strong risk factor for developing AUD. Genetic factors may explain some individual and group differences in AUD prevalence based on genetic differences in alcohol metabolization, impulsivity, and behavioral disinhibition. Some of the key genetic variants relevant for AUD that you may be asked about on the board examination include:

- **ADH1B**: Codes for ADH, responsible for metabolizing alcohol to acetaldehyde. The ADH1B*2 variant is common among East Asians and is associated with a more rapid alcohol metabolism to acetaldehyde.
- **ALDH2**: Codes for ALDH. A common variant among East Asians is ALDH2*2, which is less metabolically active than wild-type ALDH and leads to accumulation of acetaldehyde.
- **AUTS2**: Autism susceptibility candidate 2 gene; the major variant is associated with greater alcohol consumption than the minor variant.
- **GABRA2**: Encodes the α2 subunit of the GABA-A ionotropic receptor and is associated with alcohol dependence.

Know This:

Alcohol flush reaction is common among individuals of East Asian descent because of a higher frequency of both the ADH1B*2 and ALDH2*2 alleles, both of which lead to accumulation of acetaldehyde. Increased amounts of acetaldehyde lead to the release of histamines, which causes vessel dilatation and skin redness.

A low **sedative-ataxic response** (reflective of acute functional tolerance) is a phenotypic marker of genetic risk for AUD. Higher concentrations of BAC are frequently sedating (and thus protect against high levels of alcohol use). Individuals with a low sedative-ataxic response (measured by variables like body sway during intoxication) lack this protective effect. They can drink to higher levels while continuing to experience the euphoric effects of alcohol.

Personality Factors

AUD is significantly associated with higher neuroticism/negative emotionality, disinhibition, and low conscientiousness; it is not associated with extroversion differences, openness to experience, or agreeableness.

Psychopathological Factors

In childhood:

- Internalizing and externalizing disorders are important risk factors for the later development of AUD.
- As observed in childhood externalizing disorders, definitions in behavioral regulation and inhibition share common causes with AUD.
- Childhood antisocial behaviors (including conduct disorder and oppositional defiance disorder, referred to collectively as *deviance proneness*) and attention-deficit/hyperactivity disorder are associated with later alcohol use.
- The temporal relationship between the development of alcohol and mood/anxiety disorders is more mixed. However, prospective studies have shown that anxiety in childhood and adolescence predicts the later development of AUD.

In adulthood:

- There are strong associations between AUD and drug use disorders, tobacco use disorder, major depressive disorder, bipolar I disorder, and borderline and antisocial personality disorder.
- Associations are positive but more modest between AUD and generalized anxiety disorder, posttraumatic stress disorder, specific phobia, and panic disorder.

Know This:

The "self-medication hypothesis," first posited by Edward Khantzian and supported by considerable evidence, states that alcohol is used as a coping mechanism to allay negative emotionality. This may in part explain the association between AUD and adult neuroticism and other psychiatric disorders.

EFFECTS OF EXCESS ALCOHOL USE

Excessive alcohol use is the third leading cause of preventable death in the United States, and alcohol-related mortality rates have been rising over the past 2 decades. Here we review the main long-term effects that you may be asked about on the board examination, focusing on neurologic sequelae and intrauterine effects. The long-term effects of alcohol are also reviewed in Chapter 2 (Comorbidities of Substance Use Disorders).

Neurological Effects

Between 50% and 70% of individuals with AUD have cognitive deficits on neuropsychological testing. The DSM-5 diagnosis of *alcohol-induced mild neurocognitive disorder* is defined by milder cognitive deficits in combination with a preserved capacity for independence in daily activities. These cognitive deficits are most commonly observed in verbal learning, short-term memory, abstraction, problem solving, and visuospatial abilities; with cessation of alcohol use, verbal learning is the cognitive domain that typically recovers most rapidly. The DSM-5 diagnosis of *alcohol-induced major neurocognitive disorder* is defined by more severe cognitive deficits leading to any level of interference in the capacity of independence in daily activities. The diagnosis of the alcohol-induced major neurocognitive disorder is followed by specification type: *amnestic-confabulatory* (as seen in Wernicke or Korsakoff syndrome) versus *nonamnestic-confabulatory*.

Remember the clinical signs and symptoms of Wernicke encephalopathy and Korsakoff syndrome for the board examination:

- Wernicke encephalopathy: A reversible condition caused by a severe acute deficiency of thiamine (vitamin B1). Its classic triad of symptoms includes oculomotor dysfunction, encephalopathy, and gait ataxia. Administration of glucose before thiamine replacement in persons with AUD can deplete intracellular thiamine stores and precipitate Wernicke encephalopathy.
- Korsakoff syndrome: Occurs as a chronic, irreversible sequelae of Wernicke encephalopathy among patients who did not receive adequate treatment. The most salient feature is global (anterograde and retrograde) amnesia and confabulation.

Other neurological sequelae of alcohol use include alcoholic peripheral neuropathy and myopathy. Alcoholic cerebellar degeneration can occur after prolonged excessive alcohol exposure and involves the degeneration of Purkinje cells in the cerebellum.

Know This:

According to the DSM-5, Korsakoff syndrome is diagnosed as an alcohol-induced *major neurocognitive disorder, amnestic/confabulatory type.*

Effects of Excess Alcohol Use on Other Organ Systems

- Cardiovascular: Alcoholic dilated cardiomyopathy, atrial fibrillation (a.k.a. "holiday heart"), sudden cardiac death (primarily seen in binge drinking), peripheral artery disease, and stroke
- Gastrointestinal/hepatic: Peptic ulcer disease, gastrointestinal bleeding, pancreatitis (acute or chronic), liver disease (ranging from alcoholic steatosis, alcoholic hepatitis, and alcoholic cirrhosis), hepatic encephalopathy, portal hypertension, and hepatorenal syndrome
- Pulmonary: Aspiration pneumonia and obstructive sleep apnea (owning to reduction of muscle tone in upper airways)
- Hematologic/oncologic: Anemia (typically macrocytic), leukopenia, thrombocytopenia, and increased risk of certain cancers (oropharyngeal, esophageal, laryngeal, breast, colorectal, hepatocellular, and pancreatic).

Other effects of excess alcohol use (reviewed in Chapter 2 in more detail) include type 2 diabetes, electrolyte abnormalities (hypomagnesemia, hypophosphatemia, hypocalcemia, and hypokalemia) that can predispose to arrhythmias, nutritional deficiencies (e.g., iron deficiency, beriberi from B1 deficiency, pellagra from B3 deficiency), gout, osteoporosis, and infertility. Women have a higher risk of alcohol-related liver disease, cardiovascular complications, and brain damage because of lower levels of gastric ADH and lower gastric first-pass metabolism.

Teratogenic Effects in Pregnancy

Fetal alcohol spectrum disorders (FASDs) are the leading causes of intellectual disability and are often referred to as a "hidden disability" because they are often not identified until later in life, if at all. Many of the features of FASD are shared with other developmental conditions, which can lead to delays in diagnosis, especially if the patient has only the neurobehavioral phenotype without the characteristic facial features. FASD is the umbrella term encompassing all sequelae of alcohol-induced fetal effects, which we summarize here:

- Fetal alcohol syndrome (FAS): The most clinically recognizable form of FASD. There are four diagnostic criteria: (1) two or more characteristic facial features (short palpebral fissures, thin vermillion border, or smooth philtrum), (2) growth retardation, (3) evidence of brain involvement, and (4) neurobehavioral impairments. A documented alcohol exposure in utero is not required for the diagnosis.

- Partial fetal alcohol syndrome (pFAS): Individuals with pFAS do not meet full criteria for FAS but have some or most of its features. If in utero alcohol exposure is documented, the diagnosis requires the presence of two or more characteristic facial features and neurobehavioral impairments; if no such exposure is documented, the diagnosis requires the presence of two or more characteristic facial features, neurobehavioral deficits, growth retardation, or evidence of brain involvement.
- Alcohol-related neurodevelopmental disorder (ARND): Diagnosis requires neurobehavioral impairments with documented prenatal alcohol exposure; diagnosis cannot be made in children younger than 3 years of age.
- Alcohol-related birth defects (ARBD): Requires alcohol exposure documentation with at least one major malformation associated with alcohol exposure.
- Neurobehavioral disorder associated with prenatal alcohol exposure (ND-PAE): ND-PAE is listed in the appendix of the DSM-5 under "conditions for further study." Requires documentation of alcohol exposure with neurobehavioral impairments and onset in childhood. Facial features, growth retardation, and evidence of brain involvement are not necessary for the diagnosis.

Know This:

The diagnoses of FAS and pFAS do not require documentation of prenatal alcohol exposure.

Accidents, Trauma, Suicides, and Homicides

Alcohol is associated with an increased risk of accidents, traumatic injuries, suicides, violent deaths, and interpersonal violence. Globally, 29% of alcohol-attributable deaths were caused by injuries such as traffic accidents, self-harm, or violence.

- Risk of motor vehicle accidents increases by a factor of 5 with a BAC greater than 0.08 (the legal limit in most U.S. states), and by a factor of 27 if younger than 21 years of age with a BAC greater than 0.08.
- Alcohol is estimated to be involved in over 50% of homicides and violent assaults, as well as 25% of sexual assaults.
- Nearly 50% of patients admitted to trauma centers have a positive BAC.
- Individuals with AUD have a higher odd of suicidal ideation (odds ratio [OR] = 1.9), suicide attempts (OR = 3.1), and completed suicide (OR = 2.6).

Know This:

The U.S. Federal Aviation Administration has established a BAC offense level of 0.04 mg/dL or more owning to evidence that even a low BAC can impair flying ability.

TREATMENTS FOR AUD

Among persons with AUD, fewer than one-third receive any treatment, and less than 10% receive any medication. Here we review pharmacologic and psychosocial treatments for AUD, as well as research studies that you should know for the board examination.

Pharmacotherapy

Currently available pharmacologic interventions for AUD typically function by producing aversive effects when alcohol is consumed or by reducing the reinforcing effects of alcohol through actions on the reward system. The four available U.S. Food and Drug Administration (FDA)-approved medications are naltrexone (oral and long-acting intramuscular [IM] formulations), acamprosate, and disulfiram.

1. **Naltrexone (oral):**
   - Antagonist at μ- and κ-opioid receptors, and to a lesser extent at δ-opioid receptors.
   - Blocks opioid pathways projecting to the ventral tegmental area and nucleus accumbens, reducing alcohol-induced dopamine release and thereby reducing the positive reinforcing effects of alcohol.

- Reduces cravings, number of drinks per day, heavy alcohol use days, and rate of relapse to heavy drinking.
- Can be started while the patient is still drinking.
- Undergoes extensive first-pass metabolism, is hepatically metabolized through a non-CYP dehydrogenase and conjugated with glucuronide. Naltrexone and its metabolites are excreted in urine and should be used with caution in patients with renal impairment.
- Side effects include headache, anorexia, diarrhea, and nausea. More serious side effects include acute hepatitis, eosinophilic pneumonia, depression, and suicidality. Contraindications include acute hepatitis, liver failure, physiological dependence on opioids, current opioid use, or anticipated need for opioids.
- Once-daily dosing can present issues for patient adherence.

2. **Naltrexone (IM):**
   - For administration in gluteal muscles only.
   - Administered once every 4 weeks for improved adherence.
   - In addition to the side effects of oral naltrexone, side effects unique to IM route of naltrexone include injection site reactions.

Know This:

Polymorphisms of the OPRM1 (μ-opioid receptor) gene have been found to moderate naltrexone response in some but not all studies.

3. **Acamprosate:**
   - Acamprosate is a positive allosteric modulator of the GABA-A receptor and a NMDA receptor antagonist. It reduces glutamatergic activity and increase GABAergic activity during early abstinence and can counteract the symptoms of protracted withdrawal experienced in early abstinence.
   - Acamprosate is most effective when initiated in patients who have established abstinence.
   - Acamprosate reduces rate of relapse to drinking.
   - It is not metabolized by the body and is excreted unchanged by the kidneys. It is,

therefore, safe in patients with liver disease but should be avoided in patients who have renal impairment.
   - Because of low bioavailability, acamprosate has to be taken three times daily, which may negatively affect medication adherence.
   - Its side effects include diarrhea, nausea, anxiety, depression, and suicidal thinking. Its use is contraindicated in patients with a creatinine clearance (CrCl) less than 30 mL/min.

4. **Disulfiram:**
   - Produces a sensitivity to alcohol by irreversibly inhibiting ALDH, resulting in the buildup of acetaldehyde and leading to a highly unpleasant disulfiram–alcohol reaction.
   - The disulfiram–alcohol reaction can begin minutes following alcohol ingestion and last for several hours or until there is no more alcohol in the body. Symptoms include cutaneous flushing, head throbbing, tachycardia, palpitations, nausea, vomiting, and respiratory difficulties. Severe reactions have been reported including death from cardiorespiratory failure.
   - Patients must be warned against consuming alcohol in any form (e.g., in sauces, vinegars, cough syrups, or aftershave), and informed that a disulfiram–alcohol reaction is possible for up to 14 days after ingesting disulfiram. The half-life of disulfiram is variable (~60–120 hours) and may lead to disulfiram–alcohol reactions for as long as several weeks after ingesting disulfiram.
   - Disulfiram should only be started at least 12 hours after the patient has had their last drink.
   - Disulfiram is metabolized hepatically via glucuronidation.
   - Common side effects of disulfiram include headache and a metallic or garlic taste. More rare side effects include peripheral neuropathy, optic neuritis, cholestatic or fulminant hepatitis, rash, and psychosis. Owning to risk of drug–induced hepatic toxicity, baseline and follow-up liver function tests are recommended for patients on disulfiram. The rate of disulfiram–induced fatal hepatitis is 1 in 30,000 patients.

- Contraindications include severe myocardial disease or coronary occlusion, psychosis, or patients who are receiving alcohol or alcohol-containing products. Relative contraindications include hepatic cirrhosis or liver impairment.
- Medication compliance is frequently an issue with disulfiram, and administration is optimally supervised (e.g., by a family member) in patients who want to maintain abstinence.

Know This:

Disulfiram also inhibits dopamine-B-hydroxylase, the enzyme that metabolizes dopamine, leading to higher basal levels of dopamine in the CNS. For this reason, disulfiram is associated with neuropsychiatric side effects, including psychosis.

Other non-FDA-approved medications frequently used off-label for treatment of AUD include baclofen, topiramate, gabapentin, and ondansetron. Here we summarize key aspects about these medications:

- **Baclofen:** An antispasmodic and GABA-B agonist with mixed evidence regarding efficacy in AUD. It has limited hepatic metabolism and is largely excreted renally as an unchanged molecule. For this reason, it may be useful in patients with hepatic cirrhosis.
- **Topiramate:** An antiepileptic medication with several mechanisms of action including potentiation of currents through the GABA-A receptor and inhibition of AMPA and kainate glutamate receptors. By antagonizing glutamate, topiramate is thought to reduce dopamine release in the nucleus accumbens. It reduces drinking days and alcohol cravings. Common side effects include anorexia, word-finding difficulties, metabolic acidosis, nephrolithiasis, angle-closure glaucoma, and increased intraocular pressure.
- **Gabapentin:** A structural analog of GABA that reduces neuronal excitability through inhibition of alpha-2-delta-1 subunit of voltage-gated calcium channels. It does not act directly on the GABA receptor or modulate GABA activity. Gabapentin is not metabolized in the liver and is renally excreted. It has demonstrated efficacy for increasing rates of abstinence and reducing

number of heavy drinking days. It has low bioavailability and requires 3 times per day dosing.
- **Ondansetron:** A 5-HT3 receptor antagonist that also regulates release of dopamine. Ondansetron has been found to reduce drinking days and drinks per day in patients with early-onset AUD.
- **Sertraline:** Selective serotonin reuptake inhibitors have overall shown little efficacy for treatment of AUD except for patients with a concomitant depressive disorder. In one study, sertraline was found to be helpful in patients with Babor type A (lower risk/lower severity), but not type B AUD. In fact, sertraline appeared to worsen alcohol use among patients with type B AUD.

Know This:

For pregnant patients with AUD, pharmacologic treatments are generally not recommended unless it is for treatment of acute alcohol withdrawal or a co-occurring condition.

Psychosocial Interventions for AUD

The majority of patients who are treated for AUD receive psychosocial interventions without medication management. The primary psychosocial modalities for treatment of AUD are reviewed in greater depth in Chapter 13 (Psychosocial Approaches to Substance Use Disorder Management) and include the following:

- Alcoholics Anonymous (AA)
- Twelve-step facilitation (TSF)
- Motivational interviewing (MI)
- Motivational enhancement therapy (MET)
- Cognitive behavioral therapy (CBT)

Project MATCH (Matching Alcoholism Treatment to Client Heterogeneity): Recall the results of Project MATCH reviewed in Chapter 2 ("Matching alcoholism treatments to client heterogeneity," 1998). It is a multisite clinical trial comparing CBT, MET, and TSF for treatment of AUD. The main findings were that no method had a distinct advantage. Subgroup analysis found that MET was superior for angry patients and those with lower initial motivation, CBT was superior for patients with less severe AUD, and TSF was superior for patients with little social support for abstinence and those with more severe AUD.

Combined Pharmacotherapies and Behavioral Interventions (COMBINE) study: This is a multicenter, randomized placebo-controlled trial comparing different combinations of three interventions for AUD (Anton et al., 2016). Two of the interventions were medication management (MM) with naltrexone and/or acamprosate, and the third was a combined behavioral intervention (CBI). Patients received 16 weeks of treatment and were followed for 1 year; the primary outcomes were percent of days abstinent and time to first heavy drinking day. Patients were randomized to one of nine groups evaluating different combinations of MM and CBI. Drinking was reduced in all groups. Acamprosate was not associated with reduced drinking compared with placebo when given alone or in combination with naltrexone and/or CBI. The group performing most poorly received CBI without MM (including placebo). The best treatment outcomes were observed among patients receiving MM with naltrexone with or without CBI, and among patients receiving CBI and MM with placebo. At 1-year follow-up, there were no discernible differences between any of the treatment groups.

REFERENCES

Anton, R. F., O'Malley, S. S., Ciraulo, D. A., Cisler, R. A., Couper, D., Donovan, D. M., Gastfriend, D. R., Hosking, J. D., Johnson, B. A., LoCastro, J. S., Longabaugh, R., Mason, B. J., Mattson, M. E., Miller, W. R., Pettinati, H. M., Randall, C. L., Swift, R., Weiss, R. D., Williams, L. D., & Zweben, A. COMBINE Study Research Group. (2006). Combined pharmacotherapies and behavioral interventions for alcohol dependence: the COMBINE study: a randomized controlled trial. *JAMA, 295*(17), 2003–2017.

Matching alcoholism treatments to client heterogeneity. (1998). Project MATCH three-year drinking outcomes. *Alcoholism, Clinical and Experimental Research, 22*(6), 1300–1311.

Sullivan, J. T., Sykora, K., Schneiderman, J., Naranjo, C. A., & Sellers, E. M. (1989). Assessment of alcohol withdrawal: the revised clinical institute withdrawal assessment for alcohol scale (CIWA-Ar). *British Journal of Addiction, 84*(11), 1353–1357.

SUGGESTIONS FOR FURTHER READING

Grant, B. F., Goldstein, R. B., Saha, T. D., Chou, S. P., Jung, J., Zhang, H., Pickering, R. P., Ruan, W. J., Smith, S. M., Huang, B., & Hasin, D. S. (2015). Epidemiology of DSM-5 alcohol use disorder: results from the National Epidemiologic Survey on alcohol and related conditions III. *JAMA Psychiatry, 72*(8), 757–766.

Reus, V. I., Fochtmann, L. J., Bukstein, O., Eyler, A. E., Hilty, D. M., Horvitz-Lennon, M., Mahoney, J., Pasic, J., Weaver, M., Wills, C. D., McIntyre, J., Kidd, J., Yager, J., & Hong, S. H. (2018). The American Psychiatric Association practice guideline for the pharmacological treatment of patients with alcohol use disorder. *American Journal of Psychiatry, 175*(1), 86–90.

Woodward, J. J. (2019). The ASAM principles of addiction medicine. In S. C. Miller, D. A. Fiellin, R. N. Rosenthal, & R. Saitz (Eds.), *Pharmacology of Alcohol* (6th ed., pp. 107–124). Wolters Kluwer.

REVIEW QUESTIONS

1. You are seeing a new patient for intake. She is a 32-year-old woman with no significant medical history. You ask her about her alcohol use. She tells you that each week she consumes about 10 standard drinks and that at most she will have three drinks at a time, typically on weekends when she is out with friends. She has no medical or functional sequelae of alcohol use. Based on the NIAAA guidelines, you tell her that:
   A. Her alcohol use is considered at-risk because she is drinking more than the accepted weekly amount for women.
   B. Her alcohol use is considered at-risk drinking because she is binge-drinking, although her weekly amount is within the accepted range for women.
   C. Her alcohol use is not considered at-risk because she has no medical or functional sequelae of her current alcohol use.
   D. Her alcohol use is not considered at-risk because she is not exceeding the weekly accepted amount for women.

2. A 50-year-old man with well-controlled hypertension and type 2 diabetes presents to your outpatient clinic for alcohol detoxification. He reports he has been drinking for the past 2 years and currently drinks a 6-pack of beer daily. He has a history of mild alcohol withdrawal symptoms but denies past alcohol-related seizures or DTs. He lives alone in a single-room occupancy and has no family in the area. He has a heart rate

of 96 and a blood pressure of 139/94 on presentation; he appears mildly tremulous without tongue fasciculations and breathalyzer shows a BAC of 0.02%. His initial CIWA is 12, indicating moderate withdrawal. He asks you if you think he can do the detox as an outpatient. You recommend that he undergo an _____ detoxification, because _____.
- A. Outpatient; he has no history of complicated withdrawal
- B. Outpatient; his CIWA score is too low for inpatient detoxification
- C. Outpatient; his presenting BAC is too low for inpatient detoxification
- D. Inpatient; he has hypertension and type 2 diabetes
- E. Inpatient; his CIWA score is too high for outpatient detoxification
- F. Inpatient; he has no social supports involved in his treatment

3. Acamprosate was one of the treatments studied in the COMBINE research study for AUD. Which of the following statements best summarizes the study's outcomes at the end of the 16-week treatment period with respect to acamprosate?
- A. Acamprosate outperformed placebo but not naltrexone.
- B. Acamprosate outperformed placebo but not disulfiram.
- C. Acamprosate outperformed disulfiram but not naltrexone.
- D. Acamprosate did not outperform either placebo or naltrexone.
- E. Acamprosate did not outperform either placebo or disulfiram.

4. According to results from the COMBINE study, which of the following treatment group showed statistically superior outcomes with respect to reduction in drinking days at the end of the 16-week treatment period?
- A. Patients receiving MM (acamprosate + naltrexone) + no behavioral intervention
- B. Patients receiving MM (acamprosate) + behavioral intervention
- C. Patients receiving MM (placebo) + no behavioral intervention

- D. Patients receiving MM (naltrexone) + no behavioral intervention
- E. Patients receiving no MM + behavioral intervention
- F. No group showed statistically superior outcomes at the end of the 16-week treatment period.

5. The COMBINE research study tested different combinations of pharmacological and behavioral interventions for AUD. Treatment was administered for 16 weeks, and participants were then followed for 1 year. At 1-year follow-up, which treatment group showed statistically superior outcomes?
- A. Patients receiving MM (acamprosate + naltrexone) + no behavioral intervention
- B. Patients receiving MM (acamprosate) + behavioral intervention
- C. Patients receiving MM (placebo) + no behavioral intervention
- D. Patients receiving MM (naltrexone) + no behavioral intervention
- E. Patients receiving no MM + behavioral intervention
- F. No group showed statistically superior outcomes at 1-year follow-up.

6. One of the possible treatments for methanol intoxication is the administration of fomepizole. Which of the following best describe fomepizole's mechanism of action in reducing the toxicity of methanol?
- A. Fomepizole prevents build-up of glycolic acid through inhibition of ADH.
- B. Fomepizole prevents build-up of formaldehyde through inhibition of ADH.
- C. Fomepizole prevents build-up of acetaldehyde through inhibition of ALDH.
- D. Fomepizole prevents build-up of glycolic acid through inhibition of ALDH.

7. You are seeing a patient in the emergency room who drank a bottle of antifreeze containing ethylene glycol following a suicide attempt. Without prompt treatment, which of the following are common consequences of ingesting ethylene glycol?

A. Production of calcium oxalate crystals, leading to renal injury
B. Production of formic acid, leading to damage of the optic nerves
C. Production of acetaldehyde, leading to a severe flushing
D. Production of acetone, leading to ketosis

8. Which of the following biomarkers for alcohol consumption is a direct measure of alcohol (i.e., alcohol or one of its metabolites)?
    A. Phosphatidylethanol (PEth)
    B. Gamma-glutamyltransferase (GGT)
    C. Carbohydrate-deficient transferrin (CDT)
    D. Ethyl glucuronide (EtG)
    E. Aspartate aminotransferase (AST)

9. On average, women have a higher BAC for the equivalent amount of alcohol consumption compared with age and weight-matched men. Which of the following best explains this phenomenon?
    A. Women have a lower expression of ADH and ALDH in the liver, reducing the rate of alcohol metabolism.
    B. Women have a lower expression of ADH in the gastric mucosa, reducing first-pass metabolism.
    C. Women have a higher expression of an ALDH isotype that metabolizes alcohol more slowly.
    D. Women have a higher expression of an ADH isotype that metabolizes alcohol more quickly.

10. The CIWA-Ar is a broadly used and well-validated scale measuring the severity of alcohol withdrawal. Which of the following sign or symptom is not included among its 10 scored items?
    A. Agitation
    B. Elevated heart rate
    C. Tremor
    D. Auditory disturbances
    E. Clouding of sensorium

11. Elena is a 25-year-old woman of East Asian descent who reports experiencing facial redness,

nausea, and discomfort when she consumes even small amounts of alcohol. Her reaction is likely due to a genetic variant in the enzyme _____ that metabolizes _____ more slowly.
    A. ALDH; acetate
    B. ADH; acetate
    C. ALDH; acetaldehyde
    D. ADH; acetaldehyde

12. The majority of individuals with AUD exhibit cognitive deficits with neuropsychological testing. Which of the following cognitive domains show the earliest reversal upon establishment of abstinence?
    A. Short-term memory
    B. Abstraction
    C. Problem solving
    D. Verbal learning
    E. Visuospatial abilities

13. What is the most common cause of alcohol-related mortality in the United States?
    A. Suicide
    B. Cardiovascular disease
    C. Motor vehicle traffic injuries
    D. Liver disease
    E. Malignant neoplasms

14. Which of the following medications for AUD predominantly works by attenuating the positively reinforcing effects of alcohol?
    A. Disulfiram
    B. Naltrexone
    C. Acamprosate
    D. Sertraline
    E. Gabapentin

15. Which of the following medications for AUD is thought to work by reducing symptoms of protracted withdrawal and thereby risk for relapse in early abstinence?
    A. Disulfiram
    B. Naltrexone
    C. Acamprosate
    D. Sertraline
    E. Gabapentin

16. Which of the following is true regarding the mechanism of action of acamprosate?

A. It is a positive allosteric modulator of GABA-A receptors.

B. It is a GABA-B agonist.

C. It is a positive allosteric modulator of glutamatergic NMDA receptors.

D. It inhibits the alpha-2-delta-1 subunit of voltage-gated calcium channels.

17. Gabapentin is frequently used as a second-line agent for the treatment of AUD. Which of the following best describes its relevant mechanism of action?

A. GABA-A receptor agonist

B. GABA-B receptor agonist

C. NMDA receptor antagonist

D. Alpha-2-delta-1 subunit of voltage-gated calcium channels antagonist

E. Alpha-2 receptor agonist

18. A 10-year-old boy in foster care is brought to your clinic because of poor attention, hyperactivity, learning problems, and frequent fighting in school. His foster parents confirm that his biological mother used alcohol heavily throughout pregnancy. On examination, he has no discernible facial dysmorphisms characteristic of prenatal alcohol exposure, and he is in the 50th percentile for height, weight, and head circumference. Neurologic examination and brain imaging are normal. On neuropsychological testing, he has an IQ of 85 and clear deficits in attention and executive functioning. Which of the following is the most accurate diagnosis?

A. FAS

B. pFAS

C. ARND

D. Alcohol-related birth defect

19. Which of the following are absolute contraindications for using disulfiram for treatment of AUD?

A. Migraine headaches

B. Hepatic impairment

C. Coronary occlusion

D. Physiological dependence on opioids

E. Severe depression

20. There are several personality factors that are associated with a higher risk of AUD. These include:

A. High conscientiousness

B. High neuroticism

C. High extraversion

D. Low extraversion

E. Low openness to experience

F. Low agreeableness

21. A 46-year-old woman with a long history of an AUD, hepatitis C, and cirrhosis is referred to your clinic for treatment. She expresses a desire to discontinue her alcohol consumption. In addition to psychotherapeutic interventions, which of the following pharmacological agents is the medication of choice for treating this patient's condition?

A. Disulfiram

B. Gabapentin

C. Ondansetron

D. Acamprosate

E. Naltrexone

5 SEDATIVES AND HYPNOTICS

GENERAL CHARACTERISTICS

Sedative/hypnotics are a diverse class of central nervous system (CNS) depressants with addictive liability and a wide range of therapeutic functions. Benzodiazepines are the most widely prescribed medication among sedative/hypnotics, and they are also the most widely prescribed class of all psychotropic medications. At any given time, approximately **5% of all adults** in the United States have been prescribed benzodiazepines.

CHEMICAL STRUCTURE AND NEUROBIOLOGY

Pharmacodynamics

The primary receptor target for all sedative/hypnotic medications is the γ-aminobutyric acid (GABA) receptor. Here we review key features of GABA receptor functioning relevant for understanding the various sedative/hypnotics' biological actions.

The two primary GABA receptors are GABA-A and GABA-B. The GABA-A receptor is an **ionotropic**, ligand-gated ion channel made up of five subunits that are arranged around a central pore. The five subunits are classified into alpha (1–6), beta (1–3), gamma (1–3), delta, and epsilon. The most commonly encountered GABA-A receptor structure has two alpha, two beta, and one gamma subunit. When GABA binds to the receptor, there is a conformational change leading to an influx of chloride and hyperpolarization of the cell membrane.

The six different isoforms of the GABA-A alpha subunit that can be expressed mediate different biological effects:

- Alpha-1 subunit mediates sleep/amnestic effects.
- Alpha-2 to -3 subunits mediate anxiolytic/muscle relaxant effects.
- Alpha-1 to -3 subunits mediate anticonvulsant activity.
- Alpha-5 subunit mediates effects of benzodiazepines.
- Alpha-4 and -6 are insensitive to benzodiazepines.

In contrast to GABA-A receptor, the GABA-B receptor is **metabotropic,** and the receptor is separate from the ion channel. The binding of GABA leads to activation of second-messenger G-proteins and opening of the ion channels.

The primary mechanism of all sedative/hypnotics is through their GABAergic actions; knowing which subunits these drugs bind to can help predict their effects.

- **Benzodiazepines**: Bind GABA-A receptors at the interface between the alpha and gamma-2 subunits with roughly the same affinities for alpha-1 to -3 and -5 subunits, and increase the frequency of channel opening; they are indirect agonists and positive allosteric modulators.
- **Barbiturates**: Bind GABA-A receptors at the interface of subunits at sites distinct from benzodiazepines and increase duration of channel opening; they are indirect agonists and positive allosteric modulators. Unlike benzodiazepines, barbiturates also block isoxazolepropionic acid (AMPA) kainate glutamatergic receptors.
- **Ethanol**: Binds GABA-A receptors; ethanol is also a positive allosteric modulator similar to benzodiazepines and barbiturates; the precise molecular target on GABA-A receptors is not fully known.

- **Z-drugs, a.k.a. nonbenzodiazepines** (e.g., zaleplon, zolpidem, eszopiclone, zopiclone): Bind GABA-A at the same sites as benzodiazepines. Z-drugs have greatest effect at alpha-1 subunits and weaker activity at alpha-2 and -3 subunits, lending to its potent hypnotic effects and lesser anxiolytic effects.
- **Gamma-hydroxy-butyrate (GHB):** GABA-B receptor agonist used for narcolepsy.
- **Baclofen**: GABA-B receptor agonist used for muscle spasticity.

Know This:

Z-drugs have greatest activity at the alpha-1 receptors; benzodiazepines have greatest activity at the alpha-1 through -3 and -5 subunits. Because Z-drugs primarily bind to the alpha-1 subunit of the GABA-A receptor, they have limited anxiolytic and anticonvulsant activity.

Z-drugs are cross-tolerant for alcohol but less so than benzodiazepines and barbiturates.

Pharmacokinetics

The pharmacokinetic effects of the various sedative/hypnotics can help to predict their effectiveness, duration of action, and differential liabilities for addiction. In general, medications with faster onsets of action are considered more addictive.

Onset and Duration of Action

The structure of prototypical sedative/hypnotics is shown in Fig. 5.1. To predict the actions of benzodiazepines, you should know the relative potency, lipophilicity, and elimination half-life.

Fig. 5.1 ■ Structure of prototypical sedative/hypnotics. Benzodiazepines are composed of a benzene ring fused to a seven-membered diazepine ring; modification of the R-groups can change the compound's characteristics. Barbituric acid is the parent compound for all barbiturates. Zolpidem is shown as a prototypical nonbenzodiazepine or Z-drug.

- **Potency** refers to the number of milligrams to obtain a given action; for example, alprazolam 1 mg is considered equivalent to diazepam 10 mg, indicating that alprazolam has a higher potency. Approximate dose equivalencies for commonly used benzodiazepines are shown in Table 5.1.
- **Elimination half-life:** The half-lives of commonly used benzodiazepines are also shown in Table 5.1. Benzodiazepines with longer half-lives can be dosed less frequently.
- **Lipophilicity:** The more lipophilic a benzodiazepine is, the more quickly it will both enter and leave the CNS. High-lipophilicity benzodiazepines have a more rapid onset and include diazepam and alprazolam; low-lipophilicity benzodiazepines include lorazepam and chlordiazepoxide.

Knowing just the elimination half-life of a benzodiazepine is not a good predictor of how quickly or how long a patient will feel the medication's effect: you must also consider its lipophilicity and potency. For example, although the half-life of alprazolam is 11 to 15 hours, patients typically experience the acute anxiolytic effects of alprazolam for approximately 2 to 4 hours; this is because alprazolam is highly lipophilic and both enters

TABLE 5.1
Commonly Used Benzodiazepines, Approximate Half-Lives and Equipotent Dosages

Benzodiazepines	Elimination Half-Life (hr)	Active Metabolite	Dose Equivalency (mg)[a]
Triazolam	2–5	Inactive	0.5
Lorazepam	10–14	Inactive	1
Temazepam	8–15	Inactive	10
Alprazolam	11–15	Inactive	0.5
Chlordiazepoxide	5–30	Active[b]	10
Clonazepam	18–50	Inactive	0.25–0.5
Oxazepam	5–15	Inactive	15–30
Diazepam	50–100	Active[b]	5

[a]These doses are approximate equipotencies and are not recommended for initiation or for conversion between medications.
[b]The active metabolites of diazepam are oxazepam, temazepam, and desmethyldiazepam; those of chlordiazepoxide are oxazepam and desmethyldiazepam. The presence of these active metabolites contributes to these compounds' longer half-lives.

and leaves the CNS rapidly. The same principles regarding lipophilicity and elimination half-life apply to other sedatives/hypnotics. Concerning barbiturates, the compound with the fastest onset of action is sodium thiopental, which is highly lipophilic and used for anesthesia. It has an onset of action of less than 1 minute and a duration of action between 5 and 10 minutes.

Metabolism

- Benzodiazepines are generally metabolized by CYP3A4 oxidation followed by glucuronide conjugation. The exceptions to this are the "LOT" (lorazepam, oxazepam, and temazepam) benzodiazepines, which undergo only glucuronidation and have no active metabolites. For this reason, they are preferred in patients with hepatic impairment or to avoid drug–drug interactions. Many of the common benzodiazepines are metabolized to oxazepam (diazepam, clorazepate, chlordiazepoxide, and temazepam). Alprazolam, lorazepam, and clonazepam do not share this metabolic pathway.
- Barbiturates are generally metabolized by CYP3A4, 3A5, and 3A7; they also induce CYP2D6, 2C9, and 3A4 and can, therefore, decrease serum levels of medications metabolized by these enzymes.
- Zolpidem and zopiclone are metabolized by CYP3A4; zaleplon is metabolized by aldehyde oxidase. There are significant sex differences in the metabolism of zolpidem. In 2003, the U.S. Food and Drug Administration (FDA) required lower recommended doses of zolpidem for women to reduce the risk of next-day activities that require alertness, such as driving. Men metabolize the standard 10-mg formulation approximately twice as quickly as women; females have also been found to have higher peak concentration of zolpidem than men.

Know This:

Most benzodiazepines are metabolized by CYP3A4 enzymes. Any medication that induces or inhibits CYP3A4 (e.g., ketoconazole, macrolides, oral contraceptives) may, therefore, affect drug levels. Exceptions to this are lorazepam, oxazepam, and temazepam, which do not undergo metabolism by CYP enzymes.

Lorazepam and diazepam are prepared in solutions with propylene glycol when administered intravenously. There have been cases of iatrogenic propylene glycol toxicity with repeated administration of intravenous benzodiazepines.

TOXICOLOGY TESTING

Toxicology testing for benzodiazepines is covered more extensively in Chapter 12. Recall that the standard toxicology test for benzodiazepines detects the presence of compounds that are metabolized to oxazepam—this includes diazepam, chlordiazepoxide, clorazepate, and temazepam. Several of the very commonly prescribed benzodiazepines (clonazepam, alprazolam, and lorazepam) have a different metabolic pathway and are frequently missed by standard toxicology tests.

SEDATIVE/HYPNOTIC MEDICAL INDICATIONS AND ADVERSE EFFECTS

Sedative/Hypnotic Medical Indications

- **Benzodiazepines:** FDA-approved indications include panic disorder, generalized anxiety disorder, social phobia, insomnia, and status epilepticus/seizures; non-FDA-approved uses include agitation, alcohol withdrawal, muscle spasms, restless leg syndrome, and presurgical medication. Benzodiazepines are classified by the Drug Enforcement Agency (DEA) as Schedule IV controlled Substances.
- **Barbiturates:** Previously widely used for sleep and anxiety but largely replaced now by benzodiazepines. They are still used as anticonvulsants, in general anesthesia, and physician-assisted suicide. The majority of barbiturates are classified by the DEA as Schedule III or IV.
- **Baclofen:** FDA-approved for spasticity, and off-label use for alcohol use disorder. Baclofen is not classified as a controlled substance.
- **GHB**: FDA-approved for narcolepsy as sodium oxybate, the sodium salt of GHB. Currently classified by the DEA as Schedule III when prescribed as sodium oxybate, and Schedule I for any other use.
- **Z-drugs:** FDA-approved for short-term treatment of insomnia. Classified by the DEA as Schedule IV.

Sedative/Hypnotic Adverse Effects

Major adverse effects of benzodiazepines include:

- **Sedation**: Can occur more frequently in patients taking benzodiazepines with longer half-lives. Individuals on stable doses of benzodiazepines will typically build tolerance to the sedative effects over time.
- **Psychomotor impairment**: Increased risk of falls, impairment of driving skills, ataxia, and muscle weakness. Older adults are more sensitive to the psychomotor impairments associated with benzodiazepine use; risk of falls is increased with higher doses and use of benzodiazepines with shorter half-lives.
- **Cognitive impairment**: Anterograde amnesia (the induction of anterograde amnesia accounts for the efficacy of midazolam for presurgical medication), impairments in attention and episodic memory. Cognitive impairments are independent of sedative effects. Even after long periods of benzodiazepine use, tolerance does not develop to their memory-impairing effects.
- **Paradoxical disinhibition**: Aggression, hostility, and increased excitability can occur, particularly in children, the elderly, and individuals with developmental disabilities.
- **Pregnancy effects**: Benzodiazepines cross the placenta. If used during pregnancy, they double the risk of cleft palate, decrease muscle tone in the newborn (a.k.a "floppy baby syndrome"), and result in neonatal withdrawal. Some studies have identified a risk for preterm delivery and low birth weight associated with benzodiazepine use.
- **Rebound insomnia:** Following discontinuation even after brief durations of administration for insomnia, patients can experience worsened sleep compared with baseline.
- **Physiologic dependence and withdrawal**: Most individuals treated with benzodiazepines for less than 1 month do not develop physiologic dependence; however, it is seen in 50% of patients treated for 4 months.
- **Abuse potential**: All compounds with GABA-A agonist effects have some abuse liability; however, most patients who are prescribed benzodiazepines do not find them reinforcing and will not develop a use disorder. Approximately 10% of patients who try benzodiazepines once will develop a use disorder.
- **Respiratory depression**: Occurs more commonly when benzodiazepines are taken in combination with other agents, such as alcohol or opioids; risk of respiratory depression in benzodiazepines is less than that compared with barbiturates.
- **Increased mortality:** According to a large study performed among primary care patients in the United Kingdom, the age-adjusted mortality hazard ratio for individuals taking benzodiazepines was **3.46** after adjustment for a range of confounders; a dose-response association has also been identified for Z-drugs (Weich et al., 2014). The FDA has issued a **black box warning** for benzodiazepines taken together with opioids owning to increased risk of respiratory depression, oversedation, and death.
- **Suicide risk:** According to a recent meta-analysis, benzodiazepines increase the odds of attempting or completing suicide by three to five times. Possible mechanisms include increased impulsivity, withdrawal symptoms, or overdose toxicity (Dodds, 2017).

Many of the common side effects of Z-drugs and barbiturates are similar to benzodiazepines. Z-drugs, however, carry the risk of complex sleep-related behaviors that include sleepwalking, night-time amnestic binging, and sleep driving. Because these effects can cause serious injuries or death, the FDA required that Z-drugs include a **black box warning** for complex sleep-related behaviors.

SEDATIVE/HYPNOTIC TOXICITY: PRESENTATION AND MANAGEMENT

Presentation of Sedative/Hypnotic Toxicity

The benzodiazepine intoxication syndrome resembles that of alcohol: symptoms include ataxia, amnesia, slurred speech, loss of inhibition, delirium, and CNS depression. Patients frequently present to the emergency room with **CNS depression but normal vital signs**. Patients with severe benzodiazepine toxicity can present stuporous or comatose; however, it is rare that someone ingesting benzodiazepines alone can reach this state.

Barbiturate toxicity is far less common today than it was during the 1960s and 1970s when they were more commonly prescribed. Barbiturates have largely been replaced by benzodiazepines due to their dangerousness in overdose and narrow therapeutic window. One unique complication of barbiturate-induced intoxication is bullous lesions, frequently seen on the hands.

The **differential diagnosis** of patients presenting with suspected sedative/hypnotic intoxication is broad. Many of the sedative/hypnotics share similar features in overdose. If patients present with altered mental status, other life-threatening medical etiologies should be ruled out such as hypoglycemia, carbon monoxide exposure, stroke, encephalitis, or head trauma. Remember that benzodiazepine overdose in isolation rarely causes life-threatening respiratory depression or coma, so evaluation for co-ingestion of substances should always be performed.

Management of Sedative/Hypnotic Toxicity

Treatment of benzodiazepine toxicity or overdose is mainly supportive. It includes evaluating and managing the ABCs (Airways, Breathing, and Circulation), oxygen therapy, and intubation if needed, with or without flumazenil. Given the frequency of benzodiazepine overdose involving another substance (e.g., alcohol or opioids), it is reasonable to give naloxone.

Flumazenil competitively antagonizes the GABA-A receptor at the benzodiazepine binding site and can reverse benzodiazepine overdose. Flumazenil can be used to reverse benzodiazepine-induced general anesthesia. However, its use for reversing benzodiazepine overdose is more controversial because it can precipitate seizures in patients who are benzodiazepine dependent. Activated charcoal is generally not recommended in cases of benzodiazepine toxicity, given the risk of aspiration.

Treatment of barbiturate toxicity is like that of benzodiazepines; it is primarily supportive. Unlike benzodiazepines, there is no antidote such as flumazenil for barbiturate overdose. Alkaline diuresis and/or hemodialysis are options for severe cases.

Other sedative/hypnotic toxidromes to know:

■ **GHB**: GHB is approved for narcolepsy but has much wider use illicitly as a recreational and date-rape drug. Adverse effects include bradycardia, respiratory depression, obtundation, stupor, coma,

vomiting, ataxia, and death. GHB has a steep dose-response curve, and the LD50 is approximately five times the typical recreational dose. Treatment includes ABCs, atropine for bradycardia, and potential intensive care unit admission.

■ **Flunitrazepam** (brand name Rohypnol): a fast-acting benzodiazepine that has also been used to facilitate date rape. It is no longer available in the United States, the United Kingdom, or Canada. It responds to flumazenil in overdose.

Know This:

Flumazenil competitively antagonizes the GABA-A receptor at the benzodiazepine binding site. Given its mechanism of action, it can reverse both benzodiazepine and Z-drug overdose but not barbiturate or alcohol poisoning.

SEDATIVE/HYPNOTIC WITHDRAWAL: PRESENTATION AND MANAGEMENT

Sedative/Hypnotic Withdrawal Presentation

Benzodiazepine withdrawal is among the most dangerous withdrawal syndromes because it is often missed, and it frequently occurs on top of other substances. In most ways it is similar to alcohol withdrawal; however, it differs from alcohol withdrawal in that there is an increased likelihood of seizures, and both the time course and duration of symptoms are much more variable. The occurrence and timing of benzodiazepine withdrawal depends on the dose, duration, and half-life of the drug involved; onset of withdrawal can vary from days to weeks. Similar to alcohol withdrawal, benzodiazepine withdawal occurs following loss of GABAergic tone in chronic use and excess cortical activity when benzodiazepines are abruptly reduced or discontinued.

Z-drugs do not typically have a dangerous withdrawal syndrome, although cases of severe withdrawal and seizures have been reported with long-term use of supratherapeutic doses. Supratherapeutic doses of Z-drugs may saturate alpha-2, alpha-3, and alpha-5 GABA-A subunits and more closely resemble benzodiazepine withdrawal with discontinuation.

Sedative/Hypnotic Withdrawal Management

For patients who have been on benzodiazepines long-term, it is generally recommended to perform a gradual taper (i.e., over months) to reduce rates of rebound anxiety and insomnia and increase tolerability. Factors to consider include duration of use and dosage; the longer the person has taken the benzodiazepine, the longer the recommended taper.

There are several approaches for performing a slow taper, which include:

- Converting to an equivalent dose of a benzodiazepine with a longer duration of effect and longer half-life (e.g., from alprazolam to clonazepam), stabilizing for several weeks, then gradually decreasing dose. Ancillary medications can be used to assist with anxiety and sleep (e.g., hydroxyzine, carbamazepine, pregabalin, trazodone).
- In some cases, you may wish to discontinue the benzodiazepine quickly and manage the withdrawal syndrome with GABAergic anticonvulsants with a better safety profile. This strategy entails starting high-dose valproic acid, carbamazepine or gabapentin, then tapering benzodiazepine by one-third each day until discontinuation. The anticonvulsant can be continued for 1 month or longer. Serum levels of valproic acid and carbamazepine should be monitored routinely. Other medications may be considered for initiation for treatment of anxiety and sleep (e.g., selective serotonin reuptake inhibitors [SSRIs]). Note that these guidelines for benzodiazepine tapers using anticonvulsants have been derived from case studies and not randomized controlled trials.

The addition of therapy has been shown to increase the rate of success with outpatient tapers; therapy can promote self-efficacy and build coping skills for managing anxiety. One study conducted among primary care patients on chronic benzodiazepines in Spain (Vicens et al., 2006) showed that patients undergoing taper were nearly five times as successful with the addition of biweekly therapy.

For patients presenting to hospital settings in acute benzodiazepine withdrawal, the management approach is similar to that for alcohol withdrawal. Keep in mind that benzodiazepine withdrawal is often variable in onset and is frequently missed, especially in patients who present with other primary complaints. Benzodiazepine withdrawal is typically treated with a benzodiazepine with a longer duration of effect (e.g., intravenous diazepam) until withdrawal symptoms are eliminated, then the benzodiazepine can be tapered gradually as an outpatient.

EPIDEMIOLOGY OF SEDATIVE/HYPNOTIC USE

Key points:

- Benzodiazepines are the most widely prescribed class of all psychotropic medications.
- Benzodiazepine prescriptions have increased dramatically since 1996: between 1996 and 2013, the number of adults filling a benzodiazepine prescription has increased 67%, with a tripling of the volume of benzodiazepine dispensation between these time points.
- Benzodiazepine-related mortality between 1996 and 2013 has increased fivefold; opioids were involved in 75% of benzodiazepine-related overdose deaths. Conversely, the National Institute of Drug Abuse (NIDA) estimates that 30% of opioid overdoses involve benzodiazepines.
- At any given time, approximately 5% of all adults in the United States are prescribed a benzodiazepine.
- Benzodiazepine use is twice as frequent in women as it is in males.
- The proportion of long-term benzodiazepines increases with age, from 15% in 18- to 35-year-olds to 31% in 64- to 80-year-olds.
- Emergency room visits for sedative/hypnotics made up 34% of all visits related to nonmedical use of pharmaceuticals (2011), making it second only to pain relievers (46%); alprazolam was implicated in one-third of those visits.
- Lifetime prevalence of sedative/hypnotic use disorder is estimated at approximately 1%.

SEDATIVE/HYPNOTIC USE DISORDER

Risk factors for developing a sedative/hypnotic use disorder include:

- Younger age
- Lower level of education

- Nonnative cultural origin
- Longer duration of benzodiazepine use
- Higher dose of benzodiazepine
- Psychiatric illness
- Other substance use disorders

As mentioned previously, approximately 10% of individuals who use benzodiazepines once will develop a substance use disorder. However, the majority do not find them reinforcing and do not develop problematic use. Benzodiazepine abuse is rarely the sole or primary substance of abuse; most benzodiazepine abuse is along with other substances, most commonly opioids. One study conducted by NIDA found that 73% of heroin users use benzodiazepines more often than weekly. When used illicitly, benzodiazepines are reported to "boost" the effects of opioids, alleviate withdrawal syndromes from other substances, and manage stimulant highs.

Signs of a burgeoning use disorder include rapid development of tolerance with frequent requests for dose increases, requests for early refills, using a higher dose and using more often than prescribed, escalating use despite negative consequences, using medication for euphoric high, using medication when feeling upset, preoccupation with medication, reported inability to function without it, and use of other drugs or unhealthy use of alcohol.

Know This:

You may be asked about "**pseudoaddiction**" on the board examination, which is the notion that patients treated with inadequate doses may repeatedly request increases in dosages; these patients may incorrectly be seen as drug-seekers. Pseudoaddiction has most widely been discussed in pain management and opioid medications but applies to benzodiazepines as well. In the context of benzodiazepines and treatment of anxiety, these patients' approaches include increasing the dose or frequency of dosing or considering a longer-acting agent.

Treatment of Co-Occurring Psychiatric Illness

Patients with a sedative/hypnotic use disorder have high rates of psychiatric comorbidity. Approximately half of patients have a psychiatric illness, which is higher than the comorbidity rates for other substance use disorders. In patients presenting with sedative misuse, it is especially important to evaluate for other psychiatric conditions. Common co-occurring conditions include panic disorder, mood disorders, and personality disorders. In patients with a current substance use disorder and a psychiatric illness, it is preferable **not** to initiate treatment with a benzodiazepine given their higher risk of developing a use disorder.

To choose an appropriate alternative agent to a benzodiazepine, one should perform a thorough psychiatric evaluation, determine and treat the patient's specific subtype of anxiety disorder or other psychiatric condition. Patients should be educated about the onset of action of antidepressants or other medications that are utilized and that effects will not be felt as immediately as with benzodiazepines. Therapy should be integrated into the treatment plan as needed.

Some key points:

- SSRIs and tricyclic antidepressants work about as well for generalized anxiety disorder as benzodiazepines; buspirone also has proven efficacy in multiple controlled trials.
- Alpha- and beta-adrenergic agents (such as clonidine and beta-blockers) and second-generation antipsychotics (risperidone, quetiapine, olanzapine) have reported efficacy in treatment of acute anxiety in patients in which one wishes to avoid benzodiazepines.
- There are many nonbenzodiazepine agents that can be used for treatment of insomnia including trazodone, amitriptyline, doxepin, and ramelteon. Treatment of insomnia should also include psychoeducation around sleep hygiene.

REFERENCES

Dodds, T. J. (2017). Prescribed benzodiazepines and suicide risk: a review of the literature. *The Primary Care Companion for CNS Disorders, 19*(2), 16r02037. https://doi.org/10.4088/PCC.16r02037.

Vicens, C., Fiol, F., Llobera, J., Campoamor, F., Mateu, C., Alegret, S., & Socías, I. (2006). Withdrawal from long-term benzodiazepine use: randomised trial in family practice. *British Journal of General Practice: The Journal of the Royal College of General Practitioners, 56*(533), 958–963.

Weich, S., Pearce, H. L., Croft, P., Singh, S., Crome, I., Bashford, J., & Frisher, M. (2014). Effect of anxiolytic and hypnotic drug prescriptions on mortality hazards: retrospective cohort study. *BMJ (Clinical research ed.), 348*, g1996. https://doi.org/10.1136/bmj.g1996.

SUGGESTIONS FOR FURTHER READING

Bachhuber, M. A., Hennessy, S., Cunningham, C. O., & Starrels, J. L. (2016). Increasing benzodiazepine prescriptions and overdose mortality in the United States, 1996-2013. *American Journal of Public Health*, *106*(4), 686–688. https://doi.org/10.2105/AJPH.2016.303061.

Bisaga, A., & Mariani, J. J. (2015). Benzodiazepines and other sedatives and hypnotics. In M. Galanter, H. D. Kleber, & K. Brady (Eds.), *The American Psychiatric Association Publishing textbook of substance abuse treatment* (5th ed.). American Psychiatric Association Publishing.

Olfson, M., King, M., & Schoenbaum, M. (2015). Benzodiazepine use in the United States. *JAMA Psychiatry, 72*(2), 136–142. https://doi.org/10.1001/jamapsychiatry.2014.1763.

Soyka, M. (2017). Treatment of benzodiazepine dependence. *New England Journal of Medicine, 376*(12), 1147–1157. https://doi.org/10.1056/NEJMra1611832.

REVIEW QUESTIONS

1. Z-drugs are sedative/hypnotics with potent hypnotic and limited anxiolytic effects in comparison with benzodiazepines. The action of Z-drugs at which of the following sites best accounts for these effects?
   A. Alpha-1 subunit of GABA receptor
   B. Gamma-2 subunit of GABA receptor
   C. Alpha-1 through -3 and -5 subunit of GABA receptor
   D. N-methyl-D-aspartate (NMDA) glutamate receptor
   E. Alpha-amino-3-hydroxy-5-methyl-4-isoxazolepropionic acid (AMPA) glutamate receptor

2. Barbiturates and benzodiazepines have similar pharmacodynamic characteristics, although benzodiazepines have largely replaced barbiturates in clinical practice. In which of the following ways does the pharmacodynamics of barbiturates differ from benzodiazepines? Barbiturates:
   A. Are agonists at the AMPA receptor
   B. Are agonists at the kainate receptor
   C. Are antagonists at the GABA receptor
   D. Increase duration of GABA channel opening
   E. Increase frequency of GABA channel opening

3. A 49-year-old woman is taking fluoxetine (a 2D6 inhibitor) and verapamil (a 3A4 inhibitor). She is started on lorazepam. Which of the following CYP-related drug–drug interactions with lorazepam should you monitor for?
   A. Higher-than-expected serum concentrations of lorazepam owning to 2D6 inhibition
   B. Lower-than-expected serum concentrations of lorazepam owning to 2D6 inhibition
   C. Higher-than-expected serum concentrations of lorazepam owning to 3A4 inhibition
   D. Lower-than-expected serum concentrations of lorazepam owning to 3A4 inhibition
   E. There are no significant drug–drug interactions.

4. A 32-year-old woman with panic disorder on sertraline 200 mg daily and clonazepam 0.5 mg twice daily who has recently become pregnant presents to your office. She is concerned about pregnancy and fetal complications. Which of the following does benzodiazepine use increase the risk of during pregnancy?
   A. Neonatal abstinence syndrome
   B. Placenta previa
   C. Stillbirth
   D. Cleft palate
   E. Preeclampsia

5. Which of the following pharmacologic characteristics best explains why alprazolam has a short duration of clinical effect despite having a long elimination half-life?
   A. High potency
   B. High lipophilicity
   C. Lack of active metabolites
   D. GABA-B receptor agonism
   E. NMDA receptor antagonism

6. Which of the following benzodiazepines is not identified on a routine urine drug screen for benzodiazepines?
   A. Chlordiazepoxide
   B. Lorazepam
   C. Oxazepam
   D. Temazepam
   E. Diazepam

7. In 2019, the FDA placed a black box warning on three Z-drugs: zolpidem, zaleplon, and eszopiclone. The black box warning indicates that these Z-drugs carry a risk of:
   A. Mortality when combined with opioids
   B. Complex sleep-related behaviors
   C. Suicidal ideation
   D. Arrhythmia
   E. Respiratory depression

8. A 42-year-old woman who has been prescribed alprazolam 2 mg three times daily for 5 years. Which of the following side effects of alprazolam is she least likely to build tolerance to?
   A. Anticonvulsant effects
   B. Sedation
   C. Memory impairment
   D. Falls
   E. Impaired driving

9. A 49-year-old man who has been prescribed lorazepam 0.5 mg three times daily for the past 6 years for generalized anxiety disorder. He wants to discontinue taking lorazepam because of concerns about long-term side effects but has experienced intolerable anxiety, irritability, and sleeplessness whenever his previous doctors attempted to taper the lorazepam. Which of the following options is the next best step?
   A. Transition patient from lorazepam to clonazepam and perform a slow taper
   B. Transition patient from lorazepam to alprazolam and perform a slow taper
   C. Start a SSRI while performing a rapid taper of lorazepam
   D. Start a SSRI while performing a slow taper of lorazepam
   E. Start a SSRI and discontinue lorazepam

10. A 37-year-old man with a history of posttraumatic stress disorder is brought to the emergency room following a suicide attempt by overdosing on prescription alprazolam. On arrival, the patient is obtunded and is unable to provide a history. Respiratory rate is slowed, and he has an oxygen saturation of 86%. Administration of which of the following medications or procedures would be the immediate next best step?
    A. Flumazenil
    B. Flurazepam
    C. Naloxone
    D. Activated charcoal
    E. Hemodialysis

6

OPIOID USE DISORDER

BRIEF HISTORY OF THE CURRENT OPIOID EPIDEMIC

Beginning in the early 1800s, opium and morphine use became widespread; opiate-containing "patent medicines" were heavily marketed for several medical conditions, especially toward women. Morphine prescribing peaked in 1890, and in 1898, Bayer started marketing heroin as a treatment for morphine addiction. In 1914, changes in domestic and international policy, spurred in part by the Opium Wars in China, led to the passage of the Harrison Act (discussed in Chapter 12). This act banned physicians from prescribing opioids for the treatment of opioid use disorder (OUD) and made any medicinal use of heroin illegal.

The current opioid epidemic is not the first in this nation's history. The roots of the current opioid crisis began in the 1990s, when prescription opioid prescribing was greatly expanded along with pharmaceutical marketing of these agents as "minimally addictive." Opioid prescribing reached a zenith in 2010 when there were an astounding 81 opioid prescriptions per 100 people. Other causal factors for the current opioid epidemic include declining economic opportunities and the rise in self-reported psychological distress. Because of the alarming rates of opioid-related overdoses, the United States declared a public health emergency because of the opioid epidemic in 2017.

One critical factor in the current opioid epidemic was the change in clinical practice toward the treatment of pain (see Chapter 11). Treatment of chronic pain became an important research focus, particularly pain caused by cancer. Several articles and small retrospective studies were widely circulated in support of the claim that treatment of chronic pain with opioids rarely led to the development of a substance use disorder. In 1995, the American Pain Society launched a campaign to standardize the treatment of pain symptoms and promoted pain as "the fifth vital sign." The Federation of State Medical Boards, the Drug Enforcement Agency, and the Joint Commission also issued statements promoting pain assessments and analgesic treatment. Physicians were now pressured to provide aggressive pain control, as hospital administrations were under pressure to assess and treat pain to receive federal health care funds. Starting in 1996, OxyContin, an extended-release oxycodone, was heavily marketed by the pharmaceutical industry and its use for the treatment of noncancer chronic pain skyrocketed. The United States subsequently saw an extraordinary increase in the prescription and consumption of opioid medications.

Know This:

One important feature of the current opioid epidemic is that many new opioid users initially used prescription opioid medications (prescribed to oneself or to others) and then transitioned to the use of heroin. This transition was largely driven by reduced access and restrictiveness around opioid medication prescribing following the early rise of opioid-related deaths and OUDs, and higher cost compared to heroin.

EPIDEMIOLOGY OF OPIOID USE

Key facts to remember:

- The rate of drug overdoses has increased more than threefold between 1999 and 2017 from 6.1 per 100,000 standard population to 21.7, according to data from the Centers for Disease Control and Prevention (CDC).

- In 2017, drug overdoses were the leading cause of accidental death among people aged 15 to 64 years.
- In 2018, the prevalence of past-year illicit drug use from prescription pain relievers in people aged 12 years and older was 3.6%; it was the second most commonly used drug following marijuana. Of people aged 12 years and older, 2.1% have used heroin at some point in their lives (NSDUH, 2018).
- According to the CDC, the overdose rate from synthetic opioids (including fentanyl and its analogues) was 12 times higher in 2019 than in 2013. Between 2018 and 2019, overdose deaths from synthetic opioids increased by 16%.
- Close to half of people on chronic opioid therapy meet the criteria for an OUD.
- Age: The average age of first heroin use is in the early 20s, with the 25 to 34 age group experiencing the most opioid overdose deaths in 2019.
- Sex: Even though woman are prescribed opioid medication more frequently than men, men have 1.5-fold the risk of prescription opioid misuse and threefold the risk of heroin use. Between 1999 and 2010, overdoses from prescription opioid medication increased four times in women and over two times in men according to data from the CDC; however, men are still more likely to die from a prescription opioid overdose.
- Race: Among racial/ethnic groups, the highest opioid overdose rates are among Native Americans and non-Hispanic Whites. Approximately 90% of new heroin users in the past decade are non-Hispanic Whites.
- Geography: Between 1999 and 2015, although the greatest proportion of drug overdoses occurred in the metropolitan areas, the rate of increase in overdose deaths has been greatest in nonurban areas (nonurban: 325%; urban: 198%).

Know This:

The current opioid epidemic is demographically distinct from prior epidemics in that it has predominantly impacted non-Hispanic Whites, a greater proportion of women, and individuals living in rural and suburban areas. Previous opioid epidemics between the 1950s and 1980s were centered in urban minority communities, predominantly heroin use among young men.

KEY REGULATIONS, POLICIES, AND GUIDELINES

Narcotic Addiction Treatment Act of 1974

This act legitimizes and regulates the use of methadone to treat OUD and states that it must be dispensed in opioid treatment programs (OTPs) registered with the Drug Enforcement Administration, the federal Substance Abuse and Mental Health Administration (SAMHSA), and the home state's methadone agency.

Drug Addiction Treatment Act of 2000 (DATA 2000)

DATA 2000 permits physicians who meet the qualifications to treat up to 30 patients with OUD in an office-based setting with buprenorphine. Before enacting DATA 2000, the use of opioid medications to treat OUD was permissible only in federally approved treatment programs, such as a methadone clinic. The DATA 2000 requires prescribers to complete an 8-hour training course to receive an X-waiver to prescribe buprenorphine for OUD.

Ryan Haight Online Pharmacy Consumer Protection Act of 2008

The Drug Enforcement Administration is responsible for the implementation and enforcement of this act. Under this act, a health professional cannot prescribe a controlled substance without seeing that patient in-person. This requirement for in-person visits was waived until the end of 2021 because of the COVID-19 pandemic to enable continued treatment of patients with OUD.

Comprehensive Addiction and Recovery Act (CARA) of 2016

This act was signed into law in response to the opioid crisis. It allocates grants for the expansion of prevention and treatment programs, especially evidence-based treatments for OUD. It temporarily authorizes nurse practitioners and physician assistants to become trained and waivered to prescribe buprenorphine.

SUPPORT for Patients and Communities Act of 2018 (SUPPORT Act)

The Substance Use-Disorder Prevention Promotes Opioid Recovery and Treatment for Patients and Communities (SUPPORT) for Patients and Communities

Act of 2018 (SUPPORT Act) expands the ability to treat up to 100 patients (from 30 patients under DATA 2000) in the first year of waiver receipt if practitioners satisfy one of the following two conditions: the practitioner holds a board certification in addiction medicine or addiction psychiatry, and the practitioner provides medication-assisted treatment in a qualified practice setting under the act.

Federal Guidelines for OTPs

OTPs dispense opioid agonists on-site for the treatment of OUD and provide a number of other medical and psychosocial services. OTPs are expected to follow federal standards as outlined in Title 42 of the Code of Federal Regulations Part 8 (42 CFR § 8). Naltrexone, an opioid antagonist used for treatment of OUD, can be offered in an OTP and it is not subject to the same regulations as methadone or buprenorphine. Certification of these programs is overseen by SAMHSA.

Know This:

Methadone can only be dispensed in an OTP when prescribed for the treatment of OUD. Buprenorphine can be offered in either an office-based opioid treatment clinic or an OTP; if used in an OTP, it must be dispensed by the clinic similar to methadone.

Prescription Drug Monitoring Programs

Prescription drug monitoring programs (PDMPs) are electronic databases that track controlled substance prescriptions in a state in real-time. Pharmacies have to report to the PDMP whenever a prescription for a controlled substance is dispensed to a patient. Some states have policies requiring the provider to check the state's PDMP before prescribing controlled substances.

PDMPs enable state health departments to better understand physician and patient behavior and evaluate interventions to reduce inappropriate prescribing of controlled substances.

OPIOID PHARMACOLOGY

In this section, we review the pharmacology of opioid medications used to treat pain. A note on terminology: although they are distinct, the terms "opioids" and "opiates" are frequently used interchangeably. "Opiates" refers specifically to natural or semisynthetic opioids derived from the poppy plant, which include opium, morphine, heroin, and codeine. "Opioids" refers to all natural, synthetic, or partly synthetic molecules, such as hydrocodone, fentanyl, and methadone that act on opioid receptors. Synthetic and semisynthetic molecules, such as oxycodone, hydrocodone, hydromorphone, methadone, tramadol, and fentanyl, are not found in nature.

Opioids exert their effects through several molecular pathways on the level of both the peripheral and central nervous system. The family of opioid receptors consist of three G protein-coupled receptors: the mu, delta, and kappa receptors. The mu-opioid receptors mediate the analgesic properties of opioids and their euphoric properties, as well as tolerance and physical dependence. The role of delta-opioid receptors is linked to reducing chronic pain, drug reward regulation, inhibitory control, and learning. Kappa receptors are the most abundant opioid receptors in the brain and have functions related to the modulation of stress, anxiety, and emotional reactions. These effects are mediated by dynorphins and not by enkephalins, which predominantly bind to delta- and the mu-opioid receptors.

Opioid intoxication causes the following physiological and psychological effects:

Physiological	Psychological
▪ Meiosis	▪ Poor decision making
▪ Head nodding	▪ Lowered motivation
▪ Sedation	▪ Anxiety attacks
▪ Hypokinesis	▪ Slurred speech
▪ Hypothermia	▪ Sleeping more and feeling tired
▪ Hypotension	
▪ Bradycardia	▪ Mood swings
▪ Abdominal pain	▪ Euphoria or dysphoria
	▪ Irritability

Opioid use is associated with adverse effects including:

▪ Respiratory depression: This is the most concerning opioid side effect and the hallmark of opioid overdose. Sedation occurs before the onset of significant respiratory depression and, therefore, is a warning sign. It is caused by the opioid's effects on the medullary respiratory center and is marked by impaired breathing, decreased tidal volume, and minute ventilation. Opioid-related respiratory depression causes a right-shift CO_2 response, hypercapnia, hypoxia, and decreased oxygen saturation.

- Constipation: Opioid-related constipation is not dose-dependent and needs to be anticipated as it is probably one of the most common opioid side effects. If severe, it can be managed using laxatives, bowel stimulants, or switching to a different opioid (avoid bulking agents because of the increased risk for bowel hypomotility).
- OUD (see later).
- Nausea and vomiting can be managed by using antiemetic agents or switching to a different opioid.
- Pruritus: This occurs because of mast cell release of histamines. Use an antihistamine, preferably a nonsedating one, to treat it.
- Decreased libido: Caused by the hypothalamic–pituitary–adrenal axis dysfunction with suppression or reduction in sex hormone production.

The CDC published the following general principles for safer opioid prescribing for chronic pain:

- The initial course of treatment should be viewed as short term (<60 days)
- Start low and titrate cautiously
- Do not start extended-release or long-acting formulations in opioid naïve patients
- Avoid daily doses of more than 90 mg morphine milligram equivalent (MME)
- Individualize opioid selection and dosing based on the patient's age and health status
- Consider patients' previous exposure to opioids and their risks for opioid tolerance

Know This:

The doses of pain medications, especially opioids, should be lower in patients with renal failure, hepatic failure, or age older than 65 years.

When prescribing opioids, the following measures can be taken to mitigate the associated risks:

- Safe storage and disposing of the prescriptions (e.g., storage in a lockbox)

- Educating family members
- Having the poison control number handy
- Naloxone distribution for overdose reversal
- Setting realistic function-based goals for pain management
- Optimizing the use of nonopioid therapies
- Meaningful discussions on the benefits and risks of using opioids with the patients
- Carefully evaluating the risk of harm or misuse by checking the PDMP data
- Performing periodic urine drug screenings

Screening tools for opioid use behaviors are helpful at assessing one's potential for adverse effects and/or potential for prescription opioid misuse and risk for developing OUD. Screening tools cannot be used in isolation but should be combined with standardized clinical examination and, when indicated, urine drug screening and risk assessment tools. Commonly used tools include:

- Current Opioid Misuse Measure (COMM): For patients on chronic opioid therapy
- Opioid Risk Tool (ORT): To assess the risk of opioid misuse
- Patient Medication Questionnaire (PMQ): For patients already taking opioid medications for pain
- Screener and Opioid Assessment for Patients with Pain-Revised (SOAPP-R): Used before the initiation of long-term opioid therapy

In the next section, we review some commonly encountered (and assessed in board examination) prescribed opioids.

Morphine

Morphine is a mu-, kappa-, and delta-opioid receptor agonist, with strongest affinity for the mu-opioid receptor. It is glucuronidated to two metabolites with potentially significant differences in efficacy, clearance, and action: morphine-6-glucuronide (M6G) and morphine-3-glucuronide (M3G). The M3G metabolite of morphine lacks analgesic activity but has neuroexcitatory effects and may be responsible for opioid-induced hyperalgesia. The M6G metabolite has analgesic effects but less than the parent molecule. Morphine is not recommended for use in patients with advanced chronic kidney disease.

Know This:

- All opioids are generally cross-compared to one another by their MME doses.
- Excessive morphine can cause pulmonary edema.
- Tolerance to opioids is more likely to occur at doses of opioids more than 90 mg MME.

Codeine (3-Methylmorphine)

Codeine is a prodrug with weak analgesic effects; its analgesic properties are primarily exerted by its metabolites, morphine and codeine-6-glucuronide. It is metabolized by the CYP2D6 system. It is typically used as a combination product with nonopioid analgesics because of its low potency.

Know This:

- Codeine can cause spasm of the sphincter of Oddi and should be used with caution in patients with biliary tract disease.
- CYP2D6 inhibitors decrease or hold the conversion of codeine to morphine.
- Nicotine can increase codeine analgesic effects by the induction of CYP2D6 and central activation of codeine to morphine.

Methadone

Methadone is a long-acting full mu-opioid receptor agonist. It has a long, variable, and very unpredictable half-life of 20 to 120 hours and a stable concentration reached within 5 to 7 days. Its concentration in the lungs, liver, and kidneys is much higher than in blood because of its binding to albumin and other plasma and tissue proteins. Its side effects are similar to those associated with other opioid drugs, including the prolongation of the QT interval, which can lead to torsade de pointes arrhythmias. Methadone is metabolized by CYP3A4. Its most important metabolites are 2-ethylidene, 1,5-dimethyl-3,3-diphenyl-pyrrolidine (EDDP), and 2-ethyl-5-methyl-3,3-diphenyl-1-pyrrolidine (EMDP), both of which are inactive.

As such, CYP3A4 inducers (such as rifampicin, phenytoin, carbamazepine, oxcarbazepine, phenobarbital, dexamethasone, and certain HIV medications) can produce withdrawal symptoms. In contrast, CYP3A4 inhibitors (such as amiodarone, erythromycin, diltiazem, antifungals, fluoxetine, fluvoxamine, isonicotinic acid hydrazide, atazanavir, clarithromycin, indinavir, ketoconazole, nefazodone, nelfinavir, ritonavir, telithromycin, diltiazem, erythromycin, cimetidine, fluconazole, fosamprenavir, grapefruit juice, and verapamil) can produce methadone toxicity.

Know This:

Although methadone has a long half-life, administering methadone twice or three times daily enhances the analgesic effect of the medication.

Oxycodone

Oxycodone is a semisynthetic opioid metabolized by CYP3A4 to nor-oxycodone and by CYP2D6 to oxymorphone. It has an average plasma half-life of 3 to 5 hours.

Hydromorphone

The primary metabolite of hydromorphone, hydromorphone-3-glucuronide, has neuroexcitatory potential similar to the M3G metabolite of morphine.

Tramadol

Tramadol is a dual-mechanism opioid medication with weak mu-opioid agonist and is a norepinephrine and serotonin reuptake inhibitor. It undergoes both CYP3A4- and CYP2D6-mediated metabolism. Its use is associated with a higher risk for seizures, substance use disorder, and serotonin syndrome risk (particularly when combined with other serotonergic agents).

Fentanyl

Fentanyl is a synthetic opioid agonist with analgesic and anesthetic properties. It selectively binds to and activates the mu-receptor in the central nervous system and has a half-life of 3 to 8 hours. Fentanyl is metabolized almost completely in the liver to multiple metabolites, including norfentanyl, hydroxy-propionyl-fentanyl, and hydroxy-propionyl-norfentanyl.

Buprenorphine

Buprenorphine is a partial agonist at mu-receptor and an antagonist at kappa and delta receptors with a half-life of 24 to 42 hours. It will be discussed in more detail later.

Meperidine

Meperidine is a mu- and kappa-opioid receptor agonist with a half-life of 2 to 5 hours. Its metabolism produces normeperidine, which has a longer half-life of 15 to 30 hours and has been linked to seizures and renal failure. Transdermal preparations are a unique but unusual formulation for use in primary care and pain management.

Know This:

- Fentanyl is approximately 50 times more potent than heroin and 100 times more potent than morphine.
- Carfentanil, an extremely potent fentanyl analog, is estimated to be 10,000 times more potent than morphine.

OPIOID OVERDOSE PRESENTATION AND MANAGEMENT

The use of large amounts of opioids can lead to an opioid overdose, particularly in medically compromised individuals or in combination with other sedatives, such as benzodiazepines. Overdoses are marked by the following triad of symptoms:

- Altered mental status (sedation)
- Respiratory depression
- Miotic pupils

Untreated overdoses can be lethal or cause irreversible brain damage because of prolonged hypoxia. In addition to using naloxone for overdose reversal, the management of opioid overdose requires airway support, breathing (ventilation), and cardiovascular support (hypotension should be managed with intravenous fluid).

Naloxone is a potent opioid receptor antagonist and as such carries no abuse potential. It is administered parenterally (intranasally, intravenously, or intramuscularly) to rapidly reverse opioid-related sedation, respiratory depression, and opioid overdoses within 2 to 3 minutes. Given that naloxone has a short half-life and duration of action that range from 30 to 90 minutes, the symptoms of the opioid overdose may recur, particularly if the used opioid causing the overdose is long-acting.

Know This:

Oral naloxone has poor systemic bioavailability but blocks intestinal opioid receptors and mitigates opioid-related constipation.

CLINICAL CONSIDERATIONS OF OUD

MULTIPLE internal and external factors can contribute to the development of an OUD, including:

- A personal history of a substance use
- Comorbid psychiatric disorders
- Initiation of opioid use at a young age
- Lacking social support
- A history of trauma
- A family history of substance use disorders
- A history of legal involvement

According to the *Diagnostic and Statistical Manual of Mental Disorders*, Fifth Edition, the diagnosis of OUD is established based on the diagnostic criteria listed in Chapter 1. Tolerance to opioids refers to a decreased sensitivity to the effects of opioids that develops in individuals with long-term opioid use. Tolerance develops with chronic opioid use, but the timeframe is variable between individuals. Individuals who have developed tolerance to opioids will require an increased opioid dosage of medication to achieve the same intoxicating or analgesic effect.

Know This:

- Although tolerance develops to many of the side effects of opioids, tolerance typically does not develop for constipation or miosis.
- Methylnaltrexone is an opioid antagonist with high bioavailability in the gastrointestinal tract. It is used to treat opioid-induced constipation.

The use of opioid agonists leads to inhibition of cyclic adenosine monophosphate phosphorylation (cAMP) signaling pathways in cells of the locus coeruleus, leading to a reduction of noradrenergic release and symptoms such as sedation. However, chronic activation of opioid receptors leads to an adaptive upregulation of the cAMP signaling pathway. In settings of opioid discontinuation, cAMP signaling increases and leads to noradrenergic overactivation in the locus coeruleus and the classic symptoms of opioid withdrawal.

On discontinuation of opioid use, the onset of opioid withdrawal symptoms depends on the half-life of the specific opioid used. In persons using short-acting opioids, such as heroin, oxycodone, morphine, hydrocodone, and fentanyl, withdrawal symptoms typically appear within 8 to 12 hours with a peak in symptoms within 1 to 3 days and can persist for up to 7 days. Withdrawal symptoms from long-acting opioids, such as methadone, typically first appear 1 to 2 days following opioid discontinuation and can persist for more than 14 days.

The Clinical Opiate Withdrawal Scale (COWS) is the most commonly used tool for the assessment and monitoring of opioid withdrawal in inpatient or outpatient settings. It is based on the Clinical Institute Withdrawal Assessment of Alcohol (CIWA-A) Scale used to measure alcohol withdrawal. Alternatively, the Finnegan scoring system can be used to assess opioid and nonopioid withdrawal.

Opioid withdrawal syndrome is marked by the following physiological and psychological signs and symptoms:

Physiological	Psychological
▪ Bone pain	▪ Physical agitation
▪ Muscle aches	▪ Poor decision-making
▪ Hyperthermia	▪ Abandoning responsibilities
▪ Agitation	
▪ Shivering	▪ Slurred speech
▪ Abdominal pain	▪ Sleeping more or less than usual
▪ Restlessness	
▪ Nausea/vomiting	▪ Changes in mood
▪ Diarrhea	▪ Irritability
▪ Excessive tearing	▪ Depression
▪ Runny nose	▪ Lowered motivation
▪ Tachycardia	▪ Anxiety
▪ Hypertension	▪ Insomnia
▪ Hyperreflexia	
▪ Diaphoresis	

Although generally not life threatening, opioid withdrawal causes significant distress and discomfort and can lead to relapse. Supervised medical withdrawal treatment includes the use of mu-opioid receptor agonists (e.g.,

methadone, tramadol, and buprenorphine) or alpha2-adrenergic receptor agonists (e.g., clonidine, tizanidine, and lofexidine). Adrenergic agents are effective for the treatment of opioid withdrawal symptoms by targeting noradrenergic hyperactivity in locus coeruleus neurons but may cause hypotension.

Know This:

- COWS are commonly used during buprenorphine inductions. Patients must be experiencing moderate opioid withdrawal before administration of the first buprenorphine dose, equivalent to a COWS score of 8 to 11.
- Transcutaneous electrical acupoint stimulation (electrical acupuncture) has been used for opioid detoxification because of reduced cravings via endorphin release.
- Detoxification is not a treatment for OUD. Without subsequent maintenance treatment, it carries a risk of overdose and decreased retention rates to care.

PHARMACOLOGIC TREATMENT OF OUD

Know This:

- Untreated OUD is associated with unintentional overdose and death, HIV, hepatitis C, other infectious diseases, legal issues, and a decrease in social functioning.
- Many adolescents do not receive treatment despite the evidence supporting the use of medication-assisted treatment.

Methadone

Methadone is a long-acting full mu-opioid receptor agonist that is approved by the U.S. Food and Drug Administration (FDA) for the treatment of pain and OUD maintenance. When used for OUD, it may only be dispensed in a licensed OTP. Although it is approved for treating OUD in people older than 18 years of age, it may be used to treat adolescents ages 16 to 18 years with parental consent and documentation of two drug-free treatment and psychosocial intervention failures. Research data indicate that methadone maintenance with doses greater than 80 mg per day are associated with superior clinical outcomes. Methadone maintenance leads to marked reductions in illicit opioid use, including injection opioid use, fewer HIV or hepatitis C infections, increased employment rates, and decreased likelihood of criminal justice involvement. Data are mixed regarding the effect of methadone maintenance on the use of illicit drugs other than opioids.

Know This:

Patients receiving methadone maintenance should receive an electrocardiogram at the onset of treatment and within 30 days because methadone causes QTc prolongations.

Buprenorphine

Buprenorphine is a long-acting partial agonist at mu-opioid receptors and an antagonist at kappa and delta receptors that is approved by the FDA for the treatment of pain and OUD maintenance in patients aged 16 years and older. When used for OUD, it can be offered in either an office-based opioid treatment clinic or in an OTP. As a highly potent mu-opioid receptor partial agonist, it can precipitate withdrawal if given too soon after the last use of a mu-opioid receptor agonist. Because of its ceiling effect at high doses on some opioid agonist effects, for example respiratory depression, buprenorphine is safer compared to full mu-opioid agonists with respect to overdose risk.

Know This:

- Buprenorphine is commonly administered sublingually. Newer formulations include long-acting injectables and require additional Risk Evaluation and Mitigation Strategy (REMS) training and approval for placement and removal.
- Buprenorphine is combined with naloxone to reduce its risk of abuse by injection (because naloxone is not absorbed if ingested orally alongside buprenorphine).

Naltrexone

Naltrexone is an opioid antagonist at mu-opioid receptor that is approved by the FDA for the maintenance treatment of OUD (and alcohol use disorders; see Chapter 4). It is available in daily oral tablets or as a long-acting injectable. It has been associated with hepatocellular injury particularly when used in doses much higher than 50 mg daily, although it may still be used in patients with hepatic impairments in consultation with the patient's gastroenterologist. Recent studies of naltrexone have focused on pharmacogenetic predictors of treatment response, namely the mu1-opioid receptor (OPRM1) gene.

Know This:

Naltrexone produces some pupillary constriction by an unknown mechanism.

OUD AND PREGNANCY

Opioid use is not uncommon among pregnant women in the United States. Opioids can cross the placenta and the blood–brain barrier, thereby posing risks for fetuses and newborns exposed to opioids in utero. Such risks include spontaneous abortion, premature rupture of membranes, preeclampsia, abruption placentae, fetal death, congenital heart defects, neural tube defects, gastroschisis, oral clefts, ventricular/atrial septal defects, and spina bifida.

The treatment of OUD during pregnancy with methadone, buprenorphine, or naltrexone reduces opioid use during pregnancy and improves treatment retention. Naltrexone is not a first-line treatment, primarily because detoxification and an opioid-free period are required.

Opioid use in pregnancy increases the risk of stillbirth, neonatal opioid withdrawal syndrome (NOWS) or neonatal abstinence syndrome (NAS), low birth weight, meconium aspiration, and microcephaly. NOWS or NAS refers to a neonatal withdrawal syndrome seen in babies of mothers who used opioids during their pregnancies. Babies with NAS present with:

- Central nervous system excitability causing seizures, hypertension, poor sleep, and a high-pitched cry
- Autonomic instability causing sweating, sneezing, tearing, and hyperthermia
- Gastrointestinal symptoms with feeding difficulty, vomiting, and diarrhea
- Respiratory distress with increased secretions, tachypnea, cyanosis, and apnea

Signs and symptoms of NAS occur 48 to 72 hours post-birth following discontinuation of prenatal opioid exposure, and the syndrome duration depends on the half-life of the opioids used. NAS is treated using deodorized tincture of opium or oral morphine. Barbiturates can be used as second-line treatment for severe withdrawal, including withdrawal seizures, or if maximum safe doses of morphine or deodorized tincture of opium have already been used.

Women who are on treatment for OUD and on a stable dose of methadone or buprenorphine should be encouraged to breastfeed unless specifically contraindicated. A study of neonates prenatally exposed to methadone or buprenorphine for a minimum of 30 days found that breastfed neonates had significantly shorter lengths of hospital stay and need for pharmacotherapy for NAS.

Know This:

- The Maternal Opioid Treatment: Human Experimental Research (MOTHER) study was a large-scale trial comparing maternal and neonatal outcomes in pregnant women with OUD randomly assigned to methadone or buprenorphine pharmacotherapy during pregnancy. It showed that OUD treatment using buprenorphine is associated with shorter treatment duration, less medication needed to treat NAS symptoms, and shorter hospitalizations for neonates. The buprenorphine-exposed group of neonates showed less motor activity suppression and a longer movement duration. The methadone-exposed fetuses were found to have a higher incidence of intrauterine growth restriction than buprenorphine-exposed fetuses. They were also more likely to have an abnormal nonstress test and fewer fetal heart rate accelerations.
- The Pregnant and the Reduction of Opiates: Medication Intervention Safety and Efficacy (PROMISE) study found that the amount of opioid-agonist medication administered to treat NAS in methadone-exposed neonates was three times greater than for buprenorphine-exposed neonates. Similarly, the length of hospitalization was shorter for buprenorphine-exposed than for methadone-exposed neonates.

REFERENCE

Center for Behavioral Health Statistics and Quality. (2019). *2018 National Survey on Drug Use and Health Final Analytic File Codebook*. Substance Abuse and Mental Health Services Administration, Rockville, MD.

SUGGESTIONS FOR FURTHER READING

American Psychiatric Association. (2013). *Diagnostic and statistical manual of mental disorders* (5th ed., p. 541). American Psychiatric Association.

American Society of Addiction Medicine. (2016). *Sample office-based opioid use disorder policy and procedure manual*. American Society of Addiction Medicine.

Faggiano, F., Vigna-Taglianti, F., Versino, E., & Lemma, P. (2003). Methadone maintenance at different dosages for opioid dence. *Cochrane Database Syst Rev*, (3), CD002208.

Food and Drug Administration. (2017). *Appropriate use checklist: Buprenorphine-containing transmucosal products for opioid dependence*. Food and Drug Administration.

Jones, H. E., Johnson, R. E., Jasinski, D. R., O'Grady, K. E., Chisholm, C. A., Choo, R. E., Crocetti, M., Dudas, R., Harrow, C., Huestis, M. A., Jansson, L. M., Lantz, M., Lester, B. M., & Milio, L (2005). Buprenorphine versus methadone in the treatment of pregnant opioid-dependent patients: effects on the neonatal abstinence syndrome. *Drug and Alcohol Dependence, 79*(1), 1–10.

Kosten, T. R., & Baxter, L. E. (2019). Review article: Effective management of opioid withdrawal symptoms: a gateway to opioid dependence treatment. *American Journal on Addictions, 28*(2), 55–62.

Substance Abuse and Mental Health Services Administration. (2015). *Clinical use of extended-release injectable naltrexone in the treatment of opioid use disorder: A brief guide*. Substance Abuse and Mental Health Services Administration. HHS Publication No. (SMA) 14-4892R.

Substance Abuse and Mental Health Services Administration. (2016). *Pocket guide: Medication-assisted treatment of opioid use disorder*. Substance Abuse and Mental Health Services Administration. HHS Publication No. (SMA) 16-4892PG.

REVIEW QUESTIONS

1. A 35-year-old woman is being started on metha-
    done after 2 years of intravenous heroin use.
    What is the lowest dose range of methadone
    that is considered adequate to suppress opioid
    urges?
    A. 10 to 30 mg
    B. 40 to 60 mg
    C. 60 to 80 mg
    D. 80 to 100 mg
    E. 100 to 120 mg

2. A 19-year-old woman in her third trimester of preg-
    nancy presents to the emergency room because of
    confusion and respiratory depression. Per her boy-
    friend, she has been receiving treatment at the local
    methadone clinic for the past 5 months. Her chart
    indicates she was recently started on a new medica-
    tion. Which of the following medications is most
    likely responsible for her presentation?
    A. Carbamazepine
    B. Methadone
    C. Fluconazole
    D. Saquinavir
    E. Naltrexone

3. Which of the following is the typical time frame
    when peak methadone levels occur after taking
    an oral dose?
    A. 15 to 45 minutes
    B. 2.5 to 4 hours
    C. 8 hours
    D. 12 hours
    E. 24 hours

4. A 19-year-old man with a history of major depres-
    sive disorder and OUD on buprenorphine pres-
    ents to your office with a urine drug toxicology
    test that is positive for both buprenorphine and
    opiates. He is adamant that he has not been using
    any opiates for the past 6 months. Which of the
    following could potentially cause a false-positive
    result for opiates on a standard urine drug screen?
    A. Buprenorphine
    B. Morphine

C. Clonidine
D. Dextromethorphan
E. Sertraline

5. A 67-year-old woman with a long history of gas-
    trointestinal adhesions and chronic renal disease
    presents to the emergency room with stomach
    pain. The patient was given medication for pain.
    Minutes later, she has a tonic-clonic seizure.
    Which of the following opioid analgesics is most
    likely to have caused this patient's presentation?
    A. Naltrexone
    B. Meperidine
    C. Codeine
    D. Morphine
    E. Oxycodone

6. A 24-year-old man is referred to your office for the
    assessment and treatment of OUD. He was first
    prescribed oxycodone for a back injury over a year
    ago. He currently endorses cravings to use, miss-
    ing work because of substance use, using more
    than intended, and spending much of his time ob-
    taining the substance illicitly. He is now interested
    in starting injectable naltrexone after not liking
    how buprenorphine made him feel. Which of the
    following is most likely to be a potential disadvan-
    tage of naltrexone for this patient?
    A. High rates of naltrexone discontinuation
    B. Interaction with ibuprofen for chronic pain
    C. The requirement for 7 days of abstinence
       from opioids before naltrexone initiation
    D. Need to always try the oral formulation of
       naltrexone first
    E. Need for at least mild opioid withdrawal
       with first use of naltrexone

7. In the case above, the patient meets the criteria
    for what type of OUD?
    A. OUD, in partial remission
    B. OUD, in full sustained remission
    C. OUD, mild
    D. OUD, moderate
    E. OUD, severe

7 TOBACCO AND OTHER NICOTINE PRODUCTS

NICOTINE PHARMACOLOGY

Chemical Structure and Mechanism of Action of Nicotine

The nicotine molecule is a tertiary amine alkaloid with pyridine and pyrrolidine rings, and it exists in two enantiomeric forms. The S-enantiomer is a more potent agonist at the nicotinic acetylcholine receptor compared to the R-enantiomer. Nicotinic acetylcholine receptors are ionotropic ligand-gated ion channels found throughout the central and peripheral nervous systems. As a nicotinic receptor agonist, nicotine activates the ventral tegmental area dopaminergic neurons in the mesolimbic dopamine system and the glutamatergic neurons that innervate ventral tegmental area dopamine neurons. Nicotine may also indirectly activate endogenous opioid pathways.

Nicotine acts as a stimulant at lower doses and a sedative at higher doses. It causes vasoconstriction, increased blood pressure, increased cerebral blood flow, tachycardia, decreased appetite, and skeletal muscle relaxation. As such, nicotinic agonists have been found to improve performance on attention and memory tasks (Table 7.1). Nicotine has been studied for its effects on cognitive enhancement in patients with some types of dementia, psychoses, and attention deficit disorders.

Nicotine Pharmacology

- Mucosal nicotine absorption is pH-dependent and is marked by decreased absorption with a more acidic, lower pH.
- Inhaled nicotine reaches the brain within 20 seconds.

- Nicotine is metabolized predominantly in the liver through CYP2A6 into cotinine (and to a lesser extent in the lungs and brain).
- The half-life of nicotine is about 2 hours. In contrast, the metabolite cotinine has a half-life of 16 hours. Because of its longer half-life, cotinine is more useful as a biomarker of nicotine use.
- Individuals of African and Chinese descents metabolize nicotine at a slower rate than Whites because of an increased prevalence of hypoactive CYP2A6 alleles.
- Women and persons taking exogenous estrogen are faster metabolizers of nicotine because of higher levels of estrogen, which induce CYP2A6. At the same time, cigarette smoking can reduce the efficacy of estrogen and estrogen's ability to prevent osteoporosis and cardiovascular disease.
- CYP2A6 inducers such as estrogen, phenobarbital, and rifampicin increase the rate of nicotine metabolism.
- Older adults metabolize nicotine more slowly because of reduced CYP2A6 activity.
- The polycyclic aromatic hydrocarbons in tobacco smoke are believed to be responsible for the induction of the isoenzyme CYP1A2, possibly affecting plasma levels of medications metabolized by this isoenzyme. CYP1A2 activity is higher in heavy smokers than in nonsmokers, and quitting can normalize the CYP1A2 activity. Individuals using nicotine replacement products will not experience alterations in CYP1A2 activity.

TABLE 7.1
Nicotine Effects via Neurotransmitter Receptors

Nicotine Effects Via	Effect During Intoxication	Effect During Withdrawal
Serotonin	Mood elevation; poor appetite	Depressed mood
GABA	Anxiety relief	Anxiety
Acetylcholine	Arousal and cognition	Insomnia
Endorphins	Reduction in tension	Irritability
Glutamate	Learning and memory	Poor concentration
Norepinephrine	Arousal; poor appetite	Decreased heart rate
Dopamine	Pleasure; poor appetite	Increased appetite; craving

Know This:

The rate of nicotine metabolism is a key factor influencing risk for addiction, cigarette smoking behavior, and efficacy of pharmacologic treatment for tobacco use disorder. Individuals with a faster metabolism on average have a higher risk of addiction and lower success with quit attempts.

Nicotine Product Additives

- The majority of the adverse medical consequences of nicotine are caused by other additives and compounds. Keep in mind that although nicotine is the addictive component of tobacco, it has not been found to be carcinogenic. A cigarette contains about 1 mg of nicotine as well as 7000 other chemicals, including known carcinogens such as nitrosamines, polycyclic aromatic hydrocarbons, and many others.
- Beta-carotene, vitamin E, and alpha-tocopherol are added as antioxidants to counteract the carcinogenic effects in some tobacco products.
- Menthol is added to provide anesthetic activity and to make cigarettes less harsh to smoke, although they are no safer than regular cigarettes and may in fact be more addicting. It may inhibit the CYP2A6, decreasing the metabolism of nicotine. Menthol

cigarettes were recently banned by the European Union and the United Kingdom.
- Eucalyptol is an antimicrobial additive believed to increase the mucociliary clearance of some of the chemicals in cigarettes, protecting the lungs from tobacco exposure.

Know This:

- The 15q25 locus, *CHRNA3*, and *CHRNA5* are some of the genes with variants that encode for the α5, α3, and β4 nicotinic receptor subunits associated with altered smoking behaviors in European Americans.
- Of the more than 7000 chemicals in tobacco smoke, at least 250 are known to be harmful, including hydrogen cyanide, carbon monoxide, and ammonia. At least 69 of these can cause cancer.
- Tobacco affects sleep during withdrawal but not during intoxication (most other substances affect sleep both during withdrawal and intoxication).

EPIDEMIOLOGY OF TOBACCO USE DISORDER

- More than one-fifth of those who experiment with cigarettes will meet nicotine and tobacco use disorder criteria in their lifetime.
- Individuals with low socioeconomic status, indigenous populations, persons with serious mental illness, the homeless, prisoners, and youth are more vulnerable to dangerous smoking behaviors.
- Nicotine use disorder has been correlated with alcohol use disorder.

Nicotine Use and Women

- Tobacco is a modifiable risk factor for heart disease and the leading cause of death in women in the United States.
- Smoking is directly responsible for four out of five lung cancer deaths in women in the United States.
- Women smokers carry a 20-fold increased risk of death from chronic respiratory conditions.
- The antiestrogen effect of tobacco can cause premature menopause and increase the risk of heart disease as well as bone fractures.
- Smoking in postmenopausal women causes decreased bone density.

- Women who smoke have an increased risk for hip fractures.
- Nicotine concentration can be twice as high in breast milk compared to blood concentration in lactating women.

Secondhand Smoke

- Many of the chemicals that smokers inhale directly are also found in secondhand smoke.
- Secondhand smoke is associated with premature death in nonsmoking people.
- According to the Centers for Disease Control and Prevention, secondhand smoke exposure increases the risk of heart disease and stroke by more than 20%.
- Secondhand smoke exposure during pregnancy is associated with low birthweight, preterm birth, spontaneous abortion, and other adverse pregnancy outcomes.
- Infants exposed to secondhand smoke have a higher risk of sudden infant death syndrome.
- Children exposed to secondhand smoke have a higher risk of asthma, bronchitis, pneumonia, and ear infections.

Tobacco Use Disorder

The diagnosis of a tobacco use disorder is given to a person who has a pattern of problematic use of nicotine products. It leads to the inability to reduce consumption, cravings to use nicotine-containing products, continuing to use nicotine despite adverse consequences, and needing to use increased amounts of nicotine to achieve the desired effect. According to the *American Psychiatric Association's Diagnostic and Statistical Manual, 5th Edition*, the diagnosis of tobacco use disorder is established based on the diagnostic criteria listed in Chapter 1. Nicotine withdrawal symptoms include anxiety, irritability, decreased concentration, restlessness, insomnia, decreased heart rate, and depressed mood.

Know This:

- Tobacco use is strongly associated with psychotic disorders. Nicotine has been linked to a reduction in the negative symptoms in psychosis as well as the sedating side effects of antipsychotic medications.

- The Fagerström Test for Nicotine Use Disorders is a standard instrument for assessing the intensity of physical dependence to nicotine. The higher the total Fagerström score, the more intense is the patient's physical dependence on nicotine. The results correlate with smoking cessation outcomes.
- The 5 A's of smoking cessation: Ask, Advise, Assess, Assist, Arrange

TREATMENT OF TOBACCO AND OTHER NICOTINE PRODUCTS DISORDER

Nicotine Replacement Therapy

- There are currently five nicotine replacement therapy (NRT) products: transdermal patch, nasal spray, inhaler, lozenge, and gum.
- NRT can be used during pregnancy and while breastfeeding.
- Combination NRT consists of using both the nicotine patch (a long-acting form of NRT) and a short-acting NRT of the patient's choice.
- Nasal spray is the NRT with the highest abuse potential.
- The nicotine patch, but not gum or nasal spray, has short-term efficacy for adolescents.
- Relapse after discontinuation of NRT remains elevated.
- Use NRT with caution in patients with cardiovascular disease and in patients under the age of 18.
- Nicotine absorption from the gums or lozenges is reduced in acidic environments.

Varenicline

- Varenicline is a partial agonist for the α4β2 subtype and a full agonist at the α7 unit of the nicotinic acetylcholine receptors.
- Analogous to the mechanism of action of buprenorphine for opioid use disorder, varenicline will block the effects of nicotine while providing partial agonist effect at the level of the nicotinic acetylcholine receptor.
- Varenicline reduces nicotine withdrawal and reduces the reinforcement and reward from nicotine use.

- Varenicline is typically started at least 1 week before the quit date.
- Common side effects are nausea, sleep disturbances, constipation, and flatulence.
- Caution should be used for:
  - Individuals with severe renal impairment (dosage adjustment is necessary)
  - Pregnancy and breastfeeding, due to limited data on safety
  - Adolescents
  - Individuals at elevated risk for cardiovascular events

Bupropion

- Bupropion is a dopaminergic and norepinephrine reuptake inhibitor approved for the treatment of smoking cessation. It also antagonizes brain nicotinic acetylcholine receptors and blocks the reinforcing effects of nicotine.
- It improves nicotine withdrawal, reduces craving, prevents weight gain, and improves co-occurring depression.
- It is contraindicated in people with a seizure disorder or those that are predisposed to seizures. Only 0.1% of patients on bupropion get seizures, but caution is recommended.
- Common side effects are dry mouth, insomnia, tremor, skin rash, headache, and urticaria.

Second-Line Pharmacological Agents

Nortriptyline, cytisine, and clonidine are considered a second-line medication for smoking cessation but are not approved by the FDA for this indication.

Know This:

- Do not use NRTs in patients with recent (≤2 weeks) myocardial infarction or those with underlying severe arrhythmias or angina pectoris.
- The Evaluating Adverse Events in a Global Smoking Cessation Study (EAGLES) trial evaluated the safety and efficacy of varenicline, NRT (nicotine patches), and bupropion and found that varenicline had slightly better abstinence rates than bupropion or NRT.
- A black box warning was placed in 2009 on varenicline for increased suicidal ideation and agitation, but it was removed in 2019 after the EAGLES trial findings did not substantiate these assertions.

SUGGESTIONS FOR FURTHER READING

Goniewicz, M. L., & Delijewski, M. (2013). Nicotine vaccines to treat tobacco dependence. *Human Vaccines & Immunotherapeutics, 9*(1), 13–25.

Hopkins, R. J., & Young, R. P. (2016). Gene by environment interaction linking the chromosome 15q25 locus with cigarette consumption and lung cancer susceptibility–are African American affected differently? *EBioMedicine, 4*, 13–14.

Mooney, M. E., Reus, V. I., Gorecki, J., Hall, S. M., Humfleet, G. L., Muñoz, R. F., & Delucchi, K. (2008). Therapeutic drug monitoring of nortriptyline in smoking cessation: A multistudy analysis. *Clinical Pharmacology and Therapeutics, 83*(3), 436–442.

National Center for Chronic Disease Prevention and Health Promotion (US) Office on Smoking and Health. (2014). *The health consequences of smoking—50 years of progress: A report of the surgeon general.* Centers for Disease Control and Prevention (US).

Siu, A. L., & U.S. Preventive Services Task Force. (2015). Behavioral and pharmacotherapy interventions for tobacco smoking cessation in adults, including pregnant women: U.S. preventive Services Task Force recommendation statement. *Annals of Internal Medicine, 163*(8), 622–634.

REVIEW QUESTIONS

1. A 41-year-old woman who smokes close to 15 cigarettes per day presents to your office. Recently, a family member was diagnosed with lung cancer. This event has motivated her to quit smoking. She has tried several times to quit without success. Which of the following treatment options has been shown to have the greatest efficacy in achieving abstinence in individuals with tobacco use disorder?

   A. Buspirone
   B. Varenicline
   C. Clonidine
   D. Bupropion
   E. NRT

2. Which of the following is a symptom of nicotine withdrawal?
   A. Abdominal cramps
   B. Hypersomnia
   C. Decreased appetite
   D. Decreased heart rate
   E. Tremor

3. A 21-year-old woman was brought to your office by her mother. She has been smoking close to 10 cigarettes a day. You discussed NRT to which she agrees. What dose of nicotine patch would you prescribe to the patient?
   A. 7 mg every 12 hours
   B. 14 mg every 12 hours
   C. 14 mg every 24 hours
   D. 21 mg every 24 hours
   E. 2 patches of 21 mg every 12 hours

4. Which of the following is recommended to decrease side effects when using nicotine patches as NRT?
   A. Not wearing the patch during nighttime
   B. Apply the patch once a day, ideally at different times each day
   C. Wear the patch over clothing
   D. Use two patches if the patient smokes more than five cigarettes per day
   E. Use the same patch for more than 24 hours

5. Which of the following Nicotine Replacement Therapy option has a higher risk of being abused?
   A. Inhalers
   B. Nasal spray
   C. Lozenges
   D. Gum
   E. Patch

6. Which one of the following medications can increase the odds of quitting smoking?
   A. Paroxetine
   B. Duloxetine
   C. Nortriptyline
   D. Fluoxetine
   E. Desvenlafaxine

CANNABIS USE DISORDER

GENERAL CHARACTERISTICS

Cannabis is the most commonly illicitly used drug in the United States, as well as globally. The cannabis plant contains over 100 different cannabinoids, molecules that share their chemical structure with delta-9-tetrahydrocannabinol (THC) and cannabidiol (CBD), the two major psychoactive components of the cannabis plant.

CHEMICAL STRUCTURE AND NEUROBIOLOGY

The Cannabis Family

There are over 700 different types of plants within the Cannabis family; the two main subspecies are *Cannabis indica* and *Cannabis sativa*. *Cannabis sativa* has a higher ratio of THC to CBD, whereas *Cannabis indica* has a higher ratio of CBD to THC. Different cannabis plants are engineered to have different properties; "hemp" plants, for instance, are legal in a number of US states and are cannabis plants with high concentrations of CBD and negligible THC. The concentration of THC and CBD varies throughout different parts of the cannabis plant and is highest in female plants' flowering tops. These areas produce high numbers of *trichomes*, fine glandular outgrowths that produce THC, CBD, and other cannabinoids.

Cannabis potency is considered high if it contains greater than 10% of THC by dry weight. The average potency of cannabis has steadily increased over time as cannabis plants have been selectively bred for higher THC content.

A note on terminology: There is no such thing as the "marijuana plant," all forms of plant-based cannabis are subsumed under the cannabis family. Although marijuana and cannabis are commonly used interchangeably, "marijuana" is a term created during the Great Depression to mark cannabis as a drug mainly used by Mexicans.

Cannabinoids

Cannabinoids refer to the family of molecules which share the 21-carbon structure of THC and include plant-based, endogenous, and synthetic cannabinoids. See Fig. 8.1 for a side-by-side comparison of their molecular structures.

- **Plant-based cannabinoids:** More than 100 plant-based cannabinoids have been identified, but the main cannabinoids to know are **THC** and **CBD**. Both molecules have long aliphatic chains responsible for their hydrophobic, lipophilic properties and perfusion into adipose tissue (Fig. 8.1).
- **Endogenous cannabinoids: Anandamide** and **2-arachidonoylglycerol** are the main endogenous

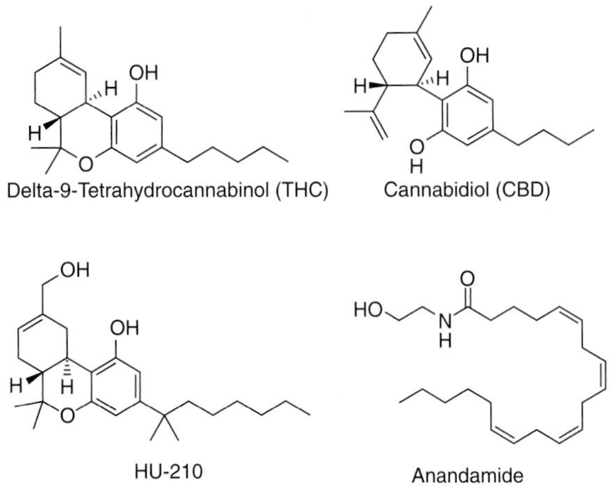

Fig. 8.1 ▪ Chemical structure of select cannabinoids.

cannabinoids to know and are the key ligands for endocannabinoid receptors (CB1 and CB2) expressed widely in the central nervous system (primarily CB1) and the periphery (primarily CB2).

- **Synthetic cannabinoids:** These are a heterogeneous family of ever-evolving, laboratory-produced cannabinoids that share structural homology with THC, although they are misleadingly marketed for their "natural" high and at times for their "legal" high. The prototypical synthetic cannabinoid is **HU-210** (for Hebrew University, where the first synthetic cannabinoid was created). Synthetic cannabinoids are known and sold by many names, including K2 and spice.

Know This:

For the board examination, you should be able to identify the chemical structure of delta-9-THC. You can easily remember it by its long aliphatic chain.

Standard urine drug screens (UDSs) cannot detect synthetic cannabinoids for THC because of its inexact homology with THC. This property can be exploited by individuals who want to evade urine drug screens.

Dronabinol is synthetically produced delta-9-THC and will cause a positive urine drug screen for THC because it is structurally identical. *Nabilone* is a synthetic analog of THC, and it has minimal euphoric effects.

Cannabinoids: Pharmacology and Mechanism of Action

For the board examination, it is important to know the differing receptor properties and mechanisms of action for THC, CBD, and synthetic cannabinoids.

THC:

- Partial agonist at CB1 and CB2 (CB1>CB2)
- Modulates beta-2-adrenergic receptors
- Modulates mu- and delta-opioid receptors
- Metabolized by CYP3A4, inhibits CYP2C9, induces CYP1A2
- Rapidly metabolized to 11-hydroxy-THC (psychoactive), then to THC-carboxylase (not psychoactive)
- Elimination half-life ranges from 25 to 36 hours and is longer for regular cannabis users (in part due to storage in fat reserves)
- Predominantly eliminated via feces (>65%) and urine (20%)

CBD:

- Low affinity for CB1 and CB2
- Modulates mu- and delta-opioid receptors
- 5-HT1A partial agonism
- Modulates psychotomimetic effects of THC
- Suggested to have anticonvulsant, antipsychotic, antianxiety properties
- Does not have euphoric, intoxicant effects
- Metabolized by CYP3A4, it inhibits CYP2D6 and CYP2C9

Synthetic Cannabinoids (e.g., K2, Spice, HU-2010):

- Full agonists at CB1
- Have much higher receptor affinity (approximately 100×) for CB1 compared with THC

Know This:

CBD modulates the psychotomimetic effects of THC. Cannabis strains that have higher THC-to-CBD ratios are therefore more psychotomimetic.

Synthetic cannabinoids have greater psychotomimetic properties compared to plant-based THC because it has greater receptor affinity and is a full agonist at CB1, in addition to lacking any CBD.

Rimonabant is a CB1 receptor antagonist and has been studied to treat cannabis use disorder and weight loss.

The Endocannabinoid System

THC was first isolated in 1965. Subsequent decades of research and interest in the effects of THC led to the discovery of the endocannabinoid system. Here we review the structure and function of the endocannabinoid system as well as cannabinoid receptors.

The endocannabinoid system regulates a wide variety of physiological properties, including pain, appetite, mood, immune system modulation, gastrointestinal tract function, the cardiovascular system, and stress regulation. For the board examination, the two key receptors of the endocannabinoid system to know are cannabinoid receptors 1 and 2 (CB1 and CB2), although there are others under investigation. Both CB1 and CB2 are G-protein receptors, and CB1 is the most abundant G-protein receptor expressed in the CNS. CB1 is widely expressed in various brain regions as well as in most tissues and organs in the periphery. Centrally, the highest concentrations can be found in the hippocampus and the basal ganglia. CB2 receptors, however, are largely expressed in immune cells but are also expressed in the CNS. Endogenous ligands for CB1 and CB2 include anandamide and 2-arachidonyl glycerol, both lipid-based retrograde neurotransmitters.

An important property of CB1 is that it co-localizes and dimerizes with a number of other receptor types in the CNS and the periphery. These include the mu-, kappa- and delta-opioid receptors, orexin-1 receptors, A2A adenosine receptors, and the beta-2-adrenergic receptors.

Know This:

The highest concentration of CB1 receptors is found in the hippocampus and basal ganglia. However, CB1 receptors are expressed in very low density in the brain stem, explaining why cannabis has little to no effect on the respiratory drive.

CB1 receptors co-localize with beta-2-adrenergic receptors, which is postulated to cause its adrenergic-like effects (e.g., tachycardia or panic attacks in cannabis intoxication).

The combination of cannabinoids with anticholinergic drugs can lead to marked tachycardia.

TOXICOLOGY TESTING

UDSs include immunoassays that test for the presence of delta-9-THC metabolites, typically THC carboxylase. The elimination half-life of THC ranges from 25 to 36 hours but is longer in regular cannabis users and can have an unpredictable elimination due to storage and release of THC from adipose cells. A UDS will stay positive for occasional users for about 1 to 2 weeks, but it can remain positive for heavier users for more than 1 month.

Know This:

Although commonly claimed, passive inhalation does not produce a positive urine drug screen for THC.

False positives are rare due to the unique chemical structure of THC but have been reported with efavirenz, proton pump inhibitors, hemp seed oil, and nonsteroidal anti-inflammatory drugs. Dronabinol causes a positive test because it is structurally identical to delta-9-THC.

CANNABIS INTOXICATION AND WITHDRAWAL

Here we review the physiological and psychological signs and symptoms of cannabis intoxication, which are commonly tested on board examinations. It is important to contextualize these findings with the reported desirable effects of cannabis, including euphoria, enhancement of sensory experiences (taste, colors, sights, smells, sounds), relaxation, easy laughter, and enhanced creativity.

Cannabis Intoxication

The signs and symptoms of cannabis intoxication are summarized in Table 8.1. Recall that CB1 receptors co-localize with beta-2-adrenergic receptors and therefore can cause a number of adrenergic-like effects, including tachycardia, blood pressure variability, and tachypnea. The cognitive effects of cannabis intoxication include short-term memory, judgment, concentration, and motor impairment; the latter effect becomes important for cannabis-related traffic accidents. The psychotomimetic effects of THC can lead to

TABLE 8.1
Cannabis Intoxication: Physiological, Cognitive, and Psychiatric Effects

Physiological effects	Adrenergic-like state (tachycardia, blood pressure variability, tachypnea)
	Dry mouth
	Conjunctival injection
	Cyclic vomiting (cannabinoid hyperemesis syndrome)
Cognitive impairments	Short-term memory
	Judgment
	Concentration
	Attention
	Reaction time
	Motor coordination
Psychiatric effects	Psychosis
	Hypervigilance
	Anxiety
	Paranoia

psychiatric effects, including anxiety, hypervigilance, and psychosis.

Cannabis hyperemesis syndrome (CHS) is a consequence of heavy cannabis use and is characterized by nausea, abdominal pain, and severe cyclic vomiting. Individuals who present with CHS are predominantly young, male, heavy and/or daily cannabis users who frequently report relief of symptoms with very hot showers. The pathophysiology is unclear, but the most effective treatments to date include cessation of cannabis use, oral dopamine antagonists (e.g., haloperidol), or topical capsaicin (applied to the abdomen). The hypothesized pathophysiology of CHS involves dysregulation of the endocannabinoid system and CB1 receptors in the hypothalamus and gastrointestinal tract.

Cannabis intoxication is not a common chief complaint for individuals who come for medical attention compared with other intoxication syndromes; among those who do present in emergency settings, it is most often for anxiety, panic, psychosis, or CHS. At doses of THC above 7.5 mg/m^2 (approximately 12 g for an average adult woman; 14 g for an average adult man), it can cause delirium, postural hypotension, myoclonic jerking, and panic attacks. For reference, an average joint contains approximately 0.5 to 1 mg of THC.

The time to onset of action, peak, and duration of effects varies greatly depending on the route of administration (oral, sublingual, smoked). Table 8.2 summarizes these differences and common side effects for each route of administration.

Know This:

The route of administration that is disproportionately associated with the greatest number of emergency room visits is **oral** (edibles), typically by inexperienced users who consume large quantities of cannabis before the onset of its acute effects.

Although commonly believed to be toxin-free, cannabis smoke in fact leads to a higher respiratory

TABLE 8.2
Cannabis Route of Administration

Route of Administration	Smoking (Joints, Pipes, Blunts)	Vaporization	Mucosal (Oils)	Edible
Toxicity	Combustion at high heat leads to production of toxic byproducts	Utilizes moderate heat—some production of toxic byproducts	No toxic byproducts or pulmonary symptoms	No toxic byproducts or pulmonary symptoms
Onset of action	Rapid onset of action (5 min), peak at 30 min, short duration (2–4 h)	Rapid onset (5 min), short duration (2–4 h)	Rapid onset of action (15–30 min)	Onset of action much longer and very unpredictable (1–3 h); duration of action 6–8 h
Side effects	Pulmonary symptoms Cough Bronchitis Frequently mixed with tobacco	Pulmonary symptoms E-cigarette or vaping product use associated lung injury (EVALI)	No pulmonary symptoms	No pulmonary symptoms

burden of carbon monoxide and tar than tobacco. This effect is independent of the concentration of THC in the cannabis plant.

Cannabis Withdrawal Syndrome

Cannabis withdrawal is a relatively recently identified syndrome following abrupt cessation of frequent cannabis use. Cannabis withdrawal is not as dangerous as alcohol/sedative-hypnotic withdrawal or as uncomfortable as opioid withdrawal but can lead to distressing symptoms that make it difficult to quit. The symptoms of cannabis withdrawal are fairly nonspecific and include anxiety, difficulty sleeping, decreased appetite, irritability, and restlessness. Most symptoms have onset within 24 to 72 hours, peak within 1 week, and last for approximately 1 to 2 weeks.

Know This:

Specific polymorphisms of the fatty acid amide hydrolase (**FAAH**) gene, which encodes the enzyme metabolizing AEA, are linked with more severe cannabis withdrawal. There is currently a FAAH-inhibitor in clinical trials for the treatment of cannabis use disorder.

EPIDEMIOLOGY OF CANNABIS USE

In terms of the overall epidemiology of cannabis use, some key facts to remember are:

- Cannabis is by far the most commonly used illicit substance both in the United States and globally.
- In 2016, the prevalence of past-year cannabis use was 13.9%, and past-month prevalence was 8.9% based on a nationally representative epidemiological survey (National Survey on Drug Use and Health [NSDUH], 2016).
- Nationally, cannabis use has been rapidly increasing; from 2007 to 2013, past-month use increased from 5.8% to 7.5% of the population; the use of most other illicit drugs over the same time frame has stabilized or declined (NSDUH, 2016).
- The *perceived risk* of cannabis has been declining since 2005 among 8th, 10th, and 12th graders and has been accompanied by an increase in cannabis use among these age groups (Monitoring the Future, 2013).

In terms of other demographic risk factors:

- Age: The highest prevalence of past-year cannabis use by age is among 18- to 25-year-olds (33%); lowest among 12- and 13-year-olds (0.5% and 2.8%, respectively), and those aged 65 years and older (3.3%) (NSDUH, 2016).
- Sex: Men are nearly twice as likely than women to use cannabis (11.3% versus 6.7%; NSDUH, 2016).
- Race: Prevalence of cannabis use varies by race/ ethnicity. From highest to lowest: Mixed race (17.7%), Native American (13.6%), Black/African American (11.1%), non-Hispanic Whites (9.0%), Hispanics (7.7%), Pacific Islanders (8.6%), > Asians (3.3%) (NSDUH, 2016).
- Pregnancy: Although pregnant women are still less likely to use cannabis compared with nonpregnant women, cannabis use has been steadily increasing. From 2009 to 2016, self-report in past-month cannabis use among pregnant women aged 15 to 44 increased from 4.2% to 7.1% according to the NSDUH.
- Low income and low education are also risk factors for increased cannabis use.

Know This:

Make sure to remember the main surveys used to estimate the prevalence of substance use in the United States: National Survey on Drug Use and Health (NSDUH), National Epidemiologic Survey on Alcohol and Related Conditions (NESARC), and Monitoring the Future (MTF) studies.

There is an inverse relationship between perceived risk and substance use; as the perceived risk of cannabis has been declining among high schoolers, cannabis use has increased. The converse is true regarding tobacco use among high schoolers. Tobacco use has reduced substantially over the past decade.

LONG-TERM EFFECTS OF CANNABIS USE

Cannabis Use Disorder

Among individuals who have tried cannabis once, about 9% will eventually develop a cannabis use disorder. This makes cannabis rank among one of the lesser addictive substances compared to heroin (24%) and cocaine (15%).

The diagnosis of cannabis use disorder is established based on the *American Psychiatric Association's Diagnostic and Statistical Manual, 5th Edition* diagnostic criteria listed in Chapter 1.

Know This:

The heritability of lifetime cannabis use is estimated at 45% based on a meta-analysis of twin studies.

The *CNR1* gene encodes the cannabinoid type I receptor. There is an AAT repeat in an unexpressed area of this gene, and individuals with increased number of AAT repeats may have a higher risk for cannabis use disorder.

Substance Use Comorbidities

Having a cannabis use disorder is associated with increased odds of having a co-occurring alcohol, tobacco, and any other drug use disorders. According to findings from two waves of survey data from the NESARC, cannabis use is also associated with increased odds of *subsequently developing* alcohol, tobacco or a drug use disorder. Keep in mind that even with these temporal findings, causality cannot be inferred between early cannabis use and later development of other substance use disorders; the relationship could alternately be explained by shared risk factors.

Know This:

Among individuals who use cannabis, concurrent alcohol use is reported at 75%. This has major public health implications for driving accidents related to co-use of cannabis and alcohol, which is increasingly common.

Psychiatric Comorbidities

Cannabis use and use disorder is associated with significant psychiatric comorbidity; cannabis use disorder is associated with increased odds of having major depression, bipolar disorder, schizophrenia, anxiety disorders, posttraumatic stress disorder, attention-deficit/hyperactivity disorder, and personality disorders. However, according to findings from two waves of NESARC survey

data, cannabis use (not cannabis use disorder) was not associated with the later development of mood or anxiety disorders, again bringing the question of causality to the forefront. Schizophrenia is discussed separately.

Association of Cannabis Use With Schizophrenia

There is no question that there is a strong positive association between cannabis use and schizophrenia. However, a debate has raged in the medical literature questioning the *direction of causality* between cannabis use and schizophrenia. Does cannabis cause schizophrenia, or do genetic risk factors increase the risk for both disorders? This debate has taken on greater urgency as cannabis (and particularly high-potency cannabis) becomes more widely available to young adults because of large-scale changes in policy and cultural norms.

Here are key points to remember regarding the association between cannabis and schizophrenia:

- There is a strong, dose-dependent association between use of high-potency cannabis use (>10% THC concentration) and later development of schizophrenia.
- Individuals who have a family history of schizophrenia and those who begin using cannabis in adolescence appear more vulnerable to develop psychosis.
- Patients with psychosis who continue to use cannabis have a worse prognosis (longer hospitalizations and more frequent psychotic episodes).
- Polymorphisms of the genes **AKT1** and **COMT** are associated with increased risk of schizophrenia with exposure to cannabis; **AKT1** is essential for cellular signaling and dopamine transmission. **COMT** encodes the enzyme responsible for the degradation of catecholamines. There is a high-risk polymorphism of the **AKT1** gene associated with a **sevenfold risk** of developing psychosis with daily cannabis use compared with those with low-risk polymorphism.

Comorbid Medical Conditions

Cardiovascular

The endocannabinoid system (including CB1 and CB2 receptors) is important in regulating the cardiovascular system, and there are components of marijuana smoke that cause cardiovascular damage on the cellular level (e.g., carbon monoxide and tar). However, the largest study to date examining cardiovascular outcomes with cannabis use, the CARDIA study (Reis et al., 2017) did not find an association between cannabis use and cardiovascular events.

Pulmonary

Pulmonary sequelae of cannabis use occur exclusively via the smoked or vaped route of administration due to the release of toxic byproducts and chemical irritants, and include cough and/or bronchitis (Table 8.2). An increasingly popular route of administration is through vaping, which involves heating a liquid containing cannabinoids via a battery-operated device. Compared with smoking cannabis through combustion, vaping releases *fewer* toxic byproducts but is still not toxin-free. In the summer of 2019, cases of acute lung injury caused by vaping were identified, called e-cigarette or vaping product use associated lung injury (EVALI). The majority of affected patients vaped THC that contained vitamin E acetate as an additive and required hospitalization. In severe cases, ventilation and/or lung transplantation were needed.

Cancer

No clear association has been found to date between cannabis use and lung cancer, although effects can be hard to separate because of common co-use of cannabis and tobacco.

Pregnancy and Cannabis Use

Cannabis is the most widely used illicit substance in pregnancy, and its use during pregnancy has been steadily increasing. Many women report using cannabis to counteract nausea or treat hyperemesis gravidarum. This increase in cannabis use occurs in parallel with the reduction in perceived risk of cannabis; studies to date indicate that most women using cannabis during pregnancy perceive little to no harm in using cannabis. Research on the effects of cannabis use during pregnancy has been limited because cannabis use in this period is typically accompanied by the use of other substances (most commonly tobacco), making it difficult to study the independent effects of cannabis on the developing fetus. In 2019, Corsi et al. published a study in *JAMA* examining the association between cannabis use and neonatal outcomes. This retrospective cohort study's strengths are that it used an enormous sample (>600,000 women in Ontario, Canada, who gave birth between 2012 and 2017) and compared mothers who self-reported cannabis use during pregnancy to matched controls who did not self-report cannabis use. This study found that cannabis use in pregnancy was associated with a significantly increased risk of preterm births (10% versus 7%) and an increased risk of the infant requiring transfer to the neonatal intensive care unit and being small for gestational age.

Know This:

Remember the results of the Corsi et. al. study. Cannabis use during pregnancy is associated with an increased risk of preterm birth, infants who are small for gestational age, or newborns who require transfer to the neonatal intensive care unit.

Prospective cohort studies have not unequivocally or consistently shown that cannabis affects child/adolescent development. It is biologically plausible that there may be developmental effects because of the importance of the endocannabinoid system to fetal development.

Cannabinoids readily cross the placenta as well as into breast milk.

Cannabis and Driving

Cannabis intoxication increases the risk of car accidents by a factor of 2 (for comparison, alcohol with a blood alcohol level >0.08% increases the risk of car accidents by a factor of 5); however, the compounded risk associated with cannabis and alcohol use is greater than either alone. Cannabis intoxication leads to delayed reaction time, poorer hand–eye coordination, and impairs automatic driving. This loss of automaticity can be compensated with higher-order cognitive strategies, but this ability to compensate is diminished with co-use of alcohol.

Cannabis and Opioid Use

Another major debate in the literature is whether cannabis use reduces the prevalence of opioid use, opioid use disorder, and opioid deaths. Given the current opioid crisis in the United States, this question has major health and policy ramifications.

A widely cited and influential study in this area is by Bachhuber et al. (2014), which analyzed state-level variables between 1999 and 2010 and showed that states that passed medical marijuana laws had fewer state-level opioid overdoses compared with those that did not; the authors hypothesize that individuals who are using medical marijuana may be substituting away from opioids. An updated study by a different group of authors (Shover et al., 2019), however, extended the same analysis to 2017 and found that the trends reversed. Ongoing research studies with individual-level data on opioid consumption for individuals using medical marijuana for pain will prove instrumental in answering this question.

Know This:

Although the jury is still out on whether medical marijuana reduces the risk of opioid overdose, medical marijuana is approved for opioid substitution and opioid use disorder in several states.

TREATMENTS FOR CANNABIS USE DISORDER

Pharmacotherapy

Currently, there are no US Food and Drug Administration (FDA)-approved medications for cannabis use disorder, although several commonly used psychiatric medications have been studied, are currently under study, or are used off-label. Agonists that have been studied for cannabis use disorder include *dronabinol* and *nabilone*. Antagonists include rimonabant, a CB1 receptor antagonist, and a weight-loss drug whose use was limited due to the adverse effect of suicidality. Rimonabant is no longer available in the United States. Other medications under active investigation include lofexidine (a centrally acting alpha-2 agonist recently approved by the FDA for the treatment of opioid withdrawal), gabapentin, and N-acetylcysteine. There are negative studies on many medications, including mirtazapine, naltrexone, nefazodone, quetiapine, baclofen, divalproex, bupropion, and buspirone.

Psychosocial Interventions

The primary evidence-based psychosocial treatments include motivational enhancement therapy (MET), contingency management (CM), cognitive behavioral therapy (CBT), and family-based treatments (see Chapter 13).

Know This:

The most effective evidence-based psychosocial intervention for cannabis use disorder is abstinence-based voucher CM with CBT; this combination is more effective than either intervention alone.

MEDICAL MARIJUANA

History and Policy

Under US federal law, cannabis is a Schedule I controlled substance. However, individual states can have medical and recreational cannabis programs because of the Justice Department's *Cole Memorandum* in 2013, which stated that states pursuing state-legal cannabis enterprises would not be prosecuted. In 2018, Attorney General Jeff Sessions rescinded the *Cole Memorandum* under President Donald Trump; despite this, in practice, the Justice Department has generally adhered to *Cole Memorandum*-era enforcement priorities.

Timeline of cannabis in the United States:

- 1700s–1890s: Hemp (from cannabis plants) is legal in most states and used to make fibers. Cannabis is used widely in the United States and Europe.
- 1910–1920s: Many states ban cannabis as part of Prohibition, but doctors still prescribe it.
- 1930s: Cannabis is renamed "marijuana" by the United States government as racial tensions against Mexicans grow during the Great Depression; propaganda films (e.g., *Reefer Madness*) suggest it causes insanity.
- 1937: The *Marihuana Tax Act* was passed, which criminalized marijuana, created new taxes on manufacturing or selling cannabis, and created additional barriers for prescribing doctors.
- 1952–1956: The *Boggs Act* of 1952 and *Narcotics Control Act* of 1956 established mandatory sentencing for cannabis possession.
- 1970s: The *Controlled Substance Act* is passed in 1970, creating mandatory sentences for marijuana possession and use. President Nixon also declares the "War on Drugs" and created the Drug Enforcement Agency (DEA) scheduling system, making cannabis Schedule I.

- 1996: California is the first state to legalize medical marijuana for approved conditions.
- 2012: Colorado is the first state to legalize recreational marijuana.
- As of 2020, 33 states and Washington, DC, allow medical cannabis.

Know This:

Remember that a Schedule I drug is defined as a drug with no currently accepted medical use, high abuse potential, and lack of accepted safety.

Clinical Uses for Medical Marijuana

Cannabis has well-established antiemetic, appetite stimulant, antiepileptic, and analgesic properties. Qualifying conditions for use of medical marijuana vary by state, but most states include the following: amyotrophic lateral sclerosis, HIV/AIDS, inflammatory bowel disease, multiple sclerosis, severe chronic pain, cancer, and posttraumatic stress disorder.

Commonly used medicinal cannabinoids that you should remember for the board examination include:

- Dronabinol: Synthetic delta-9-THC approved for chemotherapy-induced nausea/vomiting and AIDS wasting
- Nabilone: Synthetic THC analogue approved for treatment of cancer-related nausea/vomiting
- Epidiolex: Cannabis-derived CBD, which is approved for treatment of Lennox-Gastaut syndrome
- Sativex: An oromucosal spray that is 1:1 delta-9-THC:CBD that is approved in many countries but not currently in the United States; used for treatment of spasticity in multiple sclerosis

Know This:

Dronabinol, nabilone, and Epidiolex are the only FDA-approved cannabinoids. Nabilone is

Schedule II, dronabinol is Schedule III, and Epidiolex is Schedule V.

REFERENCES

Bachhuber, M. A., Saloner, B., Cunningham, C. O., & Barry, C. L. (2014). Medical cannabis laws and opioid analgesic overdose mortality in the United States, 1999-2010. *JAMA Internal Medicine, 174*(10), 1668–1673.

Reis, J. P., Auer, R., Bancks, M. P., Goff, D.C., Jr., Pletcher, M. J., Rana, J. S., Shikany, J. M., & Sidney, S. (2017). Cumulative lifetime marijuana use and incident cardiovascular disease in middle age: The coronary artery risk development in young adults (CARDIA) study. *American Journal of Public Health, 107*(4), 601–606.

Shover, C. L., Davis, C. S., Gordon, S. C., & Humphreys, K. (2019). Association between medical cannabis laws and opioid overdose mortality has reversed over time. *Proceedings of the National Academy of Sciences of the United States of America, 116*(26), 12624–12626.

SUGGESTIONS FOR FURTHER READING

Blanco, C., Hasin, D. S., Wall, M. M., Flórez-Salamanca, L., Hoertel, N., Wang, S., Kerridge, B. T., & Olfson, M. (2016). Cannabis use and risk of psychiatric disorders: Prospective evidence from a US national longitudinal study. *JAMA Psychiatry, 73*(4), 388–395.

Brezing, C. A., & Levin, F. R. (2018). The current state of pharmacological treatments for cannabis use disorder and withdrawal. *Neuropsychopharmacology: Official Publication of the American College of Neuropsychopharmacology, 43*(1), 173–194.

Gates, P. J., Sabioni, P., Copeland, J., Le Foll, B., & Gowing, L. (2016). Psychosocial interventions for cannabis use disorder. *The Cochrane Database of Systematic Reviews, 2016*(5), CD005336.

Piomelli, D. (2015). Neurobiology of marijuana. In M. Galanter, H. D. Kleber, & K. Brady (Eds.), *The American Psychiatric Publishing textbook of substance abuse treatment* (5th ed., pp. 241–250). American Psychiatric Publishing.

Welch, S. P., Smith, T. H., Malcolm, R., & Lichtman, A. H. (2019). The pharmacology of cannabinoids. In S. C. Miller, D. A. Fiellin, R. N. Rosenthal, & R. Saitz (Eds.), *The ASAM principles of addiction medicine* (6th ed.). Wolters Kluwer.

REVIEW QUESTIONS

The following vignette is linked to questions 1 and 2.

A 20-year-old pre-med college student comes to you because of trouble focusing and academic decline. He was a straight-A student all through high school and his first year of college, but this semester he is getting Bs and Cs. He wonders if he has attention-deficit/hyperactivity disorder and if stimulant medication might be helpful. He shares with you that he has smoked marijuana several times daily for the past 6 months.

1. Which of the following is a well-known effect of cannabis intoxication that is relevant to his presenting problem?
   A. Long-term memory impairment
   B. Short-term memory impairment
   C. Respiratory depression
   D. Distortion of time perception
   E. Early-onset dementia

2. His mother calls you several months after the initial appointment and says that he was taken to the emergency room by his roommate after he was found at home hearing voices and paranoid that he was being chased by cops. She states that the roommate found an empty package of K2 on his table. Compared with plant-based cannabis, which of the following properties of K2 best explains his symptoms?
   A. Lower affinity for the CB1 receptor
   B. Higher affinity for the CB1 receptor
   C. Higher affinity for the CB2 receptor
   D. Higher affinity for the D2 receptor
   E. Lower affinity for the D2 receptor

3. The prevalence of marijuana use in the United States has been increasing over the past decade among teens. Which of the following explanations best accounts for this trend?
   A. The perceived risk of marijuana use has declined among this age group.
   B. The perceived risk of marijuana use has increased among this age group.
   C. THC content in marijuana has declined, making it more palatable to naïve users.
   D. CBD content in marijuana has increased, making it more palatable to naïve users.

E. Marijuana is no longer a federally controlled substance for individuals aged 18 and over.

4. Cannabis intoxication is characterized by which of the following symptoms?
   A. Tachypnea
   B. Bradycardia
   C. Piloerection
   D. Hypersalivation
   E. Sensation of time "speeding up"

5. A 22-year-old woman in a substance use treatment program for severe cannabis use disorder. Every week that she has a negative urine toxicology, she gets a small prize such as a movie ticket or a gift card for a coffee shop. This method is a component of which evidence-based treatment for cannabis use disorder?
   A. CBT
   B. CM
   C. Motivational interviewing
   D. Alcoholics Anonymous
   E. Family-based therapy

6. Your cousin calls you and is panicking because his 18-year-old daughter told him that she tried marijuana for the first time at a party last weekend. His daughter is functioning well socially and academically. Your cousin is terrified that his daughter will now develop schizophrenia and become addicted to marijuana and asks you whether this is true. You tell him which of the following?
   A. There is a clear positive association between cannabis use and schizophrenia, and it is well-established that cannabis use is a causal factor for schizophrenia.
   B. There is a clear negative association between cannabis use and schizophrenia, and cannabis use reduces the risk of schizophrenia.
   C. There is no clear association between cannabis use and schizophrenia.
   D. The majority of individuals who try cannabis once will not develop a cannabis use disorder.
   E. The majority of young adults who try cannabis once will develop a cannabis use disorder.

7. Which of the following plant-based cannabis products has the highest THC potency?
   A. Hashish
   B. Hash oil
   C. Butane hash oil
   D. Sinsemilla
   E. Mixture of cannabis stems and leaves

8. A 54-year-old man is undergoing chemotherapy for prostate cancer. He has no history of substance use but is prescribed a cannabinoid-based medication to help manage his chemotherapy-associated nausea. On his routine employment UDS, he tests positive for THC. Which of the following medications is he most likely being prescribed that would explain his positive result?
   A. Nabilone
   B. Dronabinol
   C. Cannabidiol
   D. Epidiolex
   E. Sativex

9. A 25-year-old woman who is 2 months pregnant presents to your office. She reports severe hyperemesis gravidarum that has been unresponsive to standard medication approaches. She is wondering if she can receive medical marijuana, as she did some research online and found that many women have successfully used it, and research has shown that it is safer to use than tobacco in pregnancy. She asks for your opinion about the effects of marijuana use on the fetus. You tell her that marijuana use in pregnancy is associated with:

A. Increased risk of preeclampsia
B. Decreased risk of preeclampsia
C. Increased risk of preterm birth
D. Increased risk of neonatal abstinence syndrome
E. Increased risk of stillbirth

10. Several medications have been tested in clinical trials for efficacy in treating cannabis use disorder. Rimonabant is one such medication that was tested in clinical trials. Its mechanism of action is _____, but use was limited because of this adverse effect: _____.
    A. CB1 antagonism; seizure
    B. CB1 agonism; seizure
    C. CB1 antagonism; suicidality
    D. CB1 agonism; suicidality
    E. Alpha-2-agonism; arrhythmia

11. Your friend from high school is a daily marijuana user and works as an Uber driver. He tells you that when he smokes marijuana, he is a better driver because he drives more slowly. You tell him that the compared with drivers not under the influence of cannabis, research shows that:
    A. Cannabis use decreases the risk of driving accidents to one-fifth.
    B. Cannabis use decreases the risk of driving accidents by half.
    C. Cannabis use has no effect on the risk of driving accidents.
    D. Cannabis use increases the risk of driving accidents twofold.
    E. Cannabis use increases the risk of driving accidents fivefold.

STIMULANT USE DISORDER

NEUROBIOLOGY AND GENERAL CHARACTERISTICS

Stimulants refer to a heterogeneous class of substances with the action of stimulating the central nervous system, primarily through noradrenergic and dopaminergic effects. The stimulants discussed in this chapter include amphetamines, methamphetamines, methylphenidates, cocaine, cathinones, 3,4-methylenedioxymethamphetamine (MDMA), and over-the-counter medications such as phenylephrine and pseudoephedrine. Many stimulants share a common structure, a phenethylamine component—this is present on amphetamine, methamphetamine, cathinone, pseudoephedrine, dopamine, serotonin, and bupropion (Table 9.1).

Know This:

- Cocaine is an alkaloid that can be found in the leaves of the *Erythroxylum* genus of plants.
- Cocaine exists in two chemical forms: as a salt or base. Cocaine in powder form is typically a salt. Cocaine in base form, commonly known as "crack," is typically smoked.
- Low-potency stimulants, such as ephedrine and phenylephrine, usually act only on noradrenergic receptors in contrast to high-potency stimulants, such as cocaine and amphetamines, which act as indirect but potent dopamine and noradrenergic receptor agonists.
- Methamphetamine has two isomers, d-methamphetamine and l-methamphetamine. D-methamphetamine has stimulant effects, and l-methamphetamine affects the sympathetic nervous system but has little activity in the central nervous system.

- Methamphetamine exists in base and salt forms. It is also more lipophilic than amphetamine, crossing the brain barrier more easily and leading to a more rapid onset of action than amphetamines.
- Variable-number tandem repeats (VNTRs) in the dopamine transporter 1 (*DAT1*) gene is associated with cocaine- and methamphetamine-induced psychosis, as well as attention-deficit disorder.
- The presence of specific variants of the nicotinic acetylcholine receptor (CHRNB3-A6) locus on chromosome 8 reduces the response to nicotine and cocaine, causing desensitization and risk for cocaine and nicotine use disorder.
- Specific variants of the calcium/calmodulin kinase IV (CAMK4) are linked with a higher susceptibility for cocaine use disorder.
- Animals that lack the period circadian regulator (*PER1*) gene have abnormal locomotor sensitization and conditioned preference for cocaine.

EPIDEMIOLOGY OF STIMULANT USE DISORDER

According to the National Survey on Drug Use and Health of 2018, more than 16% of people aged 26 years or older had used cocaine in their lifetime; prevalence of past-month cocaine use was 0.6% in people aged 12 years or older. One-third of people prescribed stimulants misused their prescriptions. Based on the Treatment Episode Data Set Admissions from 2017, men are hospitalized for cocaine overdoses at nearly double the rate of women, and women show higher dropout rates and more use during treatment than men. Studies have found that the 12-month prevalence of cocaine use is significantly higher among Hispanic

TABLE 9.1

Mechanism of Action and Molecular Targets of Common Stimulants

Drug	Mechanism of Action	Molecular Target
Cocaine	Stimulates CNS by inhibiting presynaptic reuptake of dopamine and norepinephrine. Blocks neuronal sodium channels, accounting for its local anesthetic properties	DAT, neuronal plasma membrane transporters for norepinephrine and serotonin, and neuronal sodium channels
Methamphetamine	Increases release of monoamine neurotransmitters through its effects on VMAT2 in addition to some inhibition of dopamine and norepinephrine reuptake	VMAT2 DAT, and neuronal plasma membrane transporters for norepinephrine and serotonin
Amphetamine analogues	Similar to mechanism of action for methamphetamine	VMAT2 DAT, and neuronal plasma membrane transporters for norepinephrine and serotonin
Methylphenidate	Similar to mechanism of action for methamphetamine, but methylphenidate does not enhance dopamine release from synaptic vesicles	DAT, and neuronal plasma membrane transporters for norepinephrine and serotonin
Khat and Cathinones	Similar to mechanism of methamphetamine	VMAT2 DAT, and neuronal plasma membrane transporters for norepinephrine and serotonin
MDMA (3,4-Methylenedioxy methamphetamine)	Promotes release of serotonin, dopamine, and norepinephrine into synaptic clefts; prevents serotonin reuptake; acts as agonist at serotonin, dopamine, and alpha- and beta-adrenergic receptors	VMAT2, TA1-receptor (TAAR1), serotonin (5-HT1A, 5-HT2A, 5-HT2B, 5-HT2C), dopamine (D1, D2), and alpha- and beta-adrenergic receptors
Pseudoephedrine	Stimulates alpha- and beta-2-adrenergic receptors, causing vasoconstriction of blood vessels and relaxation of smooth muscle in airways	alpha- and beta-2-adrenergic receptors
Phenylephrine	Agonist at alpha-1-adrenoceptors, causing vasoconstriction of blood vessels	alpha-1-adrenergic receptors
Nicotine (discussed in detail in Chapter 7)	Agonist at nicotinic acetylcholine receptors	Nicotinic acetylcholine receptors
Caffeine (discussed in detail in Chapter 10)	Nonselective adenosine receptor antagonist and phosphodiesterase inhibitor	Adenosine-1, adenosine-2a, and adenosine-2b receptors

CNS, Central nervous system; DAT, dopamine transporter; MDMA, 3,4-methylenedioxymethamphetamine; VMAT2, vesicular monoamine transporter-2.

youth when compared to non-Hispanic youth. Death from overdose due to cocaine use is more prevalent among Black individuals.

Prescription stimulant misuse prevalence ranges from 5% to 9% in grade school- and high school-aged children and 5% to 35% in college-age individuals. Cognitive performance and an improvement in attention were the most reported reasons for misusing stimulants, and the most likely source for misuse was obtaining them from relatives or friends. Among college students, the illicit use of amphetamine-dextroamphetamine is more prevalent than the illicit use of methylphenidate formulations.

Know This:

- Speedballing is the action of using cocaine followed by an opioid, typically intravenously or by insufflation.
- Stimulant use can cause sexual dysfunctions during the intoxication period.
- Cocaine is metabolized via ester bond hydrolysis in the liver to form benzoylecgonine, which is the metabolite readily detectable by standard urine immunoassays for up to 2 or 3 days following last use.

STIMULANT INTOXICATION

Stimulants are used for their energizing and mood-elevating effects. In states of intoxication, they can cause unpleasant signs and symptoms summarized in the table below:

Physiological	Psychological
Tachycardia or bradycardia	Anxiety
Elevated or lowered blood pressure	Impaired memory
	Anhedonia
Nausea or vomiting	Irritability
Weight loss	Paranoia
Psychomotor agitation or retardation	Mood swings
	Drug-induced psychoses
Physical complications (e.g., respiratory depression, cardiac arrhythmia, cerebrovascular accident, hypertension crises, hyperthermia)	Confusion
Sexual dysfunction	

Stimulant intoxication should be managed with supportive care, hydration, and a low-stimulus environment. If severe, medications can be used. Benzodiazepines are first-line treatment for stimulant toxicity where agitation and violence are present. Antipsychotics, such as haloperidol and olanzapine, may be added if benzodiazepines are not sufficient. Caution should be used when using antipsychotic medications due to their effect on lowering the seizure threshold. Complicated intoxication states may require airway management, fluid resuscitation, or vigorous cooling measures. Remember to assess for rhabdomyolysis and, if present, manage it using alkalinized intravenous fluids with sodium bicarbonate, agitation control, and temperature regulation.

Know This:

Beta-blockers should be avoided in stimulant intoxication to prevent unopposed vasoconstriction (alpha-adrenergic effect). If needed, labetalol can be used to manage tachycardia and hypertension due to its combined beta-/alpha-blocker effects.

Methamphetamine use is associated with higher rates of xerostomia and extensive dental disease, sometimes referred to as "meth mouth."

CLINICAL MANAGEMENT OF STIMULANT USE DISORDER

Psychotherapeutic Treatment Options

Although the US Food and Drug Administration (FDA) approves no medications for the treatment of stimulant use disorder, behavioral interventions can be highly effective and should be used as first-line treatment.

These include:

- Contingency management (CM): This treatment intervention is based on the principles of operant conditioning and uses immediate reinforcements for positive behaviors to modify problem behaviors and decrease the influence of reinforcement derived from using drugs.
- Cognitive behavioral therapy (CBT): This treatment intervention teaches skills to regulate craving for stimulants and other substances of abuse.
- Family-based approaches: Therapists seek to engage the patient and family in applying behavioral strategies and skills to improve their environment and reduce substance use.

Pharmacological Treatment Options for Stimulant Use Disorder

Pharmacological Treatment Options for Cocaine Use Disorder

There are no medications approved by the FDA to treat cocaine use disorder. Several medications are showing promise in reducing cocaine use. These include bupropion, topiramate, amphetamine salts, cholinesterase inhibitors (donepezil, galantamine, rivastigmine, tacrine), N-acetylcysteine, naltrexone, prazosin, doxazosin, and lofexidine. Recent research has been investigating the use of immunotherapy with vaccination for cocaine use disorder. Anticocaine antibodies have shown to bind to cocaine in the peripheral circulation by an anticocaine monoclonal antibody, preventing its access to all sites of action in the brain.

Pharmacological Treatment Options for Methamphetamine Use Disorder

Like cocaine, there are no medications approved by the FDA to treat cocaine use disorder. Several medications are showing promise in reducing methamphetamine use. These include mirtazapine, bupropion, naltrexone (the bupropion/naltrexone combination is showing great promise), topiramate, calcium channel blockers (nifedipine, flunarizine, and diltiazem), and cholinesterase inhibitors.

STIMULANT WITHDRAWAL SYNDROME

The abrupt discontinuation of stimulant use in individuals with chronic and excessive stimulant use results in a stimulant withdrawal syndrome marked by the signs and symptoms summarized in the table below. Note that some withdrawal symptoms occur within a few hours and up to a few days after last use. Severity of symptoms is based on the amount of stimulants used.

Physiological	Psychological
Dehydration	Dysphoric mood
Fatigue	Cravings
Psychomotor retardation before agitation	Vivid dreams
	Anxiety
Weight loss or anorexia	Impaired memory
Insomnia followed by hypersomnia	Anhedonia
	Irritability

Stimulant withdrawal syndrome is not medically life-threatening but the risk of self-mutilating behaviors, suicide, and risk to others may be high during the withdrawal period and management is recommended.

Know This:

Chronic use of cocaine may lead to perforated nasal septum due to vasoconstriction and resulting ischemic necrosis.

Chronic cocaine use can damage many organs by reducing blood flow with toxic effects on the cardiovascular, neurological, and gastrointestinal systems.

PREGNANCY AND STIMULANT USE

Stimulant use during pregnancy is associated with maternal migraines, seizures, premature rupture of membranes, and placental abruption. Newborns that were exposed to cocaine prenatally are more likely to be premature, have low birth weights, smaller head circumferences, and shorter length. Methamphetamine and cocaine metabolites are excreted in the breast milk and the active use of these is a contraindication to breastfeeding.

ATTENTION-DEFICIT/HYPERACTIVITY DISORDER AND STIMULANT USE DISORDER

Attention-deficit/hyperactivity disorder (ADHD) has a high prevalence in patients with substance use disorders (SUDs) compared to the general population. Stimulant medications (amphetamine analogues and methylphenidates) are highly effective in treating ADHD and are currently the first-line pharmacologic treatment for children and adults. For patients with active SUD and comorbid ADHD, the risks and benefits of treating ADHD with stimulant medication must be weighed carefully. In patients with active SUDs, FDA-approved nonstimulant medications should be considered first-line; these include atomoxetine, guanfacine, and clonidine. Other off-label medications used to treat ADHD include bupropion, venlafaxine, and modafinil.

Individuals with SUDs and ADHD have an earlier onset of substance use than those without ADHD. Treating a patient with ADHD has not been directly linked to having higher risk of having a stimulant use disorder later in life. In fact, several studies have suggested that ADHD treatment using stimulant medications may reduce the risk of illicit stimulant use.

Know This:

Students with and without ADHD misuse prescription stimulants to:
- Promote academic performance
- Lose weight
- Increase energy and wakefulness
- Induce euphoria

SUGGESTIONS FOR FURTHER READING

Abarca, C., Albrecht, U., & Spanagel, R. (2002). Cocaine sensitization and reward are under the influence of circadian genes and rhythm. *Proceedings of the National Academy of Sciences of the United States of America, 99*(13), 9026–9030.

Colfax, G. N., Santos, G. M., Das, M., Santos, D. M., Matheson, T., Gasper, J., Shoptaw, S., & Vittinghoff, E. (2011). Mirtazapine to reduce methamphetamine use: A randomized controlled trial. *Archives of General Psychiatry, 68*(11), 1168–1175.

Grant, J. E., Odlaug, B. L., & Kim, S. W. (2010). A double-blind, placebo-controlled study of N-acetyl cysteine plus naltrexone for methamphetamine dependence. *European Neuropsychopharmacology: The Journal of the European College of Neuropsychopharmacology, 20*(11), 823–828.

Levin, F. R., Mariani, J. J., Pavlicova, M., Choi, C. J., Mahony, A. L., Brooks, D. J., Bisaga, A., Dakwar, E., Carpenter, K. M., Naqvi, N., Nunes, E. V., & Kampman, K. (2020). Extended release mixed amphetamine salts and topiramate for cocaine dependence: A randomized clinical replication trial with frequent users. *Drug and Alcohol Dependence, 206*, Article 107700.

Ma, J. Z., Johnson, B. A., Yu, E., Weiss, D., McSherry, F., Saadvandi, J., Iturriaga, E., Ait-Daoud, N., Rawson, R. A., Hrymoc, M., Campbell, J., Gorodetzky, C., Haning, W., Carlton, B., Mawhinney, J., Weis, D., McCann, M., Pham, T., Stock, C., Dickinson, R., & Li, M. D. (2013). Fine-grain analysis of the treatment effect of topiramate on methamphetamine addiction with latent variable analysis. *Drug and Alcohol Dependence, 130*(1-3), 45–51.

Newton, T. F., Roache, J. D., De La Garza, R., 2nd, Fong, T., Wallace, C. L., Li, S. H., Elkashef, A., Chiang, N., & Kahn, R. (2006). Bupropion reduces methamphetamine-induced subjective effects and cue-induced craving. *Neuropsychopharmacology: Official Publication of the American College of Neuropsychopharmacology, 31*(7), 1537–1544.

Sadler, B., Haller, G., Agrawal, A., Culverhouse, R., Bucholz, K., Brooks, A., Tischfield, J., Johnson, E. O., Edenberg, H., Schuckit, M., Saccone, N., Bierut, L., & Goate, A. (2014). Variants near CHRNB3-CHRNA6 are associated with DSM-5 cocaine use disorder: Evidence for pleiotropy. *Scientific Reports, 4*, 4497.

Schmitz, J. M., Lindsay, J. A., Green, C. E., Herin, D. V., Stotts, A. L., & Moeller, F. G. (2009). High-dose naltrexone therapy for cocaine-alcohol dependence. *American Journal on Addictions, 18*(5), 356–362.

Trivedi, M. H., Walker, R., Ling, W., Dela Cruz, A., Sharma, G., Carmody, T., Ghitza, U. E., Wahle, A., Kim, M., Shores-Wilson, K., Sparenborg, S., Coffin, P., Schmitz, J., Wiest, K., Bart, G., Sonne, S. C., Wakhlu, S., Rush, A. J., Nunes, E. V., & Shoptaw, S. (2021). Bupropion and naltrexone in methamphetamine use disorder. *The New England Journal of Medicine, 384*(2), 140–153.

Volkow, N. D., Wang, G. J., Fischman, M. W., Foltin, R., Fowler, J. S., Franceschi, D., Franceschi, M., Logan, J., Gatley, S. J., Wong, C., Ding, Y. S., Hitzemann, R., & Pappas, N. (2000). Effects of route of administration on cocaine induced dopamine transporter blockade in the human brain. *Life Sciences, 67*(12), 1507–1515.

REVIEW QUESTIONS

1. Which of the following medications, when combined with CM, has been shown to reduce cocaine use more than either treatment alone or placebo?
   A. D-Amphetamine
   B. Methylphenidate
   C. Modafinil
   D. Bupropion
   E. Disulfiram

2. A 26-year-old White male law student in his second year of law school had a long history of experimental drug use, including alcohol and psychoactive drugs. Approximately 2 years ago, he was introduced to cocaine in a social setting by friends. He has moved to a more daily pattern in the last 2 months. He has found that the inhalation of methamphetamine stimulated his performance and ability to study all night. Which of the following medications have demonstrated improvements in sustained attention, methamphetamine-associated increases in diastolic blood pressure, and self-reported feelings of anxiety in people with methamphetamine use disorder?
   A. Varenicline
   B. Modafinil
   C. Amphetamines
   D. Glutamate agonists
   E. Rivastigmine

3. You determined that your patient meets criteria for cocaine use disorder. Which of the following treatment modalities proven to treat cocaine use disorder is based on the principles of operant conditioning?
   A. CM
   B. Standard counseling
   C. Twelve-step facilitation
   D. CBT
   E. Family-based therapy

4. A 31-year-old single Hispanic woman with a history of a SUD was taken to the emergency room by her friend with new-onset paranoid delusions and agitation. Per her girlfriend, she has been smoking "something different" that a friend has been making using common household equipment, over-the-counter drugs, and some other chemicals at his place. What are some of the neurologic effects of the substance she is using?
   A. It induces intracellular dopamine-containing vesicles to release dopamine into the synaptic cleft and blocks the reuptake of dopamine.
   B. It blocks the reuptake of dopamine from the synaptic cleft
   C. It breaks down L-DOPA into dopamine
   D. It competitively binds to adenosine receptors.
   E. It induces extracellular dopamine-containing vesicles to release dopamine into the synaptic cleft.

5. An antagonist of the noradrenergic alpha-2 receptor and the 5-HT2A/C and 5-HT3 receptors has demonstrated efficacy in reducing the rewarding effect of illicit stimulant use. Which compound has this pharmacological profile?
   A. Fluoxetine
   B. Cannabis
   C. Glutamate
   D. Mirtazapine
   E. Bupropion

6. A 21-year-old woman was brought to urgent care by a friend. The friend states that she has been extremely anxious today. On examination, she has dilated pupils, tachycardia, and diaphoresis. She is talking in complete sentences and denied the use of any substance. She denies nausea, vomiting, or changes in appetite. Use of which of the following substances is most likely to explain the patient's presentation?
   A. Heroin
   B. Naloxone
   C. Amphetamine
   D. Alcohol
   E. Tobacco

7. Specific variants in which of the following genes would increase the risk of having a cocaine use disorder?
   A. ADHD1
   B. DAT1
   C. VNTR
   D. CAMK4
   E. ADH1

8. Which of the following is an adverse effect of MDMA use?
   A. Lacrimation
   B. Miosis
   C. Vomiting
   D. Bruxism
   E. Weight gain

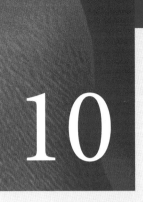

10

DISSOCIATIVE DRUGS, HALLUCINOGENS, CAFFEINE, INHALANTS, AND OTHER SUBSTANCES OF ABUSE

DISSOCIATIVE DRUGS

This section discusses ketamine, phencyclidine (PCP), and dextromethorphan (DXM). Nitrous oxide is an inhalant with dissociative properties and is discussed in greater detail later in the chapter. All four of these substances share the pharmacological property of being N-methyl-D-aspartate (NMDA) receptor antagonists. Recall that the NMDA receptor is an ionotropic glutamate receptor that is important for memory and synaptic plasticity.

Ketamine

- Ketamine is a noncompetitive antagonist of the NMDA receptor. At the NMDA receptor, ketamine prevents the influx of calcium and sodium ions. Currently, it is used as an anesthetic and for the treatment of pain and depression. Ketamine is also being investigated for the treatment of PTSD and cocaine use disorder.
- Ketamine is a derivative of PCP; laboratory investigation of PCP led to the discovery of ketamine.
- Ketamine exists in two enantiomers: S-ketamine and R-ketamine. Esketamine, which is U.S. Food and Drug Administration (FDA)-approved for depression and available as an intranasal spray, is made up of only the S-enantiomer, which has more potent NMDA antagonism than the R-enantiomer. Intravenous ketamine is a racemic mixture of both enantiomers.
- At higher doses, individuals consuming ketamine enter what is popularly known as the "K-Hole"— a dissociative state commonly described as an out-of-body experience.

- The acute effects of ketamine intoxication include amnesia, dilated pupils, nystagmus (although less than PCP), and increased heart rate and blood pressure.
- Ketamine can be found in different compounds like in a white powder, liquid, and pill form.
- Ketamine overdose can lead to respiratory depression, apnea, and death, although the lethal dose is about 50 times higher than the typical recreational dose.
- It is used as a dissociative anesthetic and for the treatment of pain and depression.

Know This:

Lamotrigine inhibits glutamate release and may reduce the physiological and cognitive effect of ketamine abuse or misuse.

PCP

- It is an NMDA antagonist and a dopamine type 2 receptor partial agonism.
- PCP-induced psychosis resembles schizophrenia in both positive and negative symptoms. In fact, PCP animal models are used to study medications for schizophrenia.
- The effects of PCP include dissociation, hallucinations, paranoia, analgesia, and violence. Other signs and symptoms of PCP intoxication include hypertension, nystagmus, and ataxia. An overdose with PCP can lead to coma, seizures, and death.
- Repeated PCP administration can cause a disruption in glutamate transmission and γ-aminobutyric

acid function in the prefrontal cortex, causing symptoms similar to schizophrenia.

- PCP was used as an intravenous human and veterinary anesthetic, but it was replaced by ketamine due to its adverse effect of prolonged delirium.
- PCP's false-positive urine screens can occur with tramadol, dextromethorphan, alprazolam, clonazepam, carvedilol, and diphenhydramine.

DXM

- It is an over-the-counter cough suppressant. It is frequently sold in combination with other medications like chlorpheniramine or acetaminophen. Cough syrups with DXM are widely abused for their dissociative and euphoric effects (a.k.a. "robotripping"), mainly by teenagers and young adults.
- In addition to being an NMDA antagonist, DXM is also a sigma-1-opioid receptor agonist and a nonselective serotonin reuptake inhibitor.
- DXM is a synthetic analog of levorphanol, which is an opioid that is structurally similar to morphine.
- At low doses, DXM has opioid-like effects (which account for its efficacy as a cough suppressant); at higher doses, it acts as a dissociative and hallucinogen.
- DXM intoxication signs and symptoms include dilated pupils, tachycardia, hallucinations, psychosis, serotonin syndrome, seizure, and rhabdomyolysis.
- Bromism, or abnormally elevated bromide levels from hydrobromide ions in cough syrups, can occur in DXM intoxication. Symptoms include fatigue, headache, and memory loss. Bromism will cause an anion gap and elevated chloride levels.
- In DXM overdose, can give charcoal and, at high doses, naloxone. Because DXM products frequently contain acetaminophen, one must also evaluate for acetaminophen overdose and hepatotoxicity. No specific antidote exists for DXM toxicity.

Know This:

Elevated bromide levels from hydrobromide ions in cough syrups can occur in DXM intoxication. Symptoms include fatigue, headache, and memory loss.

HALLUCINOGENS

Hallucinogens can be classified as tryptamine-based (lysergic acid dimethylamine [LSD], psilocybin, and dimethyltryptamine [DMT]), phenethylamine-based (mescaline and certain designer hallucinogens, e.g., 2CI), and other atypical hallucinogens (*Salvia divinorum*, hyoscine).

All hallucinogens (except *S. divinorum* and hyoscine) exert their effects through agonism or partial agonism at the serotonin 5-HT2 receptor. Hallucinogen perceptual effects include visual illusions, distortion of time and space, intensification of colors, and synesthesia. The time course of these effects depends on the drug used and route of administration. Emergency room visits for hallucinogen intoxication are primarily due to anxiety or panic attacks, and treatment is generally supportive. Serotonin syndrome can occur with hallucinogen use, typically in combination with other substances or medications.

Tryptamine Hallucinogens

Tryptamine is a chemical structure that is shared by LSD, psilocybin, DMT, and the neurotransmitter serotonin.

- Ayahuasca (*Banisteriopsis caapi*) is a plant that naturally contains both N,N-dimethyltryptamine (DMT) and monoamine oxidase inhibitors (MAOIs). Due to naturally occurring MAOIs, ayahuasca carries a higher risk of serotonin syndrome when combined with other serotonergic agents. The plant is used as a traditional spiritual medicine in ceremonies among the indigenous people of the Amazon
- Psilocybin is a natural hallucinogen produced by certain species of mushrooms. Once ingested, it is metabolized to psilocin which has potent serotonergic and hallucinogenic effects.
- LSD is a synthetic hallucinogen. It acts on multiple serotonin receptors, including 5-HT2A, and has D2 receptor agonism that sets it apart from other hallucinogens.
- Morning glory: Seeds from some of its species have hallucinogenic effects. The seeds contain lysergic acid amide, a chemical like LSD.

Phenethylamine Hallucinogens

Mescaline and some designer hallucinogens are substituted phenethylamines. Recall that the phenethylamine structure is typical in psychoactive compounds, including many stimulants, hallucinogens, and neurotransmitters.

- Mescaline is a natural hallucinogen found in cacti, including peyote and the San Pedro cactus.
- Several so-called "research chemicals" have been synthesized and are phenethylamine derivatives with hallucinogenic effects. These include 2CB, 2CE, 2CI, and others. 2CI is one of the better-known research chemicals and was popularized in a book by Dr. Alexander Shulgin and Anne Shulgin, who synthesized 2CI and many other phenethylamine-based compounds

Atypical Hallucinogens

S. divinorum and hyoscine have hallucinogenic effects but differ from classical hallucinogens in that serotonergic receptors do not mediate their effects.

- *S. divinorum* is the name of the plant from which salvinorin A, a potent hallucinogen, is derived. Salvinorin A is a kappa-opioid agonist and does not share a structural similarity with any synthetic or naturally occurring opioid.
- Hyoscine, also known as scopolamine, is found in several plants in the nightshade family and has antimuscarinic anticholinergic activity. An overdose can present with delirium, hallucinations, and anticholinergic features.

Know This:

Some individuals continue to experience flashbacks and reexperiencing of hallucinations (primarily visual) well after the intoxicant effects of the hallucinogen have ended. These flashbacks can occur weeks or even years later from the last use. This phenomenon is referred to as hallucinogen persisting perception disorder and has been most frequently described following use of LSD.

GAMMA-HYDROXYBUTYRATE

Gamma-hydroxybutyrate (GHB) is a neurotransmitter and both a precursor and metabolite of GABA. Given its similarity to GABA, GHB is a central nervous system (CNS) inhibitor and considered a sedative-hypnotic. GHB acts at both GABA-B and specific GHB receptors. The effects of GHB include relaxation, tranquility, and sensory and sexual enhancement; low doses resemble the effects of mild alcohol intoxication.

- GHB is also abused by bodybuilders. Although there is limited evidence for this, GHB is believed to increase fat metabolism and release of growth hormone.
- It has a half-life of 30 to 60 minutes.
- GHB has amnestic effects and is known for its use as a date-rape drug. Because of its short half-life and lack of a rapid toxicology test, its presence is difficult to detect.
- Signs and symptoms of GHB intoxication include respiratory depression and bradycardia; overdose is a medical emergency and can lead to stupor, coma, and death.
- GHB dependence and withdrawal syndromes can develop with chronic use; withdrawal symptomatology can be treated with benzodiazepines or barbiturates.
- Therapeutically, GHB is used for the treatment of narcolepsy with cataplexy and is available as the Schedule III medication sodium oxybate.

FLUNITRAZEPAM

Flunitrazepam, also referred to as "roofies," is a benzodiazepine with rapid onset and a half-life of 20 hours. It causes anterograde amnesia and is commonly used as a date-rape drug. It is no longer available in the United States.

ANABOLIC ANDROGENIC STEROIDS

Anabolic androgenic steroids (AAS) are hormones that include testosterone and its analogues. They bind to the androgen receptor producing their anabolic and androgenic effects, and have psychoactive effects through allosteric modulation and enhancement of the GABA-A receptor. Steroid abuse is more common among males, with an average age of onset of 20 years old, with up to one-third using steroids chronically and developing dependence. The most common reasons for abusing these compounds are for physical or performance enhancement. Anabolic steroids are available in different formulations, including as oral medications, topical gels, intramuscular injections, and transdermal patches.

Adverse Effects

- Anabolic steroid use can lead to weight gain, kidney failure, alteration in serum lipids, liver damage, heart disease, and increased risk of coagulopathy and stroke.
- In males, AAS use can lead to baldness, gynecomastia, smaller testes and lower sperm count. In females, it can lead to increased facial and body hair, an enlarged clitoris, deepening of the voice, and menstrual cycle irregularities.
- Long-term changes in the brain can lead to mood changes and behavior, including paranoia, delusions, and aggression.

Know This:

- The 17-alpha-alkylated anabolic steroid, a commonly abused AAS, is associated with a higher incidence of hepatotoxicity and hepatic tumors.
- Testosterone is metabolized to dihydrotestosterone (DHT) by 5-alpha-reductase and then to estradiol by aromatase. Estradiol causes gynecomastia in men, whereas DHT leads to male pattern baldness.
- Body dysmorphic disorder is common comorbidity among those abusing and misusing AAS.

INHALANTS

Children and adolescents commonly abuse inhalants and solvents to achieve an altered mental state. The peak age of inhalant abuse is between the ages of 14 and 16 years. Inhalant abuse is more common in individuals from minority and marginalized populations because of their low price, legal status, and widespread availability. There is usually a rapid pulmonary absorption, as these are highly lipid-soluble compounds, reaching the brain in seconds. The initial effects of these substances are similar to those of anesthetic agents. Methods of abusing inhalants are listed in Table 10.1.

Routine urine drug screenings do not detect inhalants, so detection relies on the clinical diagnosis. Some laboratory findings include an elevation of liver enzymes. There is no FDA-approved psychopharmacological treatment for inhalant abuse, and recommended treatments include individual and family therapy.

TABLE 10.1
Methods of Abusing Inhalants

Method of Use	Action
Sniffing or snorting	Directly inhaling fumes
Bagging	Inhaling fumes from substances sprayed or deposited inside a bag
Huffing	Spraying or soaking the substance on a rag or cloth to then holding it over the mouth or nose
Glading	Inhaling an air freshener aerosol
Dusting	Spraying aerosol cleaners directly into the mouth or nose

Aliphatic, Aromatic, and Halogenated Hydrocarbons

These are common chemical components in fumigants, solvents, and insecticides. They are found in paint and varnish, textiles, rubber, plastics, and dry-cleaning products. Some examples are:

- N-Hexane and methyl N-butyl ketone
  - Pure N-hexane is a highly flammable colorless liquid.
  - Use of these substances can cause axonal swelling and relative loss of myelinated fibers leading to progressive neurologic decline similar to multiple sclerosis. Other adverse effects include hearing loss, memory loss, liver damage, and brain damage.
- Toluene
  - It is a colorless, water-insoluble liquid that is found in many industrial solvents.
  - Intoxication presents similarly to an alcohol or other sedative intoxication.
  - Toluene intoxication can present with hypokalemia, metabolic acidosis, distal renal tubular acidosis, rhabdomyolysis, and muscle paralysis.
  - Long-term adverse effects on the nervous system are severe and include dementia, ataxia, cerebral and cerebellar atrophy, and vision loss.

Nitrous Oxide

- Although classified as an inhalant, nitrous oxide (NO) is an NMDA antagonist and dissociative. NO is clinically used as a general anesthetic in humans and animals.

■ When abused, it is typically inhaled from balloons or "whippet" canisters to make whip cream. Long-term effects of NO abuse include neuropathy from B12 deficiency because NO converts B12 into its inactive form.

Volatile Alkyl Nitrites

■ The most commonly used are amyl-, butyl-, isobutyl-, or isopropyl-nitrite.
■ These substances are commonly referred to as "poppers."
■ Poppers are inhaled, or the vapors from the liquid form are sniffed.
■ Side effects include nausea, nosebleeds, and dizziness; regular exposure can cause headaches. If swallowed, amyl nitrate can be fatal.

Know This:

Phosphodiesterase-5-inhibitors (e.g., sildenafil or tadalafil) are commonly abused in combination with poppers to enhance sexual performance.

CAFFEINE

Caffeine (1,3,7-trimethylxanthine) is the world's most commonly used psychoactive substance and is classified as a stimulant. It can be found in coffee beans (the seeds of the *Coffea* genus of plants), cacao beans, and a number of teas, and it can be consumed in powder or liquid form in a wide variety of products. Caffeine belongs to the methylxanthine category of alkaloids and is structurally similar to adenosine, lending itself to its primary pharmacological effects mediated through adenosine receptors in the CNS.

Caffeine is a nonselective adenosine-1, -2a, and -2b receptor antagonist. Antagonism of the adenosine-2a receptors promotes wakefulness by reducing GABA release in nuclei of the brain that induce arousal. Caffeine does not directly affect dopamine, but the adenosine-2a receptor is believed to form a heteromer with dopamine receptors, which indirectly mediates caffeine's dopaminergic effects. Caffeine also causes sleep dysregulation by inhibiting adenosine-A1 receptors on ascending cholinergic neurons of the basal forebrain. Like other xanthine derivatives (e.g., theophylline), caffeine is also a nonspecific phosphodiesterase inhibitor.

Other characteristics of caffeine:

■ Eighty percent of caffeine (1,3,7-trimethylxanthine) is metabolized to paraxanthine by CYP1A2.
■ It has a half-life of 4 to 6 hours.
■ Caffeine withdrawal, which includes symptoms such as fatigue, headache, and irritability, can begin between 20 and 50 hours after last use and can last between 2 and 9 days.
■ Chronic consumption of caffeine leads to tolerance through upregulation of the adenosine A1 receptor.
■ Caffeine crosses the placenta, and high levels of consumption have been associated with low birth weight, spontaneous abortion, and stillbirth.

"Caffeine use disorder" is not an official DSM-5 diagnosis and is listed as a condition for further study, although caffeine intoxication, caffeine withdrawal, and other caffeine-induced disorders (e.g., anxiety) are included (American Psychiatric Association, 2013). The DSM-5 proposed diagnostic criteria for caffeine use disorder are similar to those of other substance use disorders (see Chapter 1); the estimated prevalence for caffeine use disorder in the United States is approximately 9%.

Adverse effects of caffeine include:

■ Restlessness and feeling anxious or irritable
■ Increased body temperature
■ Increased respiratory rate
■ Increased heart rate
■ Headache
■ Dehydration

Symptoms of a caffeine overdose can include:

■ Irregular heartbeat
■ Nausea or vomiting
■ Confusion
■ Shortness of breath

Caffeine overdose is rare and often related to the consumption of energy drinks or caffeine supplements. The cause of death is typically due to ventricular fibrillation and cardiac arrest. If someone presents with a caffeine overdose, medical treatment is necessary, including intravenous fluids, administration of activated charcoal, and cardiac monitoring. There is no FDA-approved psychopharmacologic treatment for caffeine use disorder, and treatment recommendations do not differ much from those used to treat other addictive behaviors. These treatments include individual and family therapy.

REFERENCE

American Psychiatric Association. (2013). *The diagnostic and statistical manual of mental disorders* (5th ed.). American Psychiatric Association.

SUGGESTIONS FOR FURTHER READING

Boot, B. P., McGregor, I. S., & Hall, W. (2000). MDMA (ecstasy) neurotoxicity: Assessing and communicating the risks. *Lancet, 355,* 1818–1821.

Center for Behavioral Health Statistics and Quality. (2019). *2018 National survey on drug use and health final analytic file codebook.* Substance Abuse and Mental Health Services Administration.

Drug Enforcement Agency. (2017). Khat. In *Drugs of Abuse: A DEA resource guide: 2017 edition.* https://www.dea.gov/sites/default/files/sites/getsmartaboutdrugs.com/files/publications/DoA_2017Ed_Updated_6.16.17.pdf#page=53.

Ferré, S. (2010). Role of the central ascending neurotransmitter systems in the psychostimulant effects of caffeine. *Journal of Alzheimer's Disease, 20*(Suppl1), S35–S49.

Sanacora, G., Heimer, H., Hartman, D., Mathew, S. J., Frye, M., Nemeroff, C., & Robinson Beale, R. (2017). Balancing the promise and risks of ketamine treatment for mood disorders. *Neuropsychopharmacology, 42*(6), 1179–1181.

REVIEW QUESTIONS

1. A senior internal medicine resident reports insomnia and recurrent headaches if he does not have two cups of coffee in the morning. He will start feeling irritable, tired, and at times will experience blurry vision. He does not want to stop coffee because it may affect his performance at the hospital. Which of the following would you recommend to the resident?
   A. Drinking coffee every 2 hours
   B. Taking caffeine pills as needed for his mood
   C. Decrease the amount of coffee as tolerated
   D. Stop drinking coffee
   E. Start drinking decaffeinated coffee

2. Caffeine use increases dopaminergic activity by acting on which of the following receptors?
   A. Glycine
   B. Adenosine
   C. P450 system
   D. Dopamine
   E. Serotonin

3. A 15-year-old boy presents to the emergency department after 3 days of vomiting and weakness in both arms and legs. His mother shares that he has been spending more time in the garage with a few friends. A computed tomography scan of the head shows mild brain atrophy, and laboratory studies are significant for hypokalemia and renal tubular acidosis. Which of the following substances has this patient most likely been abusing?
   A. Cocaine
   B. Phencyclidine
   C. Toluene
   D. *S. divinorum*
   E. Heroin

4. The father of a 14-year-old boy calls your office. His son is complaining of severe headaches and feels like he "is floating in space" and that his heart is going "out of his body." They found a couple of empty cough medicine bottles under his bed. This clinical picture is most characteristic of abusing:
   A. Dextromethorphan
   B. Cocaine
   C. N-Hexane
   D. Methylone
   E. Toluene

5. Which of the following medications can be given in cases of respiratory depression associated with DXM overdose?
   A. N-acetylcysteine
   B. Dimercaprol
   C. Atropine
   D. Methylene blue
   E. Naloxone

6. A 55-year-old White man presented to the emergency room with a blood pressure of 200/150 mm Hg and a heart rate of 118 beats per minute. He is disoriented and unable to follow commands. His pupils are dilated and he has nystagmus on examination. Which of the

following is the most likely explanation for the patient's presentation?

A. Alcohol withdrawal
B. PCP intoxication
C. Cocaine intoxication
D. Dehydration
E. Dementia with Lewy body

7. A 32-year-old man with a history of major depression on fluoxetine presents to the emergency room with signs and symptoms of serotonin syndrome after ingesting a hallucinogen. Ingestion of which of the following hallucinogens is most likely to lead to this presentation?

A. Psilocybin
B. LSD
C. *S. divinorum*
D. Ayahuasca
E. DMT

11

ASPECTS OF PAIN

THE NEUROBIOLOGY OF PAIN

General Pain Pathways

These pathways are the primary components that connect, receive, and process all the pain information generated by neurons. The pain pathway comprises three orders of neurons that transmit pain signals to the brain. Sensory or afferent neurons carrying pain are the Aδ-fibers, which are myelinated, and the unmyelinated C-fibers.

Mediators of Pain

- Beta-endorphin: A metabolite of beta-lipotropin produced in the anterior lobe of the pituitary gland in response to pain. It carries mu-opioid receptors agonist properties and acts as a synaptic transmitter agent and neural hormone.
- Substance P: A chain of 11 amino acid residues with inflammatory effects in immune and epithelial cells. Substance P induces vasodilation, increases vascular permeability, and facilitates leukocyte release to the site of injury.
- Bradykinin: An inflammatory mediator that produces edema and vasodilatation in the site of injury.
- Cytokines: Involved in the initiation of pain and chronic pain by directly activating nociceptive sensory neurons and in nerve injury–induced central sensitization.
- Prostaglandins: Produced in nearly all body tissue cells and function as enhancers of other chemical mediators, such as serotonin substance P.
- Nerve growth factor: Expressed after the inflammatory lesions are formed causing mast cell

degranulation and the release of serotonin and histamine. The nerve growth factor receptors have become potential therapeutic targets in treating acute and chronic pain states.

- γ-Aminobutyric acid (GABA): The most widely distributed inhibitory transmitter in the central nervous system. It can bind to the ionotropic GABA-A receptors or metabotropic GABA-B receptors.
- Cannabinoids: Bind to CB1 receptors in the brain and spinal cord and peripheral CB2 receptors inhibiting intracellular cyclic adenosine monophosphate formation regulating pain responses.
- Norepinephrine: Synthesized from phenylalanine in the nerve terminals and directly inhibits pain through alpha-2-adrenergic receptors.

CLINICAL CONSIDERATIONS IN PAIN MANAGEMENT

Types of Pain

- Nociceptive pain: Seen after acute tissue damage and not a direct nerve injury. It presents as dull aching pain at the site of the injury. Examples include pain from arthritis, inflammation, or bone fractures.
- Neuropathic pain: Consists of direct nerve tissue injury and presents as a sharp, lancinating, burning, or electric sensation in the affected area. Some examples of neuropathic pain are carpal tunnel pain, phantom limb pain, or postviral neuralgias. Common causes of peripheral neuropathy are diabetes, vitamin B1 or B12 deficiency, and hypothyroidism.

The *Diagnostic and Statistical Manual of Mental Disorders,* Fifth Edition, and Pain

The *Diagnostic and Statistical Manual of Mental Disorders,* Fourth Edition, pain disorder diagnosis was eliminated and largely replaced by the *Diagnostic and Statistical Manual of Mental Disorders,* Fifth Edition, of somatic symptom disorder. People suffering from this disorder have a significant focus on physical symptoms that result in concern and problems functioning.

Somatic Symptom Disorder: Diagnostic Criteria

- One or more physical symptoms that are distressing or cause disruption in daily life.
- Excessive thoughts, feelings, or behaviors related to the physical symptoms or health concerns with at least one of the following:
  - Ongoing thoughts that are out of proportion with the seriousness of symptoms
  - Ongoing high level of anxiety about health or symptoms
  - Excessive time and energy spent on the symptoms or health concerns

- At least one symptom is continuously present, although different symptoms and current symptoms may come and go.

Pain Scales

- Visual analog scale: Respondents are asked to report present pain intensity or pain intensity in the last 24 hours (Fig. 11.1).
- Wong-Baker FACES Pain Rating Scale: The assessment is done by only looking at the patient's facial expressions (Fig. 11.2).

PHARMACOTHERAPIES FOR PAIN SYNDROMES

When choosing a medication to treat pain, it is essential to consider the medication's duration, the onset of action, and prior experiences. We review below some commonly used medications effective in relieving pain.

Nonsteroidal Antiinflammatory Drugs

Nonsteroidal antiinflammatory drugs (NSAIDs) inhibit cyclooxygenase enzymes involved in the production of prostaglandins, pain mediators. NSAIDs can be cyclooxygenase-2 selective (e.g., celecoxib),

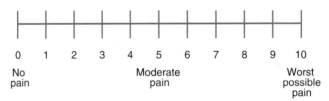

Fig. 11.1 ■ The Numeric Pain Rating Scale. The patient is asked to make three pain ratings, corresponding to current, best, and worst pain experienced over the past 24 hours. The average of the three ratings is used to represent the patient's level of pain over the previous 24 hours. (From Potter, P. A. (2016). *Pain management.* In A. G. Perry, P. A. Potter, & W. R. Ostendorf (Eds.), *Nursing interventions & clinical skills* (6th ed., p. 319). Elsevier.)

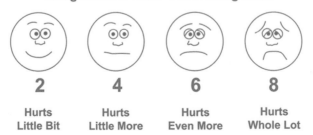

Fig. 11.2 ■ Wong-Baker FACES Pain Rating Scale. (From Wong-Baker FACES Foundation (2020). *Wong-Baker FACES pain rating scale.* Retrieved February 24, 2021 with permission from http://www.WongBakerFACES.org. Originally published in *Whaley & Wong's Nursing Care of Infants and Children.* Elsevier.)

nonselective (e.g., ibuprofen, naproxen), or partially selective (e.g., meloxicam, diclofenac). NSAIDs' side effects include ulcers and upper gastrointestinal tract bleeding, worsening congestive heart failure, aseptic meningitis, psychosis, and tinnitus. NSAID use can adversely affect the kidney by inducing sodium retention and antagonizing diuretics.

Paracetamol (Acetaminophen)

Paracetamol works by blocking cyclooxygenase-2 and inhibiting endocannabinoid reuptake in the central nervous system. It carries minor antiinflammatory activity.

Tricyclic Antidepressants

Tricyclic antidepressants block the reuptake of norepinephrine and serotonin, increasing serotonin levels, and enhancing norepinephrine activity. They function as an effective adjunctive pain management medication.

Gabapentin

Gabapentin carries direct and indirect effects on the GABA receptors and provides significant relief from neuropathic pain.

Meperidine

Meperidine is an opioid with serotonergic and anticholinergic effects. It is not an ideal choice for the management of chronic pain due to its poor oral absorption, short duration of action, and toxic metabolite (normeperidine), which can cause tremors and seizures.

Opioids

Prescription opioids are among the many options for treating severe acute pain. Opioid analgesics are not recommended for the chronic treatment of pain syndromes. Opioids are discussed in more detail in Chapter 6.

Know This:

Meperidine does not cause pinpoint pupils.

SUGGESTIONS FOR FURTHER READING

Apfelbaum, J. L., Chen, C., Mehta, S. S., & Gan, T. J. (2003). Postoperative pain experience: results from a national survey suggest postoperative pain continues to be undermanaged. *Anesthesia and Analgesia, 97*(2), 534–540.

Brennan, F., Carr, D. B., & Cousins, M. (2007). Pain management: a fundamental human right. *Anesthesia and Analgesia, 105*(1), 205–221.

Hall, J. E. (2010). *Guyton and Hall textbook of medical physiology e-book*. Elsevier Health Sciences.

Kaufman, D. M., Geyer, H. L., & Milstein, M. J. (2016). *Kaufman's clinical neurology for psychiatrists* (8th ed.). Elsevier.

Wong-Baker FACES Foundation. (2020). Wong-Baker FACES Pain Rating Scale. Retrieved from http://www.WongBakerFACES.org. Originally published in *Whaley & Wong's nursing care of infants and children*. Elsevier.

REVIEW QUESTIONS

1. A 61-year-old patient presents with low back pain. He was recommended to start taking ibuprofen as needed for his pain. He has been eating well and denied any lifestyle changes. Six weeks later, he presents to the office with 13 pounds of weight gain. Which of the following is the best explanation for the patient's weight gain?
    A. A decrease in renal function
    B. A decrease in temperature
    C. A decrease in creatinine levels
    D. An increase in the glomerular filtration rate
    E. An increase in plasma proteins

2. A 68-year-old female patient with a history of lung cancer and metastases to the lumbar spine is receiving oxycodone 10 mg three times a day. The patient's partner tells the medical resident that the patient exhibits a lack of energy and motivation, feelings of worthiness, low concentration, and reduced appetite in the past 2 weeks. What should be the next step?
    A. Start an antidepressant
    B. Physical therapy evaluation
    C. Psychiatric evaluation
    D. The patient's pain assessment
    E. Medication assisted treatment for opioid use disorder

3. A 19-year-old patient had a mechanical fall while driving his motorcycle downtown. He is complaining of a dull aching pain at the right hip. What type of pain is the patient having?
    A. Neuropathic pain
    B. Nociceptive pain
    C. Fibromyalgia
    D. Chronic pain
    E. Traumatic brain injury

12 DRUG TESTING, FORENSIC ADDICTIONS, AND ETHICS

DRUG AND ALCOHOL TESTING

Drug and alcohol testing can and should be ordered in various settings. Understanding the context for which such a thing is being ordered can help determine testing procedures. For example, for parents seeking to monitor their children's drug use, point-of-care testing at home may suffice. In contrast, when working with patients being evaluated in an emergency department setting, a urine toxicology screening test provides quick information and may guide clinical decisions. Substance use disorder (SUD) treatment providers frequently use urine toxicology screening tests followed by gas chromatography–mass spectrometry (GC-MS) confirmation of any positive screens to guide treatment regimen and monitor treatment outcomes. Persons sentenced of driving under the influence (DUI) of alcohol may be required to undergo monitoring with transdermal alcohol testing bracelets. Liver transplant evaluation frequently uses a battery of biomarkers to determine whether or not the individual abstains from alcohol. Finally, custody evaluations and other forensic assessments frequently rely on hair drug testing to assess the evaluee's drug use over the past several months. Medical Review Officers are physicians with added qualifications for interpreting toxicology testing results.

Drug Testing

Matrices

- Urine: Urine drug screening (UDS) utilizes antibody immunoassays that react to various drugs. The detection period varies based on the drug and its metabolism, ranging from 1 day to 1 month (e.g., for cannabis). The most basic UDS test is known as SAMHSA-5 assays for amphetamines, cocaine, marijuana, opiates, and phencyclidine and is used by the Department of Transportation and other federal agencies. UDS testing is typically expanded in clinical settings to include various other substances, including benzodiazepines, barbiturates, or synthetic opioids. Any positive test on a UDS should be sent to GC-MS confirmation testing. UDS uses cut-off values for screening that are typically higher than the cut-off values used for confirmation testing. UDS results are qualitative, showing whether the individual tested positive (above the cut-off value) or negative for a given drug. GC-MS confirmation results are both qualitative and quantitative, showing the metabolite concentration tested in the urine. Quantitative results should never be used to assess drug use frequency given the significant variability in urine-specific gravity and electrolyte content.
- Hair: Hair drug testing can demonstrate drug use with a detection period of up to 4 or 5 months. Testing results are both qualitative and quantitative, showing the metabolite concentration tested in hair. Unlike urine testing, quantitative results obtained from hair testing can distinguish between light, moderate, and heavy drug use. Compared to urine testing, hair testing is more expensive, takes longer for results to become available, and may miss recent drug use.
- Saliva and nails: Drug testing using saliva or nails as testing matrices are available. However, their results are not as validated and clinically useful as urine or hair testing.

Drug Testing, Drug Metabolism, and False Positives

When reading a drug testing report, it is important to understand the specific compounds tested in a given immunoassay. For example, in the SAMHSA-5 assays, the "opiates" immunoassay uses antibodies specific for morphine metabolites and, as such, detects the presence of natural and some semisynthetic opioids such as heroin, morphine, and codeine (Fig. 12.1, top panel). Detecting synthetic opioids such as tramadol, hydrocodone, oxycodone, buprenorphine, or fentanyl requires an extended opioid panel (Fig. 12.1, bottom panel). Similarly, benzodiazepine immunoassays use antibodies specific for oxazepam and detect the presence of benzodiazepines that can be metabolized into oxazepam, including diazepam, chlordiazepoxide, clorazepate, and temazepam (Fig. 12.2, top panel). Detecting the presence of clonazepam, alprazolam or lorazepam typically requires an extended benzodiazepine panel (Fig. 12.2, bottom panel). Cocaine immunoassays detect the presence of its metabolite, benzoylecgonine.

The specific substance's pharmacokinetics determines the detection period during which an individual would be expected to test positive in a UDS. Table 12.1 lists the detection periods for commonly tested substances.

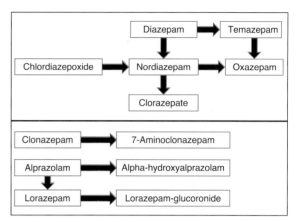

Fig. 12.2 ▪ Top panel: Metabolic pathway of benzodiazepines detected in the standard benzodiazepines immunoassay. Bottom panel: Metabolic pathway of clonazepam, alprazolam, and lorazepam.

Know This:

- Poppy seeds may cause a false-positive opiate test on UDS. Hair testing would not result in a false-positive result.
- When alcohol and cocaine are consumed simultaneously, a common metabolic pathway causes cocaethylene production (ethylbenzoylecgonine). Cocaethylene assays are commercially available for testing.
- Substances reported to cause false-positive UDSs results are shown in Table 12.2.

Drug Toxicology Validity Testing

A normal urine sample is valid for testing if:

- No gross adulterants are identified on visual examination
- Temperature between 90°F and 100°F
- pH between 4.5 and 8.5
- Nitrites less than 5mg/dL
- Urine creatinine between 2 and 20 mg/dL
- Specific gravity between 1.0030 and 1.0200

Upon review by the MROs, UDS results are reported as:

- Negative: No drug metabolites found, and all validity testing parameters listed above within normal range.

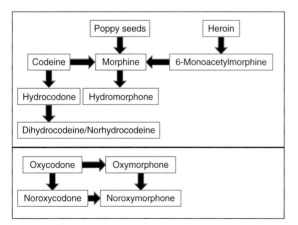

Fig. 12.1 ▪ Top panel: Metabolic pathway of natural and semisynthetic opioids detected in the standard opiate immunoassay. Bottom panel: Metabolic pathway of synthetic opioids.

TABLE 12.1

Detection Periods for Commonly Tested Substances

Substance Tested	Detection Period
Alcohol	1–12 h
Amphetamines	1–2 days
Barbiturates	1–3 days (up to 3 weeks for long-acting barbiturates)
Benzodiazepines	1–3 days (up to 6 weeks for chronic heavy use)
Cannabis	2–7 days (up to 8 weeks for chronic heavy use)
Heroin	1–2 days (6-Monoacetylmorphine)
Morphine	1–3 days
Cocaine	2–4 days
Methadone	2–4 days
Phencyclidine	7–30 days

TABLE 12.2

Substances That Cause False-Positive Urine Drug Screening Results

Drug Tested	Substance Used Causing False-Positive Urine Drug Screening Result
Amphetamines	Labetalol, ranitidine, bupropion, pseudoephedrine, ephedrine, amantadine, desipramine, selegiline, trazodone, methylphenidate, Vicks inhalers
Benzodiazepines	Sertraline
Barbiturates	Phenytoin, NSAID
Marijuana	Proton pump inhibitors, dronabinol, nonsteroidal anti-inflammatory drug
Opiates	Ofloxacin, rifampicin, poppy seeds (papaverine), fluoroquinolone
Phencyclidine	Venlafaxine, dextromethorphan, ketamine

- Negative–dilute: No drug metabolites found, creatinine concentration between 2 and 20 mg/dL, AND the specific gravity between 1.0010 and 1.0030, but all other validity testing parameters within the normal range.
- Positive with drug metabolites noted: Drug metabolites found, and all validity testing parameters within the normal range.
- Positive with drug metabolites noted–dilute: Drug metabolites found, creatinine concentration between 2 and 20 mg/dL, AND the specific gravity

between 1.0010 and 1.0030, but all other validity testing parameters within the normal range.

- Adulterated: Nitrate concentration greater than 500 mg/dL, urine pH less than 4 or greater than or equal to 11, or if the presence of chromium, halogens, glutaraldehyde, pyridine, surfactants, or any other adulterant is verified. Identifying any such compound would be evidence of tampering or adulterating urine to evade accurate drug testing.
- Substituted: Creatinine concentration less than 2 mg/dL AND the specific gravity less than 1.0010 or greater than 1.0200. For example, this is seen when urine is diluted with very large amounts of water or when artificial fluids are used in place of urine.
- Invalid: Inconsistent creatinine and specific gravity values or if urine pH is between 4 and 4.5 or between 9 and 11.

Department of Transportation rules specify that negative—dilute urine drug testing requires immediate recollection under direct observation.

Testing for Alcohol

Alcohol metabolic products and other biomarkers can be tested in urine, blood, and hair, providing an accurate assessment of its alcohol use and severity. These include:

- Ethyl glucuronide (EtG): A direct biomarker of alcohol use. It can be detected in urine for 3 to 5 days and in hair for up to 3 months.
- Eethyl sulfate (EtS): A direct biomarker of alcohol use. It can be detected in urine for 3 to 5 days and in hair for up to 3 months.
- Phosphatidylethanol (PEth): A direct biomarker of significant alcohol use. It can be detected in blood for 6 to 8 weeks.
- Carbohydrate-deficient transferrin (%CDT): A direct biomarker of significant alcohol use. It can be detected in blood for 2 to 3 weeks
- Gamma-glutamyl transferase (GGT): A liver breakdown product used as an indirect biomarker of excessive and chronic alcohol use.
- Complete blood count (CBC): An indirect biomarker of excessive and chronic alcohol use. It typically shows low hemoglobin and hematocrit values with an elevated mean corpuscular volume.

- Liver function test: An indirect biomarker of excessive and chronic alcohol use. It typically shows elevated alanine aminotransferase and aspartate aminotransferase levels.

Know This:

The Widmark equation is used to estimate blood alcohol levels (BALs). BAL = weight of alcohol used (in oz)/r × weight of the subject (in oz); r, or the Widmark factor, is approximately 0.7 for males and 0.6 for females.

MEDICAL ETHICS IN ADDICTION PSYCHIATRY AND ADDICTION MEDICINE

Ethics is a branch of philosophy that deals with personal, professional, and social values in human conduct. It provides a discussion of right and wrong, good or bad, and the motives and ends of such conduct. In the context of medical practice, the following ethical principles are identified (note that autonomy, beneficence, nonmaleficence, and justice are typically referred to as the four principles of medical ethics):

- Autonomy principle: Requires that patients are free to make their own choices as long as they are competent and have autonomy in their thought process, intentions, and actions when making medical decisions. As such, the medical decision-making process must be free of coercion or undue influence.
- Beneficence principle: Requires that any medical decision offered, or any clinical intervention performed serve to promote patients' health and welfare.
- Nonmaleficence principle: Requires that any medical decision offered, or any clinical intervention performed, does not harm the patient.
- Justice principle: Requires that health care providers make medical decisions that treat patients equally and that the burden and benefits of new or experimental interventions are distributed fairly across all patients.
- Fidelity principle: Requires that health care providers follow through with promises made to patients.

- Loyalty principle: Requires that health care providers act in a manner that benefits their patients above any other interest.

In medical practice, it is not uncommon to face situations in which there is discordance in applying the ethical principles listed above. For example, in SUD treatment, needle exchange programs can be viewed as consistent with the principle of beneficence but not of nonmaleficence. Different ethical theories can help guide clinical decision making in such situations:

- Dialectical principlism theory is based on the major moral principles and requires balancing competing principles to rich and ethically acceptable solutions.
- Deontological theory deals with the clinician's duty and moral obligation to "do the right thing."
- Utilitarianism theory aims to achieve the greatest good for the greatest number of people.
- Liberal individualism theory places paramount importance on the patient's rights and autonomy.
- Virtue theory examines whether the clinical provider intended to do good by the patient, showing good character and moral values while placing less emphasis on strictly following the rules and consequences.
- Consequentialism theory determines the moral worth of an action based on whether its outcomes or consequences are good or bad.

FORENSIC ADDICTION PSYCHIATRY AND ADDICTION MEDICINE

Forensic psychiatry is the psychiatric subspecialty in which psychiatric principles are applied in legal contexts. In the following, we review important forensic psychiatric topics relevant to SUD treatment practice.

Important SUD Legislation

Harrison Narcotic Act of 1914: Congress passed this legislation to regulate the production, importation, and distribution of opioids. The act included protections for physicians prescribing opioids "at the cost of his professional practice only." Around the time the act was passed, SUD was not considered a medical illness, and, as a result, doctors were not allowed to prescribe opioids to those with opioid use disorder. Many physicians were arrested and imprisoned for prescribing opioids to SUD patients.

Controlled Substances Act of 1970: In 1970, the federal government enacted the Controlled Substances Act, classifying various addictive drugs based on their addictive potential, the potential for harm, and therapeutic potential. The act has been amended multiple times since to include new and emerging drugs. Commonly used drugs are classified as follows:

- Schedule I: marijuana, lysergic acid diethylamide (LSD), heroin
- Schedule II: morphine, fentanyl, methadone, hydrocodone, oxycodone, amphetamine
- Schedule III: buprenorphine, ketamine, dronabinol
- Schedule IV: alprazolam, clonazepam, diazepam, zolpidem
- Schedule V: pregabalin, codeine, diphenoxylate

Drug Addiction Treatment Act (DATA) of 2000: The legislation passed by Congress allowing physicians to treat opioid use disorder with buprenorphine in an office-based setting.

42 CFR (Code of Federal Regulation) Part 2: This rule dictates privacy protection that applies for SUD treatment (it is frequently described as the Health Insurance Portability and Accountability Act [HIPAA] equivalent for SUD).

Landmark Cases in Addiction Psychiatry and Addiction Medicine

Robinson v. California (United States Supreme Court; 1962): Mr. Robinson was arrested and convicted with a misdemeanor under the California statute for being "addicted to the use of narcotics." The case was appealed to the Supreme Court, which ruled that it is unconstitutional and violated the Eighth Amendment prohibition of cruel and unusual punishment to criminalize SUD.

Powell v. Texas (United States Supreme Court; 1968): Mr. Powell was charged and convicted with public intoxication in Texas. The case was appealed to the Supreme Court, which ruled that although SUD may not be considered a state offense, it is constitutional, however, for substance-related misconduct to be subject to both civil and criminal prosecutions.

People v. Saille (California Supreme Court; 1991): In this case, the California Supreme Court ruled that voluntary intoxication may not be used as a defense in criminal procedures.

Montana v. Egelhoff (United States Supreme Court; 1996): In this case, the Supreme Court found that excluding voluntary intoxication related to a mental state in a criminal offense does not violate due process protections of the Constitution. As such, it is constitutional for states to decline excusing a crime on the basis of voluntary intoxication.

Board of Education v. Earls (United States Supreme Court; 2002): In this case, the Supreme Court ruled that it is legal to randomly drug test public school students who participate in extracurricular activities.

Know This:

- Multiple forensic issues arise in treating adolescents with SUD with multiple state-specific differences. Generally speaking, an adolescent's written consent is required to communicate with their parents, except if an imminent safety risk is identified.
- Most states do not require parental consent to provide SUD treatment to adolescents. In states where parental consent is required, the adolescent's written consent is still required for their treatment team to communicate with their parents to seek treatment.
- Unless court-mandated, drug testing in adolescents requires the patient's consent. Not unlike any other patient, adolescents may refuse drug testing.

Res ipsa loquitur is a legal term meaning "the thing speaks for itself." For example, if a surgeon is sued for malpractice because they forgot a scalpel in their patient's abdomen, forensic experts may not be required to opine because everyone would agree that leaving an instrument in a patient's body amounts to wrongdoing.

SUGGESTIONS FOR FURTHER READING

American Academy of Psychiatry and the Law. (2005). *Ethics guidelines for the practice of forensic psychiatry.* http://www.aapl.org/ethics-guidelines.

Aoun, E. G., & Kim, J. (2020). Forensic addiction psychiatry. In K. T. Brady, F. R. Leven, M. Galanter, & H. D. Kleber (Eds.), *The American Psychiatric Press textbook of substance abuse* (6th ed.). American Psychiatric Press Publishing.

Powell v. Texas, 392 U.S. 514, 88 S. Ct. 2145 (1968).

Robinson v. California, 70 U.S. 660 (more) 82 S. Ct. 1417; 8 L. Ed. 2d 758; 1962 U.S. LEXIS 850.

Swotinsky, R. B. (2014). *The medical review officer's manual: MROCC'S guide to drug testing* (5th ed.). OEM Press.

REVIEW QUESTIONS

1. Which of the following is true about SUDs among physicians?
   A. SUD prevalence rates among psychiatrists and pathologists are higher than the general population.
   B. SUD prevalence is lower for physicians than the general population.
   C. SUD prevalence rates among emergency physicians and anesthesiologists are higher than the general population.
   D. Physicians referred to physician health programs have a worse prognosis than those who do not.
   E. The prognosis of physicians with SUD is worse than the general population.

2. Which of the following statements about drug and alcohol testing is correct?
   A. Drug testing is the most effective means of detecting SUDs.
   B. A positive for-cause drug test performed indicates that the individual most likely has an SUD.
   C. A positive random drug test suggests that the individual uses the drug recreationally but does not have an SUD.
   D. A positive drug test shows recent drug use.
   E. Hair testing for biomarkers of excessive alcohol use is an effective strategy to ensure abstinence for someone who is recently charged with a DUI.

3. Which of the following clinical situations is associated with the highest risk of violence and criminal behaviors?
   A. A 34-year-old man with major depressive disorder
   B. A 26-year-old woman with cannabis use disorder
   C. A 19-year-old man with schizophrenia and phencyclidine intoxication
   D. A 24-year-old woman with cocaine use disorder
   E. A 69-year-old man with alcohol use disorder

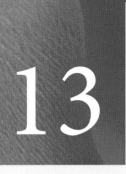

13

PSYCHOSOCIAL APPROACHES TO SUBSTANCE USE DISORDER MANAGEMENT

DEFINITIONS OF TERMS RELATING TO MODELS OF CARE

Centralized model of care: Substance use disorder (SUD) treatment is integrated and offered in a single location, frequently delivered by the primary care physician with an addiction specialist providing support.

Distributive model of care: SUD treatment is delivered with a focus on case management to maximize access to care for a wider selection of community services.

Universal programs: SUD treatment interventions designed to reach a whole section of the general population, such as interventions to get all the students in a given school district.

Family-based programs: SUD treatment interventions that are focused on addressing risk factors and protective factors for the development of SUD. Such programs involve supporting parents in how to best communicate and discipline their children to promote drug abstinence and healthy lifestyles.

Selective programs: SUD treatment interventions that target at-risk population groups. For example, interventions that target school dropouts are described as selective programs.

Indicated programs: SUD treatment interventions that target specific at-risk individuals. For example, interventions reduce subsequent drug use for a specific teenager suspended from school after LSD was found in his backpack.

LONG-TERM PSYCHOSOCIAL PROGRAMS FOR THE CARE OF PERSONS WITH SUD

The phrase "residential rehabilitation program" is not a discrete and well-defined intervention; instead, it refers to a long-term residential setting for persons with subacute SUD treatment needs in which a variety of services may be offered. Treatment programming varies widely but often follows the 28-day traditional "Minnesota Model." Residential rehabilitation programs are frequently followed by intensive outpatient programs. As discussed in Chapter 1, the American Society of Addiction Medicine (ASAM) patient placement criteria (PPC-2R) specifies which type of services and treatment settings are most appropriate for a given patient with SUD, with Level III referring to residential programs:

- Level III.1: Clinically managed low-intensity residential services
- Level III.3: Clinically managed medium-intensity residential treatment
- Level III.5: Clinically managed high-intensity residential treatment
- Level III.7: Medically monitored intensive inpatient treatment

The term "clinically managed" describes facilities with on-site skilled clinical staff but no on-site physician. Using the PPC-2R framework, individuals in need of Level III services are those with minimal withdrawal and biomedical needs who require maintenance SUD services in a 24-hour monitored recovery environment.

Therapeutic communities (TC) are a type of residential treatment facility that is traditionally longer-term (typically 6 to 12 months) and utilizes every aspect of the residential community as part of the treatment experience and an opportunity to provide services. The treatment goal is to promote resocialization of the person with SUD and use every community member, including staff and other residents, as active components of treatment. The program focuses on accountability, responsibility, and structuring a socially productive life. The TC model has been adapted to correctional settings. When combined with community-based TC on release from incarceration, such models are associated with improved substance use and criminal justice outcomes.

Overall, the clinical outcomes from residential rehabilitation treatment programs are mixed, ranging from no effect to modest or moderate benefit compared to alternative modes of treatment, such as intensive outpatient programs, and methodological issues limit many research studies. Some studies show that length of stay correlates with abstinence success rates.

Know This:

- Generally speaking, research studies have not identified any significant differences in outcome based on the length of stay in a given residential rehabilitation treatment program.
- For more severely impaired patients with limited social support and social instability, longer stays in residential rehabilitation treatment programs might be more beneficial.
- TC are generally based on Alcoholics Anonymous (AA) principles. Programming is highly structured and is often highly confrontational.
- The TC model focuses on the individual's responsibility with SUD for their behaviors and the consequences of substance-related behaviors. The therapeutic focus on "resocialization" is that isolation and dysfunctional social and interpersonal coping mechanisms precede the long-term facility presentation for many patients.

COMMUNITY MUTUAL-SUPPORT GROUPS AND 12-STEP PROGRAMS

Mutual-support groups, including 12-step programs, such as AA or Narcotics Anonymous, are peer-led groups traditionally facilitated by persons with SUD in recovery as self-directed leadership aiming to foster supportive and mentoring peer relationships. Groups are focused on a problem shared by group members, are free of charge, and encourage mutual aid. Techniques used to promote change rely on experiential learning, building structure, learning coping strategies, and strengthening social networks. The goals of such a group include promoting self-efficacy and a new identity.

We will use AA as a model for this discussion on 12-step–based mutual-support groups. AA meetings involve an opening ritual, group members sharing their experiences, and a closing ritual. Members are encouraged to "work through" the 12 steps of AA; surrender to a higher power; and select a sponsor who can provide mentorship, guidance, and support to help the member work through the steps. AA principles include taking responsibility, finding humility, and using honesty. AA uses tools based on psychological principles, including stimulus control and cue reactivity (surrounding oneself with sober social connections and avoiding people, places, and things associated with alcohol use), reconditioning (or counterconditioning: learning healthier behaviors for managing urges and substituting addictive behaviors such as seeking support from a sponsor, desensitization, assertion, and cognitive counters to irrational assertions), and positive reinforcement (offering "chips" to celebrate the duration a member has been sober).

Although many persons with alcohol use disorder find AA meetings extremely helpful, many do not. Indeed, although abstinence is not mandated to attend AA meetings, all participating members have to agree to a goal of total and complete abstinence. Setting harm reduction goals (such as reducing one's drinking rather than lifelong abstinence) is inconsistent with the AA ideology. People seeking to moderate their drinking are unlikely to benefit from AA. Similarly, persons with alcohol use disorder who cannot accept the concept of a "higher power" (loosely defined in modern AA teachings to fit a range of beliefs including a god, nature, or even the support of group fellowship) or the "alcoholic" label cannot meaningfully participate in AA.

For such persons finding AA unsuitable to their needs, organizations such as SMART Recovery, Secular Organizations for Sobriety, Moderation Management, and LifeRing serve as an alternative to the spiritually oriented AA. We will use SMART Recovery as a model for this discussion alternative to 12-step-based mutual-support groups.

Self-Management and Recovery Training (SMART) Recovery aims to teach persons with SUD coping strategies and a logical approach to thinking and acting. Groups utilize trained facilitators and seek to change maladaptive behaviors leading to substance use. The program lists four core tenets:

1. Building and maintaining motivation to abstain
2. Learning how to cope with urges
3. Managing feelings, thoughts, and maladaptive behaviors
4. Balancing immediate and long-term rewards (monetary and enduring satisfactions

SMART Recovery offers in-person and online programs, both of which are of equal effectiveness in achieving abstinence or reducing drinking and substance-related problems. Similarly, Moderation Management applies cognitive behavioral therapy (CBT) techniques in a peer-support context with a member-elected goal of either abstinence or moderation of drinking. Moderation Management promotes self-control, responsibility, choice, rational thinking, and insight into drinking behaviors.

Know This:

- Mutual-support groups provide long-term social and spiritual support to recovery and augment and cement the benefits of evidence-based treatments for SUD (such as medications or psychotherapies) but are not and should not be confused with or substituted with SUD treatment.
- Twelve-step-based programs rely on active rather than passive participation. The model views SUD as a chronic disease rather than a temporary state of excessive substance use. The principles focus on acceptance, surrendering, and actively participating in meetings and recovery activities.

The 12 steps of AA:

1. **I can't** (We are powerless over alcohol, and our lives have become unmanageable.)
2. **God can** (Power greater than ourselves can restore us to sanity.)
3. **Let God** (Turn our will and our lives over to the care of God as we understood Him.)
4. **Look within** (Made a searching and fearless moral inventory of ourselves.)
5. **Admit wrongs** (Admitted to God, to ourselves, and to another human being the exact nature of our wrongs.)
6. **Ready self for change** (Were entirely ready to have God remove all these character defects.)
7. **Seek God's help** (Humbly asked Him to remove our shortcomings.)
8. **Become willing** (Made a list of all persons we had harmed, and became willing to make amends to them all.)
9. **Make amends** (Made direct amends to such people wherever possible, except when to do so would injure them or others.)
10. **Daily inventory** (Continued to take personal inventory, and when we were wrong, promptly admit it.)
11. **Pray and meditate** (Sought through prayer and meditation to improve our conscious contact with God as we understood Him, praying only for knowledge of His will for us and power to carry that out.)
12. **Give it away** (Having had a spiritual awakening due to these steps, we tried to carry this message to alcoholics, and to practice these principles in all our affairs.)

HALT (Hungry, Angry, Lonely, or Tired) is an AA mnemonic for triggers and emotional states that promote relapse.

- Relapse prevention strategies in 12-step–based programs use Marlatt Relapse Prevention model. The model defines intrapersonal determinants of relapse as:
  - Self-efficacy
  - Outcome expectancies (beliefs about the consequences one can anticipate as a result of substance use)
  - Craving

- Motivation
- Coping
- Emotional states
- For persons with SUD in treatment, the earlier in the course of treatment that they are referred to mutual-support group meetings, the more likely they are to attend.
- Effectiveness studies show that attending AA meetings is most likely to be associated with abstinence in persons attending two or more groups per week.

SPECIFIC PSYCHOTHERAPIES

Various evidence-based psychotherapies effectively treat SUD, including CBT, motivational interviewing (MI), twelve-step facilitation (TSF), contingency management (CM), and mindfulness-based interventions.

Motivational Interviewing

This chapter will discuss MI extensively, given how frequently it is assessed on board examinations. MI is an empathic, collaborative, and client-centered approach that allows the therapist to explore and resolve in a nonconfrontational and nonjudgmental approach patients' ambivalence about the role of substances in their lives. Patients are encouraged to explore both the positive or rewarding (such as intoxication, disinhibition, socialization, and pleasure) and negative and harmful aspects of substance use, and feelings of the inability to change in those who have a strong desire to do so. During the MI process, the therapist elicits "change talk" of the patient's motivation and rationale to change and highlights the discrepancy between their behaviors (continued substance use) and their goals (abstain or reduce).

The course of MI follows broadly four therapeutic processes:

1. **Engaging:** This phase of treatment focuses on developing a collaborative relationship between the therapist and the patient setting the motivational change stage. It consists of engaging the patient in the process of self-exploration and disclosure; focusing on their concerns, interests, and hopes; and building a collaborative, trusting rapport. Patients successfully navigate the engaging process when they allow themselves to be more vulnerable and face insecurities contributing to their substance-using behaviors in a nondefensive manner.

2. **Focusing:** This phase of treatment focuses on exploring the patient's goals. For patients with more than one goal, "agenda mapping" describes the process of prioritizing goals, managing competing goals, and examining how different topics might fit together. The process is ongoing rather than set, as priorities can evolve throughout treatment. It is not uncommon for patients to present without any specific target behaviors to change. Instead, they report mood alterations, general dissatisfaction with their lives, and neurovegetative symptoms, disconnected from the impact of their substance use on these symptoms. Using a client-centered approach, the therapist can follow the patient's lead, use the focusing stage to define the problem, connect it with maladaptive substance use, and highlight strengths and possibilities.

3. **Evoking:** This third phase of MI aims to evoke the patient's perspective and motivation to change. The therapist's role is not to provide information on the harmful ways patients' substance use affects their lives or give advice on change. Indeed, it is exceedingly rare that patients are not already well aware of that. Further, being told what to do and other extrinsic motivation expressions are not motivating for patients with SUD (note that extrinsic motivation refers to the motivating factor that extend beyond the direct desire to quit using a substance, such as seeking to improve a relationship with a romantic partner. In contrast, intrinsic motivation refers to the direct motivation one has from achieving a state of recovery). Evoking focuses attention on the patient's values, preferences, hopes, and desires and inches toward long-term change by bringing out intrinsic motivation. Key tasks in the evoking phase include eliciting, focusing, and responding to "change talk," and building momentum toward change. Alternatively, when "sustain talk" comes up, the therapist accepts the patient's perspective and processes such talk in a nonjudgmental approach to prevent the patient from feeling stuck or taking a defensive stance.

MI research finds that change in talk frequency and intensity promoted one's commitment to change and increased the likelihood of successful outcomes. In eliciting change talk, the therapist ought to stimulate the patient's desires, reasons for change, and need for change.

4. **Planning:** During the fourth stage of MI, therapists provide a recapitulation of the issues, followed by asking the patient about their ideas and specific plans to operationalize change. The therapist pays extra attention to "mobilizing change talk," marking the patient's activation or plans to act on their ambivalence (for example: "I might try…"), avoids pressing for a firm commitment, and helps build momentum. The therapist can help their patients set monitoring parameters to assess their progress continually.

Motivational Enhancement Therapy (MET) refers to a specific type of MI as a manualized structured four-session program offering patients personalized risk feedback. MET is frequently used in SUD research trials.

Know This:

1. MI acronyms:
   - **OARS** (a framework of important elements guiding the therapist–patient communication):
     - **O**pen-ended questions encourage further elaboration and consideration
     - **A**ffirmations that promote positive feelings
     - **R**eflections, likely the most important aspect of MI, includes simple reflections (for example: "So you are saying that alcohol is causing a drift in your relationship."), double reflections (for example: "so on the one hand, alcohol helps you cope with stress caused by work, and on the other hand, it is causing a drift in your relationship."), or amplified reflections (for example, after a patient tells you that they enjoy drinking alcohol, you overshoot and respond: "I see, drinking alcohol has been a very positive experience in your life and you have no interest in cutting down.")
     - **S**ummary statements, extend reflections and build momentum or interest in change, redirect patients to more important aspects of their substance use to consider and solidify a commitment to change
   - **DEARS** (an overview of MI principles):
     - **D**evelop discrepancy
     - **E**xpress empathy
     - **A**mplify ambivalence
     - **R**oll with resistance
     - **S**upport self-efficacy
     - **DARN-C** (an overview of change talk in order of intensity and confidence):
   - **D**esire to change
     - **A**bility to change
     - **R**easons for change
     - **N**eed to change
     - **C**ommitment to change

2. Importance scaling can be used in the evoking phase of MI to elicit change talk. The therapist asked the patient to rate the importance of making the change on a scale from 0 to 10 and asked them why they chose that number instead of a lower number.

3. The four MI elements are partnership, acceptance (empathy), evocation, and compassion.

4. The five Rs of MI are relevance, risks, roadblocks, rewards, and repetition. These refer to guiding principles to ensure that any assertion made to the patient is consistent with the desired outcomes.

5. When initially introduced, MI utilized the stages of change as defined by the transtheoretical model of change (TTM) and viewed change as a linear, chronologic process. The third edition of the MI textbook by Miller and Rollnick (2013) presented a different behavioral change perspective. There, it is more fluid than linear. As such, rather than following the TTM stages of change, MI introduced the four stages of treatment: engaging, focusing, evoking, and planning, highlighting how a patient can transition back and forth between stages. However, the board examinations continue to assess the TTM stages of change. We review the TTM stages of change below:
   - Precontemplation: Patients in this stage are not considering change and present with active resistance. The main clinical risk during this stage is dropout from treatment.

- Contemplation: Patients in this stage are ambivalent about changing their behaviors.
- Preparation: Patients in this stage are taking steps toward changing their behaviors and present with increasing confidence in their decision to change.
- Action: Patients in this stage are overtly modifying their behaviors and factors in the environment that support continued substance use. The main clinical risk during this stage is relapse.
- Maintenance: The goals for this stage include sustaining changes, consolidating gains, learning alternative coping strategies, and recognizing triggers.
- Relapse and recycling: This stage is not inevitable. During this stage, patients' main clinical risk is to feel stuck in their old ways. As such, the primary goal of treatment is avoiding becoming stuck and redefining the relapse as an opportunity for further self-improvement.
- Termination: Patients in this stage have reached their ultimate goals and can exit the cycle of change without fear of relapse.

Cognitive Behavioral Therapy

The CBT model in SUD treatment relies on the same fundamental principle that thought processes, emotional responses, and behavioral reactions are interconnected. As adapted for SUD, CBT is based on the Relapse Prevention model by Marlatt (and Gordon) based on social learning theory and operant conditioning principles. The model posits that relapse follows immediate determinants of substance use (such as triggering people, places, and things; coping strategies; or outcome expectancies) and covert antecedents to substance use (factors that indirectly increase the likelihood of a patient using substances, including lifestyle factors and craving). During the course of treatment, the therapist and patient develop a functional analysis framework identifying high-risk antecedents and consequences of their use. Patients practice identifying and avoiding high-risk situations and learn specific coping strategies (including stimulus control and urge-management techniques and relapse road maps)

to enhance the patient's self-efficacy in maintaining sobriety. The therapeutic process utilizes assertiveness training and role-playing. Commonly used coping strategies include distraction, positive thought substitution, and recall of negative consequences.

Know This:

- CBT for SUD focuses on identifying high-risk antecedents and consequences of their use and promotes assertive communications, managing urges and craving.
- CBT is superior to other psychotherapeutic modalities in patients with co-occurring anxiety and SUD.

Contingency Management

For persons with SUD who are actively using, the valuation of substance use can surpass prosocial behaviors (such as going to work, maintaining a healthy lifestyle, caring for one's children). However, the introduction of alternative reinforcers that are valued more than using drugs or alcohol (such as monetary rewards, the fear of serious medical complications, or losing custody of one's children) tips the balance in favor of abstinence and helps promote recovery. CM as therapy involves positive reinforcement by rewarding patients with incentives for achieving their treatment goals such as abstinence. CM is not a stand-alone therapy and is typically used in addition to other therapeutic modalities such as MI or CBT. Using the foundation of operant conditioning, CM seeks to maximize the benefits of abstaining or reducing substance use. Incentives given to patients with nonpositive urine toxicology screens (drug testing, or ethyl-glucuronide for alcohol, or saliva testing for nicotine), including monetary reward or other valuable prizes, serve as alternative reinforcers whose value may supersede that of using drugs or alcohol.

In CM practice, patients with SUD would submit to a urine toxicology test. If they do not test positive for any substance, they get to draw from a bucket of tickets associated with monetary (vouchers or equivalent valuables) prizes. In addition to the positive reinforcement aspect of the incentives, they serve the purpose of lessening the relative impact associated with the initial stages of recovery (including changing habits, losing substance-using peers, and experiencing protracted withdrawal symptoms). The randomness of the rewards further promotes abstinence. The immediacy of the incentive delivery (directly following the nonpositive urine toxicology findings) addresses the immediate reward-seeking behavioral patterns seen in persons with SUD.

Research studies have found CM to be most effective in treating cocaine, methamphetamine, opioid, and cannabis use disorders and in traditionally difficult-to-treat patient groups, such as homeless patients or those with an antisocial personality disorder. However, discontinuation of CM often leads to reductions in abstinence rates (it does not appear that the benefits persist long when incentives are no longer provided). As a result, the maximal lasting benefit is seen in patients who participate in CM for at least 6 months.

Other Psychotherapeutic Modalities

- Twelve-Step Facilitation: TSF is not a 12-step mutual-support group; it is a manualized and structured 12-session approach that aims at promoting the patient's engagement in 12-step mutual-support groups. In TSF, the therapist encourages the patient to participate in 12-step mutual-support groups and guides them through the first four steps. Participation in TSF increases the likelihood that patients with SUD will affiliate with a mutual-support group and reduce their substance use (data supporting its effectiveness in alcohol is strongest).
- Mindfulness-Based Interventions: The goal of treatment is to minimize stress reactivity and develop affect regulation as healthy coping strategies for cravings. This, in turn, supports the patient's awareness and acceptance of their present situations and increases their ability to tolerate stressors and stress states that increase their vulnerability to relapse. One commonly used coping strategy is "urge surfing," which seeks to ground patients in the present and address their tendency to shift their attentional focus away from the present.
- Mindfulness-Based Relapse Prevention: A manualized and structured 8-week program using hybrid mindfulness and CBT approach to relapse prevention. The program focuses on recognizing early relapse triggers and using mindfulness skills to process situational cues and moderate the patient's psychological responses to such cues.
- Community Reinforcement Approach: Multidimensional intervention most effective for alcohol and stimulants commonly combined with CM. The focus is to create a sober living environment valued more than the environment in which the patient actively uses drugs or alcohol. It utilizes positive reinforcement principles and teaches new and healthy coping strategies to promote sobriety.
- Aversion Therapy (or Aversive Conditioning Therapy): This approach is based on classical conditioning theory by associating an unpleasant response with substance use and ultimately creating a negative cognitive and emotional response to the undesirable stimulus (substance use). Aversive stimuli include chemical aversion (such as with disulfiram and alcohol use), electrical shock, mechanical shocks, unpleasant smells or tastes, or negative imagery visualization. Aversion therapy is most effective for alcohol and cannabis use disorders.
- Dialectical Behavioral Therapy (DBT): When adapted to SUD, DBT uses the standard components of DBT with a focus on emotional states associated with abstinence and promoting motivation for change.
- Schema-Focused Therapy: This approach uses a CBT-based intervention to identify maladaptive cognitive schemas from adverse developmental events leading to cognitive distortions associated with the maintenance of substance use.
- Mentalization-Based Therapy: This cognitive-based approach is founded on psychoanalytic and social attachment theory. Mentalization refers to those mental activities that lead patients with SUD to perceive and interpret behavior as intentional (rather than circumstantial) mental states. This allows patients to feel in control of their decision-making processes. Deficits and impairments in mentalization contribute to maladaptive cognitive patterns associated with substance use maintenance.
- Seeking Safety: This cognitive-based approach is used for patients with comorbid SUD and posttraumatic stress disorder. The initial therapeutic

focus is to establish physical and psychological safety as a foundation for recovery.

- Network Therapy: This approach uses the support of a group of family and peers to support patients with SUD in their recovery process.

Know This:

- The Project MATCH study compared CBT, MI (MET), and TSF for patients with alcohol use disorder. Its main finding is that all three psychotherapeutic modalities produced roughly equivalent clinical improvements. Subgroup analysis found that MI was superior for angry patients and those with lower initial motivation. CBT was superior for patients with less severe alcohol use disorder. TSF was superior for patients with little social support for abstinence and more severe alcohol use disorder.
- In adolescents with SUD, family therapy appears to be superior to other psychotherapeutic modalities for SUD treatment.
- Stimulus control refers to modifying the environment to minimize cues that promote relapses and maximize cues that are consistent with recovery.
- Cognitive dissonance describes the mental tension noted when patients hold mutually exclusive beliefs. The tension resulting from such mutually exclusive beliefs affects patients' thoughts and behaviors to reduce that tension.
- Mindfulness skills used in SUD include promoting increased awareness of bodily sensations, acceptance of the craving symptoms, and the uncoupling of cravings from perceived positive reinforcements relating to the reasons one uses a substance (such as self-medicating).

SCREENING, BRIEF INTERVENTION, AND REFERRAL TO TREATMENT

Screening, brief intervention, and referral to treatment (SBIRT) refers to an evidence-based practice to identify, reduce, and prevent maladaptive substance use in primary care or other non-SUD-focused settings. SBIRT serves as a public health initiative to identify persons at risk for developing an SUD or with

an undetected SUD at the primary care level, offering those with less severe substance use simple interventions to address simple substance use problems and refer those with more complex substance use treatment needs to specialized services. SBIRT components include:

- Screening: Using screening questionnaires such as the NIDA single-question screen, AUDIT-C, or DAST (see Chapter 1).
- Brief interventions (BIs): Discussed later.
- Referral to treatment: Patients with more complex substance use or SUD require specialized treatment services.

BIs or early interventions have been developed to address persons with various maladaptive substance use. BIs are meant to be easily integrated within patient consultations in primary care settings. Although there is no overarching definition of what BI is, it generally involves:

- Assessing the quantity, frequency, and severity of substance use, followed by providing the patient with direct feedback on their health and the medico-social impact of their use. The goals of BI are generally to reduce the amount of substance used.
- Establishing mutually agreeable goals to discontinue (typically for tobacco or illicit drugs) or reduce (typically for at-risk alcohol use) substance use.
- Using behavioral modification techniques to support the patient in recognizing triggering cues or situations and developing coping techniques to deal with them.
- Providing patients with reference material on self-help strategies, mutual-help groups, and the problems associated with maladaptive substance use.
- Providing ongoing support.

Evidence supporting BI efficacy is strongest for maladaptive alcohol use. BI is particularly effective with patients with less severe alcohol use problems in which the intervention goal is typically a reduction of alcohol consumption rather than complete abstinence. BI for alcohol is associated with an overall decrease in alcohol use, drinking days, binge drinking, and alcohol-related deaths. The data are mixed on whether BI for alcohol is more effective for men than for women.

The use of BI is also effective in addressing tobacco use, with data supporting asking smokers about their tobacco use at every visit. Studies examining BI for illicit drug use found BI to be ineffective and costly, and as such, BI is not recommended to address the needs of patients with illicit drug use.

Know This:

1. The FRAMES acronym was developed to summarize the goals of BI:
   - **F**eedback (on the personal risk associated with maladaptive substance use).
   - **R**esponsibility (supporting the patient in taking responsibility for the problem).
   - **A**dvice (clear and explicit).
   - **M**enu (menu of options to support the patient in changing their behaviors).
   - **E**mpathy (empathic approach to counseling the change using an MI patient-centered and noncoercive framework).
   - **S**elf-efficacy (supporting the patient's self-efficacy in addressing change).
2. The basic approach for BI with tobacco use is summarized using the five As mnemonic:
   - **A**sk every patient about their tobacco use during every visit.
   - **A**dvise every smoking patient to quit smoking clearly and in an individualized manner.
   - **A**ssess every smoking patient's current willingness to quit.
   - **A**ssist every smoking patient in forming a smoking cessation plan.
   - **A**rrange for pharmacotherapy for tobacco use disorder if appropriate and referrals to specialized care, therapy, or counseling as needed.
3. For tobacco smoking patients who are unable or unwilling to quit, use the five Rs BI approach as an adaptation of the five As:
   - **R**elevance: The intervention should be relevant to a given smoking patient (such as co-morbid health conditions, family, and social circumstances).
   - **R**isks: Collaborate with patients to identify the risks associated with their tobacco use, focusing on their personal circumstances.
   - **R**ewards: Collaborate with patients to identify the rewards they would find in cessation.
   - **R**oadblocks: Collaborate with patients to identify potential roadblocks to discontinuing tobacco use.
   - **R**epetition: Repeat the intervention on every visit.

REFERENCE

Miller, W. R., & Rollnick, S. (2013). *Motivational interviewing: Helping people change* (3rd ed.). Guilford Press.

SUGGESTIONS FOR FURTHER READING

DeLeon, G. (2015). Therapeutic communities. In M. Galanter, H. D. Kleber, & K. T. Brady (Eds.), *The American Psychiatric Publishing textbook of substance abuse treatment* (5th ed.). American Psychiatric Publishing.

Glasner, S., & Drazdowski, T. K. (2019). Evidence-based behavioral treatments for substance use disorders. In I. Danovitch & L. J. Mooney (Eds.), *The assessment and treatment of addiction* (1st ed.). Elsevier.

Matching alcoholism treatments to client heterogeneity: Project MATCH posttreatment drinking outcomes. *Journal of Studies on Alcohol, 58*(1), 7–29.

Nace, E. P. (2018). Twelve-step programs in addiction recovery. In S. Miller, D. Fiellin, R. Rosenthal, & R. Saitz (Eds.), *The ASAM principles of addiction medicine* (6th ed.). Wolters Kluwer.

Tait, R. J., & Hulse, G. K. (2020). Brief and e-health interventions for the treatment of alcohol or other drug addiction. In B. A. Johnson (Ed.), *Addiction medicine: Science and practice* (2nd ed.). Elsevier.

REVIEW QUESTIONS

1. A rapid responder gave a 38-year-old patient naloxone after an opioid overdose from using cocaine laced with fentanyl. He was brought to the emergency room. After being monitored for a couple of hours, he requested to be discharged. The emergency physician expressed concern about the patient's substance use and offered him SUD treatment referrals. The patient declined, stating "I am fine, nothing happened." Using the TTM, which stage of change best represents this patient's state?
   A. Precontemplation
   B. Contemplation
   C. Termination
   D. Relapse and recycling
   E. Maintenance

2. You are seeing a 29-year-old female banker for cocaine use disorder. She tells you: "at first, I used to take cocaine for fun; now I take it to function, to think at work, to concentrate." She would like to address her cocaine use because her firm drug tests employees randomly but fears she will not perform at work. Using the MI framework, what statement would be most helpful to respond?
   A. It sounds like you're using cocaine for the wrong reasons.
   B. Cocaine really makes you perform worse at work. If you really care for your job, you should quit.
   C. It sounds like you are interested in quitting but are worried about how quitting may affect your performance.

   D. It is obvious to both of us that you should not be using cocaine, yet, you've been unable to stop. Why is that?
   E. Do you think you might be using cocaine to deal with depression or anxiety?

3. Which of the following is an accurate application of CM principles for parents trying to ensure that their teenage daughter abstains from marijuana?
   A. Weekly drug screens with gas chromatography–mass spectrometry (GC-MS) confirmation for positive screens.
   B. Restricting cell phone privileges every time they catch her smoking marijuana.
   C. Using a patient-centered approach to help her recognize how marijuana use is affecting her life.
   D. Using point-of-care testing at home three times a week and rewarding her with random gift certificates occasionally when she tests negative.
   E. Using point-of-care testing at home daily and rewarding her with $17 every time she tests negative.

4. Which of the following principles of 12-step–based mutual-support groups is associated with increased rates of continued abstinence?
   A. Surrendering to a higher power.
   B. Commitment to participating in 12-step–based mutual-support groups and to abstinence.
   C. Acknowledging that one is powerless over their substance of choice.
   D. Taking inventory of oneself.
   E. Making a list of all persons one harmed and seeking to make amends.

14

PRACTICE TESTS

1. A 59-year-old man with a 10-year history of gambling disorder and worsening anxiety presents to his monthly appointment; you ask him about his gambling behaviors. His reply is always the same: "I am not giving up my gambling; my brother does it every day of his life and has no issues with it." Which one of the following stages of change best describes this individual's motivational level?
   A. Action
   B. Contemplation
   C. Precontemplation
   D. Maintenance
   E. Preparation

2. A 72-year-old man with leukemia is currently undergoing chemotherapy and is emaciated from weight loss as a result of chemotherapy-related nausea and vomiting. You discuss the use of cannabis-related compounds for his symptoms, but he expresses that he tried smoking cannabis before and disliked the "high." Which of the following compounds is both U.S. Food and Drug Administration (FDA)-approved to treat his chemotherapy-related nausea and would minimize unwanted side effects?
   A. Dronabinol
   B. Nabilone
   C. Rimonabant
   D. Medical marijuana
   E. Cannabidiol (CBD)

3. A 52-year-old woman with severe opioid use disorder (OUD) and intravenous heroin use is referred to your office. The patient tells you that she is interested in being prescribed medication to treat OUD. The patient tells you that her use began 10 years ago when she was prescribed opioid pain medications for chronic and severe back pain. She continued using illicitly obtained opioid pain medication after her physician "cut her off" and ultimately transitioned to heroin use. The patient reports more than seven suicide attempts by intentional opioid overdose but denies any current suicidal thoughts or depression. The patient is hopeful that treatment will improve her condition. During your evaluation, the patient appeared to be in significant distress as a result of opioid withdrawal. What is the most appropriate next step?
   A. This patient should be sent to the psychiatric emergency room for an evaluation and consideration for inpatient hospitalization given her suicide history.
   B. Prescribe clonidine, ibuprofen and loperamide for her withdrawal symptoms and schedule her for a follow-up appointment in one week.
   C. Perform a naloxone challenge test. If no evidence of withdrawal is seen, prescribe oral naltrexone in preparation for starting long-acting injectable naltrexone.
   D. Send a patient to the emergency room to be admitted for a medically supervised opioid detoxification.
   E. Assess the severity of her opioid withdrawal and begin buprenorphine.

4. An 18-year-old man presents for an intake evaluation. He tells you that he has been using heroin and cocaine together by injection for 6 months and admits to sharing needles. During the examination, he mentions that he has been experiencing chest discomfort, low energy, and generalized fatigue. On physical exam, he is febrile, tachycardic, and normotensive. What is the most appropriate next step?
   A. Refer him to a methadone clinic.
   B. Send him to the emergency room.
   C. Obtain laboratory testing for HIV and hepatitis C virus (HCV).
   D. Refer him to a medically supervised inpatient detoxification program.
   E. Begin a buprenorphine induction as soon as he presents with moderate symptoms of opioid withdrawal.

5. A 35-year-old unmarried engineering graduate student presents with complaints of excessive betting on cricket matches for the past 2 years, sad mood, and irritability for the past 12 months. According to his parents, the patient started using methamphetamine with his friends in college. He has been treated with a variety of psychotropic strategies. When you took his treatment history, he mentioned that one treatment was associated with increased craving independent of how much methamphetamine he was using. Which of the following medications has been found to have a paradoxical effect on patients with methamphetamine use disorder?
   A. Naltrexone
   B. Thorazine
   C. Bupropion
   D. Topiramate
   E. Aripiprazole

6. A dental school dean calls your office expressing concerns about a senior student. According to the dean, the student was complaining of weakness, loss of balance, and problems breathing. Which of the following substances is the student most likely abusing?
   A. Morphine sulfate
   B. Mescaline
   C. Nitrous oxide

   D. Epinephrine
   E. Oleoresin

7. A 16-year-old patient is brought to the emergency room by his mother due to having aggression and confusion at school. Per his mother, he frequently goes to raves and works as a disc jockey 4 nights a week. The neurotoxicity associated with the drug he is most likely abusing is related to a deficit in which following neurotransmitters?
   A. Dopamine
   B. Leptin
   C. γ-Aminobutyric acid (GABA)
   D. Serotonin
   E. Choline

8. A 50-year-old man with alcohol use disorder who works in construction with few social supports presents to the emergency room after suffering a fall. He was intoxicated and is referred to you for treatment of alcohol use disorder. He expresses a willingness to stop drinking but does not feel confident that he will achieve this because everyone in his social network drinks alcohol. According to Project MATCH results, which of the following psychosocial interventions would be best suited for this patient?
   A. Motivational enhancement therapy (MET)
   B. Cognitive behavioral therapy (CBT)
   C. Twelve-step facilitation (TSF)
   D. Relapse prevention
   E. Supportive psychotherapy

9. According to the results of the Combined Pharmacotherapies and Behavioral Interventions (COMBINE) study, which of the following medications performed best in promoting abstinence from alcohol by the end of the treatment period?
   A. Acamprosate
   B. Naltrexone
   C. Disulfiram
   D. Gabapentin
   E. Topiramate

10. Disulfiram is a medication that is most widely known as a treatment for alcohol use disorder, causing an aversive reaction in the presence of any alcohol. However, disulfiram has also been studied for other conditions, including cocaine

use disorder. Which of the following mechanisms is most relevant to disulfiram's use in treating cocaine use disorder?

A. Inhibition of aldehyde dehydrogenase
B. Inhibition of alcohol dehydrogenase
C. Disulfiram's metabolite, ditiocarb, interferes with the ubiquitin-proteasome system
D. Inhibition of monoamine oxidase
E. Inhibition of dopamine-beta-hydroxylase

11. What is the theoretical basis of CBT's psychological theory as it applies to the treatment of SUD?

A. CBT involves processing unconscious drives and understanding defense mechanisms as a tool sobriety skill.
B. CBT is a collaborative and client-centered approach that aims at exploring and resolving patients' ambivalence about the role of substances in their life in a nonconfrontational approach.
C. CBT conceptualizes the interconnections between thought processes, emotional responses, and behaviors reactions in drug and alcohol use.
D. CBT utilizes alternative reinforcers that are valued more than using drugs or alcohol in order to tip the balance in favor of abstinence and promote recovery.
E. CBT aims to minimize stress reactivity and develop affect regulation as healthy coping strategies for cravings.

12. A 42-year-old woman presents to your office after her partner found her disoriented at home. On examination, she is bradycardic, in respiratory distress and disoriented. She has been treated for pain after she injured her back in a car accident over a year ago. According to her partner, she has been increasing her dose and buying extra pills from a friend. What should be administered to this patient so that her symptoms do not worsen?

A. Clonidine
B. Guanfacine
C. Naloxone
D. Naltrexone
E. Methadone

13. A 27-year-old college student is brought to the emergency room following an accidental opioid overdose. He is given naloxone and is held for a few hours to stabilize in the emergency room. The treating physician counseled this patient about the risks associated with drug use, recommended SUD treatment, and offered referral options. The patient was appreciative of the treatments he received in the emergency room but declined the referrals, stating that his drug use is rare and that he will never overdose again. Based on the transtheoretical model of change, what "stage of change" is this patient?

A. Precontemplation.
B. Contemplation.
C. Preparation
D. Action
E. Maintenance

14. A 19-year-old man with OUD presents to your office for follow-up. During your appointment, you help the patient plan for high-risk situations and build avoidance skills to reduce the likelihood of relapse after 2 months of sobriety. As his physician, you are utilizing which of the following therapy modalities?

A. MET
B. CBT
C. Dialectical behavioral therapy
D. TSF
E. Supportive therapy

15. A 16-year-old female high school sophomore presents to your office with her mother. You have noticed a drastic change in her appearance and behavior, in addition to the development of significant tooth decay. The mother expressed that she has not been herself, and you wonder about methamphetamine use. Which of the following compounds holds promise as a treatment for methamphetamine use disorder?

A. Paroxetine
B. Aripiprazole
C. Bupropion
D. Depakote
E. Carbamazepine

16. Flumazenil can reverse benzodiazepine and non-benzodiazepine hypnotic (Z-drug) overdose, but not barbiturate or alcohol poisoning. Which of the following best explains its selective therapeutic effect?
    A. Flumazenil binds directly onto benzodiazepines and Z-drugs and renders them inactive.
    B. Flumazenil binds to the benzodiazepine-binding site on the GABA-A receptor.
    C. Flumazenil binds to the alpha-4 and -6 subunits of the GABA-A receptor.
    D. Flumazenil binds to the GABA-B receptor.
    E. Flumazenil noncompetitively inhibits the GABA-A receptor.

17. Which of the following structures is delta-9-tetrahydrocannabinol?

18. Over the past several years, a 10-year-old boy with Lennox-Gastaut syndrome has tried multiple antiepileptic medications but has continued to have daily poorly controlled seizures. Which of the following compounds was recently FDA-approved for the treatment of seizures in Lennox-Gastaut syndrome?
    A. Dronabinol
    B. Nabilone
    C. Rimonabant
    D. Medical marijuana
    E. CBD

19. According to a recent study out of Colorado, cannabis-related emergency room visits were found to have increased threefold following marijuana legalization. A disproportionately large number of these visits was because of the consumption of cannabis edibles, despite the fact that edibles make up only a tiny fraction of cannabis purchases in the state. Which of the following best explains why edibles are responsible for a disproportionately large number of cannabis-related emergency room visits compared to the smoked route of administration?
    A. Edibles are frequently laced with other substances.
    B. Edibles are more likely to cause gastrointestinal irritation and bleeding.
    C. Cannabis consumed via the oral route has higher bioavailability.
    D. Cannabis consumed via the oral route has lower bioavailability.
    E. The onset of action of edibles is longer and harder to predict.

20. A 31-year-old college student with a history of stimulant use disorder presents to the emergency department with recurrent diarrhea and fever. A urine drug screening (UDS) test is positive for cocaine, and complete blood count shows an increased white blood cell count but negative blood cultures. The patient's fever resolves without the use of antibiotics. Use of cocaine adulterated with which of the following substances is most likely to explain this patient's presentation?
    A. Lansoprazole
    B. Levamisole
    C. Lamotrigine
    D. Levamisole
    E. Loperamide

21. The patient in Question 20 decided to start treatment for cocaine use disorder. Which of the following medications has the most evidence of possible benefit for increasing rates of abstinence in cocaine use disorder?
    A. Duloxetine
    B. Naltrexone
    C. Risperidone
    D. Topiramate
    E. Sertraline

22. A 41-year-old White man presents into your office complaining of financial difficulties. He has been preoccupied with getting more gambling money and needing to gamble with increasing amounts of money to get the same "reaction." He is asking you for "something" to decrease his urges. Which of the following medications is most appropriate for addressing the patient's concerns?
    A. Propranolol
    B. Pregabalin
    C. Benzoylmethylecgonine
    D. Buprenorphine
    E. Naltrexone

23. Which of the following best explains why cannabis is legally available in many U.S. states while being illegal under U.S. federal law?
    A. Cannabis is categorized as schedule I, but the judicial branch of the federal government issued a memorandum indicating the states would not be prosecuted for having a state-legal cannabis enterprise.
    B. Cannabis is categorized as schedule I but is permissible on a state-by-state basis if the state law conflicts with federal law in favor of legalizing marijuana.
    C. Cannabis was rescheduled from schedule I to schedule II, putting it in the same category as substances considered to have medical use but with high abuse potential, such as oxycodone and morphine.
    D. Cannabis was rescheduled from schedule I to schedule III, putting it in the same category as substances considered to have medical use but moderate or low abuse potential, such as buprenorphine.
    E. Cannabis was rescheduled from schedule I to schedule IV, putting it in the same category as substances considered to have medical use but lower abuse potential compared with schedule III, such as the benzodiazepines.

24. A 41-year-old man was recently hired as a federal employee. He has a history of depression, gastric reflux disease, and low back pain, for which he takes bupropion, pantoprazole, and ibuprofen. As part of his onboarding process, he underwent a routine physical and UDS test. His UDS test returns positive for THC and is confirmed by gas chromatography–mass spectrometry (GC-MS). He contests these results and states that his brother was smoking cannabis in his apartment 2 days before he submitted a sample, although he himself does not smoke cannabis. He also questions whether the result may be a false-positive result, as he takes several medications. Which of the following is most accurate regarding his UDS test result?
    A. Passive inhalation of cannabis smoke likely resulted in a positive test.
    B. It is likely a false positive from taking pantoprazole.
    C. It is likely a false positive from taking ibuprofen.
    D. It is likely a false positive from taking bupropion.
    E. Passive inhalation of cannabis smoke is unlikely to result in a positive test.

25. A 15-year-old girl is brought to the emergency room by her parents. At her friend's birthday party, she reportedly ate an entire bag of gummy bears, not knowing that they were cannabis edibles. On presentation, she is agitated, hallucinating, and keeps repeating that she is going to die. She is tachycardic and hypertensive but not in respiratory distress, and her oxygen saturation is normal. Which of the following best accounts for why cannabis overdose does not lead to respiratory depression?
    A. CB1 receptors are expressed in very low density in the brainstem.
    B. CB1 receptors are expressed in very high density in the hippocampus.
    C. CB2 receptors are expressed in very high density in the hippocampus.
    D. CB2 receptors are expressed in very low density in the brainstem.
    E. Endocannabinoids effectively regulate respiratory drive even in the presence of exogenous cannabinoids.

26. A 34-year-old man with severe OUD and comorbid major depressive disorder comes into the clinic for evaluation and consideration for treatment with

buprenorphine. The patient tells you that he has been injecting heroin at least four times daily on and off for the past 15 years. He acknowledges using illicitly obtained buprenorphine on multiple occasions to treat his OUD. During your evaluation, the patient admits that his father died of an opioid overdose 1 month ago, and as a result, he has been feeling very depressed. He adds that 1 month ago, he attempted suicide by intentionally overdosing on heroin. Which of the following is the most appropriate next step of this evaluation?

A. Order stat laboratory tests for HIV and HCV.

B. Assess the severity of the patient's depression and current suicidal thoughts.

C. Inform the patient that he is not eligible for treatment with buprenorphine because he has a history of obtaining it from illicit sources.

D. Inform the patient that he is not eligible for treatment with buprenorphine because of his recent suicide attempt.

E. Prescribe fluoxetine.

27. A 48-year-old man is currently admitted to inpatient rehabilitation for sedative/hypnotic (benzodiazepine) and alcohol use disorder. He completed detoxification 1 month ago and is complaining of persistent depressed mood, poor appetite, and insomnia. Which of the following would be the next best step in his treatment?

A. Initiate naltrexone for treatment of prolonged alcohol withdrawal symptoms.

B. Initiate acamprosate for treatment of prolonged alcohol withdrawal symptoms.

C. Readmit to detoxification owning to persistent withdrawal symptoms.

D. Perform a psychiatric evaluation for co-occurring psychiatric disorders.

E. Reassure the patient that these symptoms will likely self-resolve without any intervention.

28. A 28-year-old man with a generalized anxiety disorder on venlafaxine 225 mg daily, lorazepam 0.5 mg twice a day, and enrolled in CBT presents for a follow-up appointment. He has no other medical problems. His mother was recently diagnosed with cancer 2 months ago. Since then, he has increased his lorazepam dose on several occasions due to an increase in his anxiety. During your last visit, he was frustrated that you refused to increase his lorazepam dose. Which of the following is most accurate regarding his management?

A. The patient should be tapered off lorazepam due to evidence that he has developed a substance use disorder.

B. The patient should be tapered off lorazepam due to evidence that it is ineffective for his anxiety disorder.

C. The patient's current dose of lorazepam may be too low to adequately treat his anxiety disorder.

D. The patient's dose of lorazepam should be left as is, and he should be encouraged to address these issues in therapy.

E. The patient should be referred to the hospital for an inpatient psychiatric hospitalization.

29. A 57-year-old White man is engaged in psychotherapy to address the high cost of his gambling behavior. During therapy, he began understanding how each visit to the casino and time spent with people on the "tables" briefly improves his mood. This behavioral pattern can be best explained by which of the following learning theories?

A. Phobias of objects theories

B. Operant conditioning

C. Classical conditioning

D. Albert experiment

E. Reductionism

30. Which of the following is true regarding sex differences in alcohol use disorder?

A. Women have a higher prevalence of alcohol use disorder.

B. Women with alcohol use disorder have a higher risk of negative medical sequelae.

C. Women have a higher prevalence of binge drinking.

D. Women are more likely to begin drinking at an earlier age.

E. Women are less likely to have a co-occurring psychiatric disorder.

31. A 37-year-old transgender woman presents to treatment for OUD. During your session, she shares that what makes it hard to quit is that

using heroin "is the best feeling in the world." She states that nothing she has experienced can match the feeling of using heroin. Which two brain regions are most fundamental in mediating the experience she is describing?

A. Ventral tegmental area (VTA), nucleus accumbens (NAc)
B. NAc, prefrontal cortex
C. VTA, prefrontal cortex
D. Amygdala, prefrontal cortex
E. Amygdala, NAc

32. A 59-year-old man with alcohol use disorder finds that when he stops using alcohol, he feels anxious, irritable, and markedly dysphoric. Which of the following compounds is diminished in the amygdala during withdrawal states, leading to his symptoms?

A. Dynorphin
B. Norepinephrine
C. Neuropeptide Y
D. Corticotrophin-releasing factor (CRF)
E. cAMP response element-binding protein (CREB)

33. A 55-year-old man with a history of alcohol use disorder has been in remission for the past 20 years. He attends Alcoholics Anonymous (AA) meetings weekly and maintains contact with his sponsor. After his wife unexpectedly passes away, he becomes distraught and grief-stricken, and relapses to heavy alcohol use. Which of the following brain regions and neurocircuitry is most important in mediating his reinstatement to alcohol use?

A. Activation of corticotropin-releasing factor and norepinephrine in the amygdala and VTA
B. Activation of glutamatergic circuits involving the medial prefrontal cortex and ventral striatum
C. Basolateral amygdala with feed-forward inhibition of the prelimbic prefrontal cortex
D. Activation of dopaminergic cells in the VTA that project to the NAc
E. Inhibition of GABA-ergic interneurons in the VTA, which indirectly increases dopaminergic neurotransmission in the NAc

34. A 54-year-old man with a long history of depression, anxiety, and excessive alcohol use presents to your office reporting poor mood and anxiety symptoms in the context of ongoing drinking. The patient tells you that he is not interested in cutting down on the drinking because: "Honestly, I know it's bad, but it's the only thing that helps when I'm feeling anxious." Which of the following statements is consistent with a motivational interviewing approach?

A. A lot of people do not understand the relationship between alcohol and mood or anxiety disorder. Let me give you the facts.
B. Let's talk about the emotional states you are in right before you start drinking.
C. I will make you a deal. If you successfully quit drinking, I will consider prescribing you lorazepam to manage your drinking.
D. It is obvious to me that you were drinking is worsening your mood and anxiety symptoms. Let's talk about your past traumatic experiences that cause you to act in such self-destructive ways.
E. It sounds like you are worried that your anxiety will worsen if you stop drinking while at the same time recognizing the need to address your alcohol use.

35. A family would like to institute a recovery plan to help their teenage daughter discontinue marijuana use. Which of the following approaches is most consistent with contingency management (CM) principles?

A. Providing her with ample psychoeducation about the negative long-term consequences of marijuana use
B. Helping her recognize distorted thoughts and negative emotions that precede her marijuana use
C. Weekly drug testing at the nearest laboratory and grounding her any time she tests positive for marijuana
D. Weekly drug testing at the nearest laboratory and rewarding her with money any time she tests negative for marijuana
E. Weekly drug testing at home and rewarding her with money any time she tests negative for marijuana

36. Administration of which neuropeptide has been found to modulate the drug-seeking behavior for methamphetamines?
    A. Testosterone
    B. Estrogen
    C. Tyrosine
    D. Oxytocin
    E. Phentermine

37. A 67-year-old patient with a long history of gastrointestinal adhesions and chronic renal disease presents to the emergency room with stomach pain. The patient was given medication for pain. You noticed that he started having a seizure minutes later. Which of the following opioid analgesic metabolites could have caused this patient presentation?
    A. 6-ß-naltrexone metabolite
    B. Norpethidine
    C. Codeine-6-glucuronide
    D. Morphine-3-glucuronide
    E. 6-Acetylmorphine

38. Substance use can alter gene expression through cellular signaling pathways that change the expression of transcription factors. Which of the following transcription factors increases rapidly in the NAc with cocaine use and leads to dynorphin upregulation?
    A. Delta-FosB
    B. Neuropeptide Y
    C. CREB
    D. Myocyte-enhancing factor-2
    E. Nuclear Factor κB

39. Therapeutic communities (TC) are a type of residential treatment facility that is traditionally longer term (typically 6–12 months) and utilizes every aspect of the residential community as a treatment method and means to provide services. What does "residential community as a treatment method" mean?
    A. Having all residents of the TC living in the same building is the only way to get them to participate in group therapy sessions.
    B. Persons with SUD learn to utilize the social activities and chores to model change and rely on their new community to practice cog-

nitive and behavioral changes conducive to change and recovery.
    C. The TC staff are neutral experts in SUD.
    D. The daily social activities and chores are an integral part of the TC and play an important treatment role. TCs that incorporate gardening and dishwashing have better outcomes than those that do not.
    E. TCs are only effective for persons with SUD who are not homeless because the residential aspect of the program would be ineffective for those who are homeless.

40. The police bring a male–female couple in their 20s with methamphetamine intoxication to the emergency room. The woman's mother provides a history that the couple has been smoking methamphetamine for close to 2 years. Which of the following is most accurate regarding the gender differences in methamphetamine use and response to treatment?
    A. Women show higher dropout rates and more use during treatment than men.
    B. The average age of initiating methamphetamine use among men is 25 years old.
    C. Women initiate methamphetamine use at later ages compared to men.
    D. Men tend to have more severe methamphetamine use than females.
    E. Men show higher dropout rates and more use during treatment than women.

41. A 23-year-old woman with methamphetamine use disorder presents to the emergency room and is agitated, aggressive, and reporting visual and auditory hallucinations. She was admitted to the medical floor for observation and treatment. After 70 hours of admission, the patient becomes more restless, with vital signs showing heart rate of 110 and a blood pressure of 158/90 mm Hg. Which of the following diagnoses is most likely to account for her change in clinical status?
    A. Alcohol withdrawal
    B. Amphetamine-induced psychosis
    C. Benzodiazepine withdrawal
    D. Lithium intoxication
    E. Manic episode

42. A 33-year-old man was brought to urgent care by his girlfriend. On examination, his temperature is 104°F, heart rate is 110 beats per minute, blood pressure is 154/90 mm Hg, and his physical examination is notable for tachypnea and muscle rigidity. He has no significant medical or surgical history. He is started on supplemental oxygen via nasal cannula, and he dies 1 hour later. In this case, methamphetamine could have caused his death by which complication?

    A. Weight gain
    B. Hypotension
    C. Hyperthermia
    D. Hypervolemia
    E. Anorexia

43. A 34-year-old woman with a history of borderline personality disorder, generalized anxiety disorder, and tobacco use disorder presents to your office for psychiatric evaluation owning to recent events causing overwhelming anxiety. She is requesting lorazepam. She has made two-lifetime suicide attempts and has multiple prior psychiatric hospitalizations. She is currently taking lamotrigine, fluoxetine, and trazodone. Which of the following is essential in your consideration to prescribe or not prescribe a benzodiazepine?

    A. Benzodiazepines increase the odds of a future suicide attempt.
    B. Prescription of a benzodiazepine is contraindicated because she already has an SUD.
    C. Benzodiazepines are the most effective treatments for generalized anxiety disorder.
    D. Lorazepam has an adverse drug interaction with one of the medications she is currently prescribed.
    E. Patients who come to your office requesting any specific medication are generally drug-seeking.

44. A 35-year-old woman with a history of insomnia and no other medical problems presents to her primary care doctor. After multiple medication trials with noncontrolled medications, her primary care doctor prescribes zolpidem 10 mg to take at night. She begins taking it as directed, and several days later, she crashes her vehicle into a parked car while driving to work in the morning. Which of the following is true regarding this incident?

    A. The PCP should have prescribed a short-acting benzodiazepine instead of zolpidem.
    B. The patient should have been started on long-acting zolpidem instead of regular zolpidem.
    C. The patient have been counseled that driving following zolpidem use in the night prior is not recommended.
    D. The patient most likely co-ingested zolpidem with another substance such as alcohol, as appropriate use of zolpidem rarely results in adverse events.
    E. The patient was started on higher than the recommended dose of zolpidem.

45. Which of the following is true regarding benzodiazepine-related overdose deaths?

    A. Benzodiazepine overdose deaths have been on the decline over the past two decades in the United States.
    B. Alcohol is involved in the majority of benzodiazepine overdose deaths.
    C. Opioids are involved in the majority of benzodiazepine overdose deaths.
    D. Benzodiazepines are involved in the majority of opioid overdose deaths.
    E. Most benzodiazepine overdose deaths occur with benzodiazepines as the sole substance.

46. A 55-year-old man with a generalized anxiety disorder has been on clonazepam 1 mg three times daily for the past 15 years. He wishes to taper off owning to concerns about his long-term cognitive performance. When he tried to stop on his own before, he experienced intolerable anxiety and insomnia. Which of the following is the best strategy for helping him taper off this medication?

    A. Initiate an antiepileptic such as valproic acid or carbamazepine, then taper clonazepam over the course of days.
    B. Perform a taper with clonazepam over the course of months.
    C. Transition the patient to diazepam and taper over the course of days.

D. Transition the patient to diazepam and taper over the course of months.

E. Recommend that he be admitted to in-patient detoxification due to his previous outpatient failure.

47. A 42-year-old woman is brought to the emergency room by emergency medical services for chest pain and dyspnea. ST depressions are seen on electrocardiogram. The patient admits to using cocaine regularly, including snorting 1 g of cocaine on the day of admission. Assuming that her drug use played a causal role in her current presentation, what is the physiological mechanism of cocaine-induced ischemia?

A. Increased cardiac workload and systemic vascular resistance

B. Dilated cardiomyopathy

C. Superficial venous thrombosis

D. Severe hypotension following a vasovagal episode

E. Coronary thromboembolism

48. A 24-year-old man with a history of opioid and nicotine use disorder is admitted to the observation unit after having a witnessed seizure. He smokes two packs of cigarettes daily, appears irritable and is asking to leave the hospital so that he can smoke. Which intervention can help decrease this patient's irritability and reduce his nicotine cravings while admitted?

A. Start bupropion

B. Smoking cessation counseling

C. Start clonidine

D. Start nicotine replacement therapy (NRT)

E. Start varenicline

49. Which of the following is true of AA?

A. You have to be sober in order to participate in AA. Members who relapse are not allowed back into the meetings until they have been sober for at least 14 days.

B. AA has no dogma, theology, or creed.

C. People with alcohol use disorder are not responsible for their behavior because a higher power guides their decisions.

D. Commitment to AA and to abstinence is not important. As long as the person is able to get through 90 meetings in 90 days, the prognosis to achieve and maintain abstinence is high.

E. One does not need to be religious to benefit from AA; however, religious AA members tend to do better in long-term studies.

50. Which of the following scenarios is most likely to benefit from screening, brief intervention, and referral to treatment (SBIRT)?

A. A 43-year-old banker who has been drinking a bottle of wine daily for the past 6 months in the context of increased stress at work.

B. A homeless patient with schizophrenia and OUD who injects heroin.

C. A 67-year-old man with tobacco use disorder.

D. The 42-year-old athlete who has been using illicitly obtained opioids to perform in his games despite his ankle injury.

E. A 27-year-old man who needs to smoke methamphetamine to be disinhibited and perform sexually.

BONUS QUESTION

51. A 37-year-old patient with a long history of schizoaffective disorder has been treated with multiple medications, which he reports have been ineffective. He has been hospitalized twice in the last year for psychosis. The patient is smoking close to two packs a day and appears motivated to stop during this admission. Smoking in this patient would have a significant effect on which of the following medication plasma levels?

A. Quetiapine

B. Risperidone

C. Zotepine

D. Clozapine

E. Ziprasidone

BLOCK 2

1. Multiple psychotherapeutic approaches have been found to be effective in treating SUDs. Which of the following statements is accurate?
   A. As applied to SUD, CBT aims to establish a functional analysis framework identifying high-risk antecedents and consequences of their use.
   B. Mindfulness-based approaches involve establishing discrepancies between behaviors, values, and consequences.
   C. Motivational interviewing is not a stand-alone therapy and is typically used in addition to other therapeutic modalities.
   D. TSF describes the psychotherapeutic benefits patients describe after attending AA meetings.
   E. Mentalization-based therapy uses the support of a group of family and peers to support patients with SUD in their recovery process.

2. A 25-year-old woman of East Asian descent reports experiencing facial redness, nausea, and discomfort when she consumes even small amounts of alcohol. Her reaction is likely due to a genetic variant in the enzyme _____ that metabolizes _____ more slowly.
   A. ALDH; acetate
   B. ADH; acetate
   C. ALDH; acetaldehyde
   D. ADH; acetaldehyde
   E. ADH; ethylene glycol

3. Approximately which of the following percentages of people can be expected to meet criteria for a methamphetamine use disorder in the United States?
   A. 3%
   B. 1%
   C. Less than 0.5%
   D. Between 0.5% and 1%
   E. 5%

4. A 26-year-old man with a history of low back pain and obesity has been a daily cannabis user since high school. In the past month, he has increased his cannabis use and has been vaping high-potency cannabis and smoking several joints per day. He presents to the emergency room because of severe nausea and repeated vomiting for the past 2 weeks. He undergoes a full workup, which shows acute renal failure from dehydration but is otherwise negative. Which of the following is most accurate regarding his likely condition?
   A. It is uncommon in individuals who have been long-term daily users of cannabis.
   B. The majority of people presenting to the emergency room with this condition are women.
   C. Ondansetron can provide effective symptomatic relief.
   D. Capsaicin can provide effective symptomatic relief.
   E. Cold baths can provide effective symptomatic relief.

5. Which of the following compounds is an endogenous ligand for the CB1 receptor?
   A. Dynorphin
   B. Enkephalin
   C. CBD
   D. Anandamide
   E. Neuropeptide Y

6. A 21-year-old man with a history of depression and daily cannabis use for the past year has recently escalated his cannabis use over the past month and is now smoking several blunts a day. During his last appointment with his psychiatrist, he reported that he often feels uncomfortable and paranoid on the subway and hears people talking about him and calling him derogatory names. In the context of cannabis use, specific polymorphisms in which of the following genes increases the likelihood of experiencing symptoms such as those described by the patient?
   A. AKT1
   B. ADH2
   C. CNR1
   D. FAAH
   E. OPRM1

7. Which of the following best describes the differences between *Cannabis indica* and *Cannabis sativa*?
   A. The male plants of *C. indica* have greater THC content than the female plants.
   B. *C. indica* is typically grown by farmers for hemp fiber and has negligible THC content.
   C. *C. indica* has a higher ratio of CBD to THC.
   D. *C. indica* is federally legal in the United States.
   E. *C. indica* has the highest cannabis potency in the leaves and stems and not the flowering tops.

8. A 35-year-old woman with no significant medical problems has been vaping both nicotine and THC products for the past 3 years. She began experiencing progressive dyspnea, cough, and pleuritic chest pain over the course of a month. Upon presentation to the emergency room, her oxygen saturation was 85% and chest CT showed ground glass opacities in her lungs bilaterally. Workup for infectious etiologies was negative. She is admitted to the intensive care unit and treated with prednisone with significant improvement. Which of the following was most likely responsible for her condition?
   A. Carbon monoxide in THC aerosol
   B. Carbon monoxide in nicotine aerosol
   C. Vitamin E acetate (VEA) in THC cartridges
   D. VEA in nicotine cartridges
   E. Propylene glycol in THC cartridges

9. A 27-year-old woman with alcohol use disorder and a history of cocaine and heroin use by injection is referred to your methadone clinic. On methadone induction, she discontinues all illicit opioid use but continues to drink alcohol excessively and inject cocaine. Laboratory testing reveals that she is HIV positive. When is the most appropriate time for her to begin treatment for HIV using highly active antiretroviral treatment (HAART)?
   A. Only if she develops Kaposi sarcoma
   B. Only if she just continues all injection drug use
   C. Only if she discontinues all alcohol use
   D. When her CD4 count is less than 200
   E. Immediately

10. A 34-year-old woman is brought in by ambulance to the emergency department with a suspected overdose. She is unresponsive, cyanotic, and bradypneic. On examination, her skin is cold and her pupils are constricted. Paramedics tried using 4 mg of intranasal naloxone with no response. An overdose of which of the following substances is the most likely cause of her presentation?
    A. Acetaminophen
    B. Buprenorphine
    C. Doxepin
    D. Fentanyl
    E. Clonazepam

11. A methadone program has tabulated the methadone doses of all of the patients in the clinic with OUD. What is the right measure to estimate how much scores vary from the mean value?
    A. Median
    B. Mode
    C. Standard deviation
    D. Standard error
    E. Range

12. An 18-year-old pregnant woman presents to the clinic for a prenatal checkup. She is enrolled in a methadone maintenance program for OUD. Which of the following statements best explains the prevalence of psychiatric disorders among pregnant women with OUD?
    A. Anxiety disorders are the most common psychiatric disorders seen in this group.
    B. Mood disorders are the most common psychiatric disorders seen in this group.
    C. Pregnant women with an OUD do not suffer from mood disorders.
    D. Pregnant women with an OUD do not suffer from anxiety disorders.
    E. Schizophrenia is the most common psychiatric disorder seen in this group.

13. A methadone clinic wants to estimate how many patients are receiving false-positive results on urine toxicology screens for illicit opioids. What statistical measure should you use?
    A. Sensitivity
    B. Positive predictive value
    C. Specificity

D. Negative predictive value

E. Efficacy

14. A 45-year-old man with a history of alcohol and cocaine use disorder and recent cocaine and alcohol relapse presents to your clinic with increased heart rate, confusion, and euphoria. His last use of cocaine was over 3 hours ago. What compound is most responsible for his presentation?

A. Formation of cocaethylene

B. Formation of 2-Ethylidene-1,5-dimethyl-3,3-diphenyl pyrrolidine

C. Formation of ecgonine methyl ester

D. Formation of diacetylmorphine

E. Formation of catecholamines

15. An antagonist of the noradrenergic alpha-2 receptor and the 5-HT2A/C and 5-HT3 receptors has demonstrated efficacy in reducing different drugs' rewarding effect. What medication has been shown to have these antiaddictive properties?

A. Fluoxetine

B. Cannabis

C. Glutamate

D. Mirtazapine

E. Bupropion

16. What is the most common substance use disorder in the United States?

A. Alcohol use disorder

B. Tobacco use disorder

C. Stimulant use disorder

D. Cannabis use disorder

E. Opioid use disorder

17. Genetic polymorphisms in which of the following genes is believed to moderate the effect of naltrexone in patients with alcohol use disorder?

A. AUTS2

B. SLC6A4

C. OPRM1

D. CYP2A6

E. AKT1

18. A 59-year-old man with opioid and alcohol use disorder presents to the clinic. He has been treated with methadone in an opioid treatment program and has maintained abstinence from heroin for 10 years. However, he recently relapsed on alcohol and has been struggling to maintain abstinence. You are reviewing pharmacologic options for alcohol use disorder. He tells you that several years ago, his primary care provider prescribed a medication whose name he cannot remember and that he experienced a severe "allergic reaction." He reports that about half an hour after taking the first dose, he experienced severe nausea, vomiting, diarrhea, muscle, and abdominal cramps. He was taken to the emergency room by ambulance and was instructed not to continue taking this medication. He says he was not drinking at the time this occurred. Which medication did he most likely take?

A. Disulfiram

B. Naltrexone

C. Gabapentin

D. Baclofen

E. Acamprosate

19. A 56-year-old woman with severe arthritis and OUD comes to the office for a follow-up examination. The use of various conventional nonsteroidal antiinflammatory drugs has been ineffective. She tells you that she restarted using oxycodone 1 week ago after 7 months of sobriety. What type of intervention focuses on developing skills to manage factors that influence relapse?

A. MET

B. Behavioral couples therapy

C. CBT

D. Contingency management

E. Alcoholics Anonymous

20. A 37-year-old man is admitted to the hospital 35 minutes after being involved in a motor vehicle accident. Physical examination shows a slow response to stimuli. Neurologic examination shows no other abnormalities. A skull x-ray shows a linear, nondepressed basal skull fracture. His urine toxicology screen was positive for benzoylecgonine. What type of drug was the patient abusing before the car accident?

A. Amphetamine

B. Crack

C. Bath salts

D. Heroin

E. Lorazepam

21. Based on animal models involving opioid self-administration, which one of the following statements is true regarding the reinforcing effects of opioids?
    A. The stress responsive hypothalamic pituitary adrenal axis has been implicated.
    B. Patients experience hypocortisolemia or other disturbances of the hypothalamic–pituitary–adrenal system.
    C. Opioids have a significant impact on reinforcement mechanisms in the VTA.
    D. Contributions to reward focused on the serotonergic projection to the VTA.
    E. No disturbances of the hypothalamic–pituitary–adrenal system have been reported.

22. A 19-year-old woman with a 16-month history of OUD and hepatitis C delivered her second child prematurely and presents to your office. At the time of delivery, she received 30 mg of methadone. She was negative for HIV. There were no complications during delivery. She is interested in breastfeeding her newborn and is seeking your advice. What will you advise this patient to do?
    A. She should not breastfeed immediately.
    B. She should not be recommended to use methadone.
    C. She should start breastfeeding immediately; the benefits outweigh the risks.
    D. She should be started on naltrexone.
    E. She should wait at least 6 months to breastfeed.

23. A 21-year-old woman is brought to urgent care with heart palpitations, dilated pupils, and chest pain, which started approximately 30 minutes ago while watching the Super Bowl game at a friend's house. She appears guarded and detached from her surroundings. Her urine drug screen is negative, except for cannabinoids. Which one of the following diagnoses would be the most appropriate for this patient at this time?
    A. Cocaine-induced anxiety
    B. Alcohol withdrawal
    C. PCP syndrome
    D. Cannabis-induced anxiety
    E. Alcohol intoxication

24. A 31-year-old man is brought to urgent care by his partner owning to increased paranoia and decreased appetite. On physical examination, his pupils are dilated, and he appears suspicious. His partner reports that he was recently diagnosed with adult attention-deficit disorder and was prescribed amphetamine for it. Which one of the following is the most appropriate treatment for an amphetamine overdose?
    A. Bicarbonate
    B. Ammonium chloride
    C. Atropine
    D. Naltrexone
    E. Flumazenil

25. A 43-year-old man with a history of diabetes and tobacco use comes to the clinic with the desire to quit smoking. He has tried to stop on his own but continues to smoke and experiences strong nicotine cravings. What intervention has demonstrated a superior efficacy in smoking cessation?
    A. Recommend bupropion only
    B. Recommend varenicline and behavioral modification
    C. Recommend NRT only
    D. Behavioral modification only
    E. Recommend mirtazapine

26. A 31-year-old man and his wife have become increasingly distant because of her disappointment and hurt over his online pornography use. They have now experienced numerous financial consequences because he has reached the credit limit of two of their credit cards paying for pornography. He is not sleeping well, and it has been hard for him to go to work in the morning. Which medications have demonstrated efficacy in the treatment of sexual addiction?
    A. Naltrexone
    B. Tramadol
    C. Amphetamine
    D. Sertraline
    E. Buspirone

27. Which of the following is accurate about the effects of chronic excessive alcohol use?
    A. Brain imaging studies reveal frontal lobe hypertrophy and neuropsychological testing reveal cognitive deficits.

B. Neuropsychological testing of cognitive function does not reveal any impairments.

C. No changes are noted on brain imaging and neuropsychological testing reveal cognitive deficits.

D. Brain imaging studies revealed a loss of brain tissue and cognitive impairments are noted on neuropsychological testing.

E. Elevated concentration of serotonin is found in the cerebrospinal fluid.

28. Which of the following personality disorders has the highest rates of comorbid SUDs?
A. Borderline personality disorder
B. Obsessive compulsive personality disorder
C. Dependent personality disorder
D. Schizoid personality disorder
E. Antisocial personality disorder

29. A 38-year-old man with a history of major depressive disorder, cannabis and alcohol use disorder, obesity, and type 2 diabetes presents to your clinic. He takes sertraline, and his alcohol use disorder is currently in remission. He continues to smoke cannabis daily, and he reports that whenever he stops smoking, he feels depressed and anxious and is unable to sleep or eat. He asks you if any treatments can help him stop smoking cannabis. Which of the following statements is most accurate regarding his treatment options?
A. Rimonabant is a CB1 antagonist used for treatment of cannabis use disorder and can help him with weight loss.
B. He is experiencing a worsening of symptoms related to major depressive disorder, and his dose of sertraline should be increased.
C. There are no FDA-approved medications or evidence-based psychosocial interventions for cannabis use disorder.
D. There are off-label medications that can be prescribed to alleviate cannabis withdrawal symptoms.
E. Genetic testing can be helpful to determine the best medication approach for treating his cannabis use disorder.

30. Several medications are approved by the FDA for the treatment of OUD. Which of the following is an FDA-approved medication for the treatment of co-occurring PTSD and OUD?
A. Buprenorphine
B. Naltrexone
C. Methadone
D. Baclofen
E. None of the above

31. A 19-year-old man is brought to the emergency department by a friend after being found acting bizarrely and with a flat facial expression. His vital signs appear to be within normal limits, but he is not moving while sitting on the stretcher. You start asking a question, and he immediately becomes hostile and attempts to assault you. This patient most likely ingested which of the following drugs?
A. Heroin
B. Mescaline
C. Methamphetamine
D. Cocaine
E. PCP

32. A 24-year-old man is brought to the emergency room by friends after ingesting an unknown quantity of gamma-hydroxybutyrate (GHB) during a party. His friends tell you that they saw him vomiting multiple times and having convulsions, and then observed his breathing become shallow and labored. On arrival, he is immediately intubated and restrained. Which of the following clinical signs or symptoms is commonly observed in GHB overdose?
A. Psychosis
B. Bradycardia
C. Mydriasis
D. Tachypnea
E. Hypertension

33. A 54-year-old woman with a history of schizoaffective disorder and cocaine, alcohol, and tobacco use disorders presents to the emergency room with chest pain and is admitted for myocardial infarction. Her alcohol level on admission is 102, and her urine drug screen is positive for cocaine and negative for all other substances.

She is placed on a Clinical Institute Withdrawal Assessment for Alcohol (CIWA) protocol, which is discontinued on day 3 after she did not exhibit any signs or symptoms of alcohol withdrawal. On day 5, her heart rate and blood pressure increase, becoming more agitated and confused. Which of the following would best explain her change in clinical status?

A. Alcohol withdrawal
B. Sedative withdrawal
C. Cocaine withdrawal
D. Opioid withdrawal
E. Onset of a psychotic episode

34. The GABA-A and GABA-B receptors are the primary receptor targets for many medications and drugs of abuse. Which of the following compounds does not exert its primary effect through the GABA-A or GABA-B receptor?

A. Baclofen
B. GHB
C. Propofol
D. Gabapentin
E. Phenobarbital

35. A study is assessing the activity of a new opioid inhibitor in patients with chronic OUD. All patients enrolled in the study are informed that they would be treated with the inhibitor. They are assigned to successive dose cohorts of 20 to 50 mg/day of the medication. Approximately 10 patients are assigned to each dose. Treatment efficacy is determined based on urine toxicology screens and physical examinations conducted regularly throughout the study. This study is best described as which of the following?

A. Open-label clinical trial
B. Randomized clinical trial
C. Case-controlled study
D. Single-blind, randomized, controlled trial
E. Crossover study

36. A pain management doctor assesses a 55-year-old female patient with lumbar spine injury, the patient rates her pain as a 9 out of 10 on a numeric rating scale of 0 to 10. Which statement indicates the development of opioid tolerance in this patient?

A. She has been investing more time looking for doctors to prescribe the medication.
B. Larger doses of opioids are needed for analgesia.
C. The patient becomes anxious before the next dose.
D. The patient's constipation has improved.
E. The patient was prescribed naloxone.

37. A 17-year-old girl is brought to the physician after her mother learned that she was having sexual intercourse with various partners and using cocaine. She does not use condoms or other contraception. Of the following therapies listed, which type of treatment would use incentives to encourage sobriety in this patient?

A. Behavioral couples therapy
B. Dialectical behavioral therapy
C. CBT
D. Contingency management
E. MET

38. A 21-year-old man presents to your office with lower extremity pain for which you prescribe acetaminophen. He then returns to your office 2 days later complaining of gastrointestinal symptoms, lacrimation, and yawning. His blood pressure is high, and his pupils are dilated. Which of the following substances is responsible for his presentation?

A. Heroin
B. Cocaine
C. Alcohol
D. Phenobarbital
E. Cannabis

39. A grandmother brings her 15-year-old granddaughter to your office, as she is concerned that her granddaughter is spending excessive time online playing video games. Her school performance has decreased, and she has been more irritable, isolating herself, and not sleeping. She has spent a significant amount of her grandmother's savings downloading information and upgrading her games. Which of the following areas of her brain is being activated when she is engaged in playing video games?

A. Midbrain
B. Dorsal horn
C. Cerebellum
D. Nucleus accumbens
E. Amygdala

40. A 59-year-old man with OUD and alcohol use disorder is hospitalized for acute management of an abscess. He reports depression and sleep disturbance. Which of the following would be the best time to perform a psychiatric evaluation to determine whether he would benefit from treatment for an underlying depressive pathology?
   A. In the emergency room as soon as he arrives to the hospital
   B. After completing medically assisted detoxification but before starting maintenance treatment
   C. Upon admission and reassessed frequently thereafter
   D. After being sober from all drugs and alcohol for at least 1 month
   E. Never, this man's depression results from his heroin and alcohol use

41. A 34-year-old man with severe alcohol use disorder and cocaine and ketamine use is referred to you for chronic and severe anxiety and frequent panic attacks. His panic attacks are associated with significant avoidance behaviors, leading to him often skipping work. His panic attacks often happen in the morning. When meeting with him, he tells you that he drinks alcohol to "self-medicate his anxiety and panic attacks." Which of the following is the most likely explanation for this patient's anxiety and panic attacks?
   A. Cocaine intoxication
   B. Alcohol intoxication
   C. Alcohol withdrawal
   D. Generalized anxiety disorder
   E. Panic disorder without agoraphobia

42. In patients with comorbid SUDs and depression, which of the following factors is most strongly associated with improved response to antidepressant treatments?

A. Using SSRI antidepressants
B. Diagnosis of depression made while patient is actively drinking
C. Diagnosis of depression made at least 1 week after patient discontinue drinking
D. Using antidepressant medications without psychosocial interventions to treat depressive symptoms
E. Greater initial severity of the depressive symptoms

43. A 42-year-old man with severe alcohol use disorder is admitted into a combined program, including medically supervised alcohol detoxification followed by a long-term residential rehabilitation program. He reports that he has been drinking 8 to 10 alcoholic drinks daily for the past 6 years. Also, he describes symptoms of major depressive disorder for the past 7 months. Which of the following would be the most appropriate strategy to treat his depressive symptoms?
   A. This person's depression is caused by his alcohol use. Abstinence during the residential rehabilitation program will be curative for his depression.
   B. Because of the comorbid alcohol use disorder, antidepressant medications are not indicated. This patient's depression should be treated using intensive CBT alone.
   C. This patient's depression has lasted more than 6 months. This is consistent with a diagnosis of major depressive disorder, and he should be prescribed antidepressants medication immediately.
   D. Start an antidepressant medication after this patient completes the residential rehabilitation program if he remains symptomatic.
   E. Start an antidepressant medication after this patient completes the medically supervised alcohol detoxification if he remains symptomatic.

44. Routine UDS tests do not detect some of the most prescribed benzodiazepines. Standard UDS tests will reliably detect benzodiazepines that are metabolized to:
A. Alprazolam
B. Diazepam
C. Oxazepam

D. Lorazepam

E. Clonazepam

45. An adolescent who has been using illicit opioids 4 to 5 days a week presents to your office for an evaluation. He has been more isolative and missing multiple days of school. He appears to be aware of the problems that drugs are causing in his life. His use has been increasing slowly over the last 12 months. Which of the following is the most appropriate diagnosis?

A. OUD

B. Opioid intoxication

C. Personality disorder

D. Withdrawal syndrome

E. Tolerance

46. A 48-year-old man with OUD presents to your clinic seeking treatment with buprenorphine/naloxone. Point-of-care urine drug testing was positive for opiates. Using the following substances would most likely cause a false-positive test?

A. Rifampicin

B. Omeprazole

C. Sertraline

D. Phenytoin

E. Venlafaxine

47. Which of the following substances is the most widely used illicit drug in the United States?

A. Opioids

B. Alcohol

C. Cannabis

D. Caffeine

E. Tobacco

48. Which of the following is not a medical comorbidity of chronic and excessive alcohol use?

A. Glaucoma

B. Dilated cardiomyopathy

C. Myopathy

D. Hyperuricemia

E. Osteonecrosis of the hip

49. A 24-year-old woman is brought in by a friend to urgent care with altered mental status and visual hallucinations. Her friend said that their musical band was practicing when her friend started playing the wrong songs and acting bizarrely. On examination, the patient's blood pressure is high, and she has a low-grade fever. Which of the following is another complication of the substance likely being used by the patient?

A. Shortness of breath

B. Hypotension

C. Lacrimation and yawning

D. Pinpoint pupils

E. Distortion of senses

50. Which of the following medications for alcohol use disorder predominantly works by attenuating the positively reinforcing effects of alcohol?

A. Disulfiram

B. Naltrexone

C. Acamprosate

D. Sertraline

E. Gabapentin

BLOCK 3

1. What did the Supreme Court of California rule in 1991 in People v. Saille as it relates to alcohol intoxication as a criminal defense?

A. Alcohol intoxication is an affirmative defense in criminal proceedings if the defendant was unable to appreciate the wrongfulness of his acts at the time of the commission of the crime.

B. Alcohol intoxication at the time of the commission of the crime indicates guilt.

C. Defendants who were intoxicated with alcohol at the time of the commission of

the crime should be diverted to drug courts rather than the regular adversarial judicial system.

D. Alcohol intoxication at the time of the commission of the crime does not negate specific intent or mens rea.

E. Capital punishment for defendants who were intoxicated with alcohol at the time of the commission of the crime is unconstitutional, as it violates the ban on cruel and unusual punishment under the Eighth Amendment.

2. A 27-year-old female patient with major depressive disorder and a long history of marijuana use presents to your clinic. Her depression improved after being prescribed fluoxetine and discontinuing marijuana use "under pressure" by her psychiatrist. The patient noted that she "really wanted to be able to continue smoking marijuana, but the psychiatrist told me that if I did not stop, she would no longer treat me." In this situation, it appears that the psychiatrist prioritized (1) as a principle of medical ethics over (2).
A. (1): Nonmaleficence and (2): justice
B. (1): Non-maleficence and (2): autonomy
C. (1): Beneficence and (2): nonmaleficence
D. (1): Justice and (2): beneficence
E. (1): Beneficence and (2): autonomy

3. In the above patient situation (Question 2), it appears that the psychiatrist adheres to which of the following theories of medical ethics?
A. Dialectical principlism
B. Deontological theory
C. Utilitarianism theory
D. Consequentialism theory
E. Virtue theory

4. Which of the following scenarios is likely to result in a positive opiate test in a standard UDS test?
A. A 27-year-old homeless man injecting fentanyl
B. A 27-year-old disabled vet prescribed meperidine
C. A 27-year-old athlete prescribed codeine after a meniscal injury surgical repair
D. A 27-year-old executive receiving methadone through a methadone treatment program
E. A 27-year-old pharmacist using oxycodone recreationally diverted from work

5. Which of the following medications for alcohol use disorder works by reducing the symptoms of protracted withdrawal and thereby the risk for relapse in early abstinence?
A. Disulfiram
B. Naltrexone
C. Acamprosate
D. Sertraline
E. Gabapentin

6. Which of the following is true regarding the mechanism of action of acamprosate?
A. It is a positive allosteric modulator of GABA-A receptors.
B. It is a GABA-B agonist.
C. It is a positive allosteric modulator of glutamatergic NMDA receptors.
D. It inhibits the alpha-2-delta-1 subunit of voltage-gated calcium channels.
E. It inhibits the mu-opioid receptor.

7. Gabapentin is frequently used as a second-line agent for the treatment of alcohol use disorder. Which of the following best describes its relevant mechanism of action?
A. GABA-A receptor agonist
B. GABA-B receptor agonist
C. NMDA receptor antagonist
D. Alpha-2-delta-1 subunit of voltage-gated calcium channels antagonist
E. Alpha-2 receptor agonist

8. A 27-year-old banker is required to submit to a preemployment UDS test. At the collection center, they informed the staff that they had a poppy-seed bagel that morning and that a positive opiate test should be considered a false positive. Which of the following is accurate about poppy seeds and false-positive tests?
A. False positive or protests following the ingestion of poppy seeds is an urban legend, used to get away with opiate use.
B. The medical review officer is able to determine whether it is a false positive or a true positive based on their interview of the banker.
C. There is no way to determine whether the patient used illicit opioids or poppy seeds, and as a result, they should be asked to return a week later and instructed to avoid poppy seeds.
D. Ingesting poppy seeds would result in false-positive hair drug test, indicating opioid use.
E. Confirmation by GC-MS can help identify false positives from true positives.

9. Regarding the use of different matrices for drug testing, which of the following is true?
   A. Drug testing utilizing a blood matrix has the shortest window of detection.
   B. Hair drug testing is often accurate and should not be used in clinical situations.
   C. Urine drug testing utilizes polymerase chain reaction (PCR) technology to detect the presence of various drugs.
   D. Hair drug testing is the least expensive and most widely used drug test.
   E. The presence of PCP can be demonstrated using urine or saliva matrices but not hair.

10. A 27-year-old banker is required to submit to a preemployment urine drug screening test. No drugs were detected on immunoassay. Which of the following scenario with the medical review officer determines that the negative test result is valid?
    A. pH: 4; temperature: 98°F; urine creatinine: 18 mg/dL; specific gravity: 1.035; nitrites: 9 mg/dL
    B. pH: 6; temperature: 98°F; urine creatinine: 18 mg/dL; specific gravity: 1.007; nitrites: 4 mg/dL
    C. pH: 6; temperature: 103°F; urine creatinine: 1 mg/dL; specific gravity: 1.007; nitrites: 9 mg/dL
    D. pH: 6; temperature: 103°F; urine creatinine: 18 mg/dL; specific gravity: 1.035; nitrites: 4 mg/dL
    E. pH: 6; temperature: 98°F; urine creatinine: 24 mg/dL; specific gravity: 1.035; nitrites: 1 mg/dL

11. A 10-year-old boy in foster care is brought to your clinic due to poor attention, hyperactivity, learning problems, and frequent fighting in school. His foster parents confirm that his biological mother used alcohol heavily throughout pregnancy. On examination, he has no discernible facial dysmorphisms characteristic of prenatal alcohol exposure, and he is in the 50th percentile for height, weight, and head circumference. Neurological examination and brain imaging are normal. On neuropsychological testing, he has an IQ of 85 and clear deficits in attention and executive functioning. Which of the following is the most accurate diagnosis?
    A. Fetal alcohol syndrome (FAS)
    B. Partial FAS
    C. Alcohol-related neurodevelopmental disorder
    D. Alcohol-related birth defect
    E. Inherited FAS

12. Which of the following are absolute contraindications for using disulfiram for treatment of alcohol use disorder?
    A. Migraine headaches
    B. Hepatic impairment
    C. Coronary occlusion
    D. Physiological dependence on opioids
    E. Severe depression

13. There are several personality factors that are associated with a higher risk of alcohol use disorder. These include:
    A. High conscientiousness
    B. High neuroticism
    C. High extraversion
    D. Low extraversion
    E. High agreeableness

14. A 47-year-old man with OUD who is enrolled in a methadone maintenance treatment program (MMTP) is required to attend the MMTP 6 days a week, but he was only required to come twice weekly after 1 year of abstinence. He then has a relapse with multiple positive urine toxicologies, and subsequently, he is required to go to the clinic 6 days a week again. This treatment approach is best described by which behavioral principle?
    A. Classical conditioning
    B. Incentive salience
    C. Operant conditioning
    D. Negative reinforcement
    E. Positive reinforcement

15. A 26-year-old man with alcohol use disorder who committed arson while intoxicated is now court-mandated to your alcohol treatment program. On presentation to your program, he explains that he plans to attend the program because, after 6 months of "good behavior" on his part, the

court will reduce his requirement for treatment participation. His explanation of his motivation to attend treatment is an example of which behavioral principle?
A. Classical conditioning
B. Incentive salience
C. Operant conditioning
D. Negative reinforcement
E. Positive reinforcement

16. A 16-year-old girl with depression and cannabis use disorder who lives with her parents presents to your clinic. She has been failing several classes in high school and was recently arrested for cannabis possession. She presents to your clinic, and she has low motivation to stop using cannabis. You recommend a combination of MET and CBT. Which additional treatment modality has the strongest evidence based data for treating this patient's cannabis use disorder?
A. Psychodynamic psychotherapy
B. Supportive psychotherapy
C. Family-based treatment
D. Relapse prevention
E. Twelve-step group attendance

17. Which of the following is true regarding SUDs among physicians?
A. SUDs are extremely rare in physicians because of higher education. However, the prognosis for a physician with an SUD is extremely poor.
B. The prevalence of SUDs among physicians is similar to that in the general population. Physicians with SUDs have a good prognosis as the potential to lose one's license serves as an alternative reinforcer for sobriety.
C. SUDs among physicians do not manifest with the traditional symptoms of SUDs seen in the general population. Physicians are less likely to develop withdrawal and tolerance but more likely to be charged with driving under the influence.
D. Changes in sleep, weight, or mood are not associated with SUDs among physicians.
E. Physicians with SUDs never present with needle marks or bruises.

18. In which of the following five scenarios might the person be adjudicated not guilty?
A. A 27-year-old man with alcohol use disorder who drove while intoxicated because alcohol use caused disinhibition
B. A 27-year-old man who assaulted another patron at a bar after someone "roofied" him by surreptitiously putting flunitrazepam (Rohypnol) in his drink
C. A 27-year-old woman who committed a nonviolent crime under the influence of PCP
D. A 27-year-old banker who committed the crime under the influence of cocaine but does not meet criteria for SUD
E. A 27-year-old physician who was sexually inappropriate with a patient because they were under the influence of recreational drugs but had no intent to harm had they been sober

19. In SBIRT, which of the following tools carries the strongest evidence to screen for maladaptive alcohol use?
A. CAGE questionnaire
B. Michigan Alcoholism Screening Test (MAST)
C. Addiction Severity Index (ASI)
D. TWEAK questionnaire
E. Alcohol Use Disorders Identification Test (AUDIT)

20. A 47-year-old man with alcohol and cocaine use disorder, bipolar disorder, and multiple suicide attempts is well known in your emergency room. He self-presents to the emergency room, reporting suicidal ideation, and has an alcohol level of 380 mg/dL. Although he is agitated, yelling, and pacing around the emergency room, he shows no signs of body sway or ataxia, speaks without slurring, and is oriented to person, place, and time. Which of the following best explains why he does not exhibit symptoms that are frequently exhibited at his presenting alcohol level?
A. He is in a manic episode, which accounts for his psychomotor agitation.
B. He coingested cocaine, which counteracts the effects of his alcohol level.

C. He has developed tolerance to alcohol and can withstand higher alcohol levels.

D. There is likely a laboratory error, as his alcohol level is dangerously high.

E. He has a genetic polymorphism that allows him to rapidly metabolize alcohol.

21. Which of the following best summarizes the biological changes that account for alcohol withdrawal?
    A. Serotonergic overactivity and GABAergic underactivity
    B. Serotonergic underactivity and GABAergic overactivity
    C. GABAergic underactivity and glutamatergic overactivity
    D. GABAergic overactivity and glutamatergic underactivity
    E. GABAergic underactivity and serotonergic underactivity

22. A 42-year-old man with a history of alcohol and cocaine use disorder presents to your clinic. He began drinking at 14 years of age and has a significant family history of alcohol use disorder on both his maternal and paternal sides. He has been incarcerated multiple times for shoplifting, burglary, and trespassing. In the past several years, he could abstain from alcohol for 6 months and was temporarily employed. Which of the following clinical features is not consistent with his Cloninger typology?
    A. Onset of alcohol use prior to 25 years of age
    B. Male sex
    C. Significant family history
    D. Presence of antisocial behaviors
    E. Ability to abstain from alcohol temporarily

23. Alcoholics Anonymous (AA) meetings typically begin by reciting the serenity prayer. In it, what is the one requesting?
    A. Faith
    B. Knowledge
    C. Relationships
    D. Courage
    E. Success

24. Which step in AA involves making amends to those hurt by the person as a result of their substance use?

A. Step 1
B. Step 4
C. Step 5
D. Step 9
E. Step 10

25. Which of the following is correct regarding the relationship between the diagnosis of SUD and attention-deficit hyperactivity disorder (ADHD)?
    A. Having an ADHD diagnosis is protective against SUD.
    B. Patients with ADHD and comorbid SUD should not be treated using stimulants because it increases the risk of substance use.
    C. ADHD treatment, including the use of stimulants, does not increase the risk of SUD.
    D. Patients who are prescribed stimulants for ADHD are most likely to misuse the medication themselves.
    E. ADHD is the most common comorbid psychiatric diagnosis to SUD in women.

26. Which of the following statements is correct with respect to the treatment of patients with comorbid SUD and personality disorders?
    A. SUD is uncommon in patients with personality disorders.
    B. The manifestation of personality disorders is easily differentiated from behavioral and personality changes induced by substance use.
    C. An essential aspect of treating patients with comorbid borderline personality disorder and alcohol use disorder involves setting and maintaining strict therapeutic limits and boundaries.
    D. Dialectical behavior therapy is the most effective psychotherapeutic intervention for the treatment of SUD in patients with borderline personality disorder.
    E. Patients with antisocial personality disorder have higher prevalence rates of having SUD but better prognosis for recovery than the general population.

27. A 24-year-old woman with schizophrenia who is treated with daily risperidone is admitted for a medically supervised detoxification from alcohol. Her withdrawal symptoms are treated with

lorazepam. On completing the program, she was started on disulfiram to help maintain her sobriety. Two weeks later, she was arrested for disorderly conduct and found to be paranoid and combative. Which of the following is the most likely explanation for this presentation?

A. She relapsed to alcohol.

B. She stopped taking the risperidone.

C. Her medication regimen caused a recurrence of psychotic symptoms.

D. She is using other substances such as PCP.

E. This presentation is consistent with benzodiazepine withdrawal.

28. Which of the following best represents the relationship between alcohol use disorder and co-morbid psychiatric disorders?

A. Chronic and excessive alcohol use causes psychiatric symptoms.

B. Chronic and excessive alcohol use causes other psychiatric disorders.

C. Manifestations of chronic and excessive alcohol use may resemble symptoms of other psychiatric illnesses.

D. Alcohol use disorder may coincidently co-occur in patients with other psychiatric illnesses.

E. All of the above are possible.

29. Which of the following is not a risk factor for completed suicide?

A. Alcohol intoxication

B. Alcohol use disorder

C. Previous suicide attempt

D. Intellectual disability

E. Access to means for suicide

30. Which of the following medications would not be safe to be used for alcohol withdrawal management in patients with severely impaired liver function?

A. Chlordiazepoxide

B. Lorazepam

C. Oxazepam

D. Gabapentin

E. Temazepam

31. A 42-year-old woman presents to the emergency room with rapidly progressive renal decompensation. She requires urgent dialysis and is admitted to the intensive care unit. On evaluation, her mental status examination is consistent with delirium. Additionally, asterixis and ascites are noted. Laboratory testing revealed hepatitis C antibodies and antigens, creatinine of 5.4 mg/dL, BUN of 87 mg/dL, and a very dilute urine. Which of the following is most likely to effectively treat her condition?

A. Prescribing an ACE inhibitor such as lisinopril

B. Prescribing an antithrombotic agent such as clopidogrel

C. Lung transplant

D. Liver transplant

E. Portal vascular shunting

32. With regard to TSF, which of the following most accurately describes the goals of the psychotherapeutic intervention?

A. TSF posits meeting patients where they are at, helping them resolve their ambivalence toward attending AA meetings.

B. TSF aims to encourage attendance and meaningful utilization of 12-step meetings.

C. TSF aims to encourage patients to discuss the results of their urine drug tests at 12-step meetings.

D. TSF aims to provide an evidenced based, nonreligious alternative to AA and NA.

E. TSF is the collective name for psychotherapies utilized in AA, NA, LifeRing, or SMART recovery.

33. Which of the following is true concerning HCV infections in the United States?

A. Although HCV is mostly transmitted by blood, at least 30% of those infected with the virus contracted it sexually.

B. The HCV vaccine is only recommended for injection drug users because of its potential to cause cardiac arrhythmia.

C. HCV is most prevalent among those born between 1945 and 1965.

D. Persons with co-occurring HIV and HCV carry a significantly elevated risk of liver cirrhosis or liver-related mortality.

E. Malarial infections are protective against contracting HCV.

34. Psychiatric side effects are most common in patients using which of the following antiretroviral medication for HIV treatment?
    A. Nevirapine
    B. Zidovudine
    C. Lamivudine
    D. Efavirenz
    E. Tenofovir

35. A 27-year-old woman patient is brought into the psychiatric emergency room by emergency medical services with symptoms of psychosis. She acknowledged using phencyclidine (PCP) and was admitted to the inpatient psychiatric unit for further management and stabilization of the psychiatric symptoms. Which of the following would be most helpful for the treating psychiatrist to determine whether the patient's psychosis results from a primary psychotic illness instead of a psychosis induced by her use of PCP?
    A. A urine drug test showing the presence of PCP
    B. Using collateral information obtained from emergency medical services, as well as the patient's roommate to complement the structured diagnostic evaluation
    C. Having a family history of schizoaffective disorder
    D. Having a long history of PCP and methamphetamine use
    E. Performing multiple longitudinal psychiatric assessments

36. Which of the following is a validated single screening question for the detection of alcohol use disorder?
    A. How many times have you consumed alcohol to the point of intoxication over the past year?
    B. Have you consumed alcohol before 10 a.m. in the past year?
    C. Have you unsuccessfully attempted to cut down or discontinue your alcohol use in the past?
    D. How many times did you have 5 or more drinks in a single day for men or 4 or more drinks for women over the past year?

    E. How many times did you have 15 or more drinks in a single week for men or 8 or more drinks in a single week for women over the past year?

37. A 31-year-old man presents to the emergency room with decreased respiratory rate, slurred speech, pinpoint pupils, and disorientation. Which of the following medications should be used to counteract the patient's symptoms?
    A. Naltrexone
    B. Naloxone
    C. Buprenorphine
    D. Fluphenazine
    E. Valproic acid

38. During an annual physical examination, a 46-year-old woman informs her primary care physician that she has been drinking five alcoholic beverages three to four times every week. Laboratory testing revealed elevated transaminases three times higher than the cutoff value. Her physician discussed the relationship between her abnormal findings and her excessive alcohol use and recommended that she cut down on drinking to prevent further hepatic function deterioration. She appeared to understand and agreed to drink less. Which of the following best demonstrates this treatment approach?
    A. Motivational interviewing
    B. Brief treatment
    C. Screening and brief intervention
    D. CBT for SUD
    E. Referral to treatment

39. The use of Screening and Brief Intervention (SBI) would be expected to be most effective for which of the following patients?
    A. A 34-year-old man with cocaine use disorder who is recovering from a cocaine-induced acute coronary event.
    B. A 28-year-old woman with moderate alcohol use disorder in treatment with an addiction psychiatrist.
    C. A 28-year-old woman who is participating in a drug court program for heroin use.
    D. A 34-year-old man who drinks 5 alcoholic beverages 6 days a week seen at his primary care clinic for his annual physical exam.

E. A 17-year-old boy presenting to the emergency department with LSD-induced panic attacks.

40. The prevalence of marijuana use in the United States has been increasing over the past decade among teens and young adults. Which of the following explanations best accounts for this trend?
    A. The perceived risk of marijuana use has declined among this age group.
    B. The perceived risk of marijuana use has increased among this age group.
    C. THC content in marijuana has declined, making it more palatable to naïve users.
    D. CBD content in marijuana has increased, making it more palatable to naïve users.
    E. Marijuana is no longer classified as a Schedule I drug for individuals aged 18 years and over.

41. What is the most common cause of alcohol-related mortality in the United States?
    A. Suicide
    B. Cardiovascular disease
    C. Motor vehicle traffic injuries
    D. Liver disease
    E. Malignant neoplasms

42. Intrauterine cocaine exposure is associated with which of the following findings?
    A. Normal birth weight
    B. Placental abruption
    C. Increased weight gain
    D. Tetralogy of Fallot
    E. Marfan syndrome

43. Which of the following substances has a mechanism of action similar to ketamine?
    A. Cocaine
    B. Phencyclidine
    C. Psilocybin
    D. Naloxone
    E. Cannabis

44. A 34-year-old woman who is 32 weeks pregnant comes to your office seeking treatment for OUD. She has been using a gram of heroin intranasally every other day for the past 13 months. Which of the following is a problem associated with intrauterine exposure to opioids?

A. Low birth weight
B. Enlarged head circumference
C. Increase birth weight
D. Normal EEG patterns
E. An increase in amniotic fluid volume

45. A 21-year-old man presents to the emergency room accompanied by the police after being found sleeping in the library and becomes combative upon being awakened. He admitted using drugs to be able to concentrate in his classes. Which of the following may underlie this person's beliefs?
    A. Habituation
    B. Tolerance
    C. Being afraid of withdrawal symptoms
    D. State-dependent learning
    E. Intoxication

46. A 29-year-old woman with a history of insomnia on zolpidem 5 mg at night presents for follow-up. She complains that the medication is helpful, but she is still not sleeping through the night. You ask about side effects, and she tells you that she had one incident where she got up and cooked her favorite pasta dish in the middle of the night, although she does not have a clear recollection of her actions the following morning. What is your next best step?
    A. Increase the dose of zolpidem
    B. Lower the dose of zolpidem
    C. Transition patient from regular to long-acting zolpidem
    D. Discontinue zolpidem
    E. Continue the current dose but advise patient to remove the knobs off her stove and secure food items before bedtime

47. A 48-year-old woman with a history of chronic pain and OUD continues to endorse cravings to use heroin, is using more than intended, and spends much of her time obtaining the drug. She is now most interested in injectable naltrexone after not liking how methadone made her feel. She last received methadone 5 days ago. Which of the following is most likely to be a potential disadvantage of injectable naltrexone to treat her OUD?
    A. High rates of discontinuation
    B. The requirement for at least 7 days of abstinence before beginning treatment

C. Interaction with ibuprofen for chronic pain
D. Need to always try the oral formulation first
E. Need for at least mild withdrawal with the first use

48. Which one of the following pharmacotherapies should be considered a first-line treatment for pathologic gambling?
   A. Topiramate
   B. Lithium
   C. Naltrexone
   D. Bupropion
   E. Amphetamine

49. A 46-year-old woman with a long history of an alcohol use disorder, hepatitis C, and cirrhosis is referred to your clinic for treatment. She expresses a desire to discontinue her alcohol consumption. In addition to psychotherapeutic interventions, which of the following pharmacological agents is the treatment of choice for this patient's condition?
   A. Disulfiram
   B. Gabapentin
   C. Ondansetron
   D. Acamprosate
   E. Naltrexone

50. The majority of individuals with alcohol use disorder exhibit cognitive deficits with neuropsychological testing. Which of the following cognitive domains show the earliest reversal upon establishment of abstinence?
   A. Short-term memory
   B. Abstraction
   C. Problem solving
   D. Verbal learning
   E. Visuospatial abilities

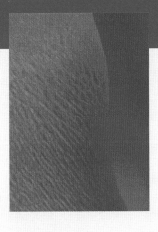

REVIEW QUESTIONS ANSWER KEY (CHAPTERS 1–13)

CHAPTER 1

1. **B.** Male gender, younger, low SES, single

   Young unmarried men of low SES carry the highest risk for developing alcohol use disorder (AUD). Generally speaking, most present with early symptoms of AUD before the age of 30. Other risk factors include having a family history of AUD, having comorbid depressive disorders, schizophrenia spectrum disorder or personality disorders and a personal history of abuse.

2. **E.** Dimension 6

   The ASAM PPC are the most commonly used standardized criteria used to attribute the appropriate level of care for patients taking into consideration their various clinical needs (dimensions). The six dimensions evaluated in the PPC are:

   - Dimension 1: intoxication and withdrawal potential
   - Dimension 2: biomedical conditions and complications
   - Dimension 3: emotional, behavioral, or cognitive complications
   - Dimension 4: readiness to change (transtheoretical model of change or stages of change)
   - Dimension 5: relapse or continued use potential
   - Dimension 6: recovery environment (including social, legal, vocational, educational, financial, housing factors)

   Dimension 6 addresses the patient's recovery environment, including barriers for their sobriety and support system. Services addressing Dimension 6 include ensuring one's ability to attend their clinical appointments (transportation, ability to take a medical leave), reside in a safe environment conducive to recovery (such as a sober house) and home cohesiveness (family members attending Al-Anon).

3. **D.** Women with SUDs experience significantly more severe adverse medical and psychological consequences than men.

   Telescoping refers to the phenomenon whereby SUD severity progresses faster for women than for men, with women more likely to seek SUD treatment and be in recovery faster than men. Women with SUD appear to be more vulnerable than men to experiencing adverse consequences of using substances.

4. **D.** Treating co-occurring psychiatric disorders leads to improved SUD outcomes.

   As noted above, the telescoping phenomenon posits that women are more likely to seek SUD treatment and be in recovery faster than men. Overall, recovery rates are equivalent between women and men. SUD treatment programs that offer comprehensive psychiatric care for women with SUD, including treatment for co-occurring psychiatric pathology, as well as addressing any abuse history, family dysfunction are associated with better outcomes. Gender-specific treatment settings have not been shown to be associated with any improved treatment outcomes.

5. **A.** Naltrexone

   There is still no FDA-approved pharmacotherapeutic treatment of gambling disorder. Studies have suggested the involvement of the μ-opioid system in the reward processes of behavioral addictions leading to the hypothesis that opioid antagonists can reduce the repetitive behaviors and the urges of addictive behaviors such as gambling. Controlled studies on naltrexone, an opioid antagonist, have shown positive results in reducing the desire to gamble. There has not been a significant difference between bupropion or mood stabilizers such as lithium, topiramate, and placebo to treat gambling disorder.

6. **C.** Telescoping Phenomenon

   Sex differences have been noticed in gambling behaviors. It has been found that females have a progression from nonproblematic to excessive engagement in gambling behaviors later in life than males. It also progresses faster from recreational to problematic. This phenomenon is described as the telescoping effect or phenomenon.

CHAPTER 2

1. **D.** Acamprosate

   The U.S. Food and Drug Administration (FDA) approved three medications to treat AUD: disulfiram, naltrexone and acamprosate. Of these, acamprosate would be the preferred medication to use in patients with hepatic insufficiency. It is excreted in urine as an unmetabolized drug. As a result, it should not be used as a first-line agent for patients with renal impairment. Naltrexone is metabolized hepatically via noncytochrome-mediated dehydrogenase and is subject to the extensive first-pass effect. Its use can be associated with increased serum transaminases, and it is contraindicated in patients with acute hepatitis or hepatic failure. Disulfiram is metabolized hepatically via glucuronidation. Its side effects include cholestatic hepatitis, fulminant hepatitis, and hepatic failure. It is relatively contraindicated in patients with hepatic cirrhosis. Gabapentin and ondansetron are used as second-line treatment options for AUD but are not FDA approved for this condition.

2. **C.** He should be screened for depression on admission and reassessed frequently thereafter

It is not uncommon for patients with SUDs to present with various co-occurring psychiatric symptoms, particularly mood and neurovegetative symptoms. It is important to assess any such symptoms seriously on an ongoing basis to determine whether the patient requires active treatments, including medications and specialized psychotherapies, and to prevent serious complications of untreated psychiatric illnesses, including profound functional decline and/or suicidal behaviors. Many patients with substance-induced mood disorders would be expected to improve after being abstinent for a few weeks. Others might suffer from independent or secondary psychiatric disorders.

3. **C.** Alcohol withdrawal

   This patient presents with a history of anxiety symptoms and panic attacks that occurs mostly in the mornings, after abstaining from any alcohol use overnight. Consuming alcohol leads to a resolution of his symptoms. This is consistent with alcohol withdrawal–related panic attacks and anxiety. Panic attacks related to substance use are seen most commonly with marijuana and LSD intoxication and alcohol withdrawal. The vignette does not provide enough information to support the diagnosis of generalized anxiety disorder or panic disorder. Further, alcohol use would not be expected to prevent panic attacks or treat anxiety in patients with a generalized anxiety disorder or panic disorder.

4. **C.** Diagnosis of depression made at least 1 week after patient discontinues drinking

   A 2008 meta-analysis of placebo-controlled trials of antidepressant medications among patients with SUD and depressive disorders by Nunes and Levin (2008) found that diagnosing depression after at least 1 week of abstinence was associated with a greater effect of antidepressant medication treatment. A depressive disorder that persists after 1 week or more of abstinence is likely independent of substance use and should be treated. For patients who cannot achieve any amount of abstinence, the meta-analysis recommended using clinical judgment in making decisions to treat the depressive disorder based on the patient's history, past episodes of independent depression, and severity of the depressive disorder. Further, most positive studies included tricyclic antidepressants or antidepressants with noradrenergic or mixed mechanisms such as serotonin and norepinephrine reuptake inhibitors. Most studies using SSRIs were negative.

5. **E.** Start an antidepressant medication after this patient completes the medically supervised alcohol detoxification if he remains symptomatic

In this clinical situation, it is unclear whether this patient's depressive symptoms are substance-induced and likely to resolve spontaneously or represent an independent depressive disorder. Given that there are no acute safety concerns reported, it is not unreasonable to hold off on starting antidepressant medications until they complete alcohol detoxification and withdrawal symptoms subside. When thinking about the psychiatric manifestations of SUD, one has to differentiate between:

- The substance's expected: Drug and alcohol intoxication or withdrawal cause psychiatric signsss and symptoms that are part of the normal toxidrome of a given substance.
- Substance induced disorders: This category refers to the presence of psychiatric symptoms that vastly exceed the expected effects of being intoxicated with or withdrawing from a substance and demonstrate symptoms of another psychiatric disorder (psychotic, bipolar, depressive, anxiety, obsessive compulsive, sleep, sexual, or neurocognitive disorder).
- Co-occurring primary psychiatric disorders: This category refers to psychiatric disorders that either preceded or followed the onset of an SUD, but neither condition played a causative role in the other's onset.
- Secondary psychiatric disorders: This category refers to psychiatric disorders that follow the onset of an SUD, with the SUD playing a causative role in the onset of the co-occurring psychiatric disorder.

6. **A.** Increased cardiac workload and systemic vascular resistance

Cocaine use is associated with significant cardiovascular pathologies that could cause angina and myocardial ischemia. Cocaine causes hypertension, increased systemic vascular resistance, and vasoconstriction. In addition to the standard protocols used for non cocaine-related cardiac events, the medical treatment of cocaine-related angina and myocardial infarction should include benzodiazepines. Benzodiazepines are necessary to manage the hypertension and tachycardia and decrease the central stimulatory effects of cocaine.

Other causes of cocaine-induced coronary artery disease involve vasculopathy and vasoconstriction. Cocaine use can also cause left ventricular hypertrophy, hyperthrombotic states, aortic dissection and rupture, and arrhythmias.

7. **B.** Assess the severity of the patient's depression and current suicidal thoughts

The most important risk factor for suicide is having a history of past suicide attempts. SUD is a major risk factor for attempted and completed suicide. Additionally, acute and severe psychosocial stressors further increase the risk. As a result, this patient presents with a very high risk for suicide and should be evaluated for current suicidal thinking. Ensuring the patient's safety if he is suicidal might require inpatient hospitalization. This patient is certainly at risk of having contracted HIV and HCV. However, laboratory testing for these infections should be offered after acute stabilization and assessment of imminent risks. Having a history of suicide attempts or of obtaining buprenorphine from illicit sources is not a contraindication for treatment with buprenorphine. This patient might benefit from treatment with an SSRI. However, it is preferable to wait until he completes a medically assisted opioid detoxification and reassess his depressive symptoms before prescribing the antidepressant medication.

8. **E.** Assess the severity of his opioid withdrawal and begin induction with buprenorphine

This patient is coming to your clinic seeking treatment using medications for opioid use disorder. Given his history of chronic pain and his ongoing pain despite the opioid use, buprenorphine might be a better therapeutic option than naltrexone because of its analgesic effect. Given that he is currently in withdrawal, you might be able to begin the office-based buprenorphine induction on the same day, maximizing the chances for his recovery. In contrast, prescribing him clonidine and other medication support for opioid withdrawal and discharging him with a follow-up appointment in 1 week will increase the likelihood that he will continue using illicit opioids after leaving your office to relieve the withdrawal symptoms. Given the information presented in the vignette, he does not appear to indicate a need for an inpatient admission for detoxification. Further, although having a history of suicide and SUD are major risk factors for suicide, the patient is not currently suicidal or depressed. There is no indication to send him to the psychiatric emergency room.

9. **B.** Send him to the emergency room

This patient should be evaluated urgently in an emergency room setting. Given his history of injection drug use, sharing needles, chest pain, fatigue, fever, and tachycardia, he is at elevated risk for infective myocarditis (endocarditis). Injecting drugs increases the likelihood of bacterial injections from nonsterile injection procedures. Additionally, drug and alcohol use are associated with behavioral disinhibition, which could further increase the risk of bacterial infections. Bacteria, most commonly *Staphylococcus*, can travel with blood and deposit as vegetations on cardiac valves (most commonly the tricuspid valve). Bacterial endocarditis is lethal if untreated. Treatment involves a long course of intravenous antibiotics and at times valve replacement.

10. **E.** Immediately

Guidelines recommend starting HAART as soon as possible. There is no recommended CD4 count cutoff at which to initiate therapy. In fact, evidence suggests that starting HAART when CD4 count is high is associated with improved long-term outcomes. HAART is associated with improved CD4 count, virologic suppression, and preserved immune function. Earlier HAART initiation may result in better immunologic responses and clinical outcomes, reductions in AIDS and non–AIDS-associated morbidity and mortality, and a significant reduction in HIV transmission risk. Although it is

certainly preferable that patients with HIV abstain from drug and alcohol use, HAART is not contraindicated in patients who are actively using it.

11. **D.** Brain imaging studies revealed a loss of brain tissue, and cognitive impairments are noted on neuropsychological testing

Persons of AUD or a chronic history of excessive alcohol use may present with neurocognitive impairment that is detected on neuropsychological testing and brain imaging. Magnetic resonance imaging studies and diffusion tensor imaging reveal a loss of brain tissue with accelerating grey matter loss. In more than half of persons with AUD, abnormalities can be seen on computed tomography imaging even in the absence of cognitive deficits. Some of these changes may be reversible with abstinence suggesting that the abnormalities might at least be in part evidence of brain tissue dehydration.

12. **E.** Antisocial personality disorder

SUDs are often comorbid with personality disorders, most commonly, antisocial personality disorder, borderline personality disorder, and schizotypal personality disorder. Of these, antisocial personality disorder is the most common.

13. **E.** None of the above

The FDA approves three medications to treat opioid use disorder: buprenorphine, methadone, and naltrexone (both as a daily oral formulation and a long-term injectable formulation). No medication is approved specifically for comorbid opioid use disorder and PTSD. In fact, no medications are approved specifically for any SUD comorbid with any other psychiatric disorder.

REFERENCE

Nunes, E. V., & Levin, F. R. (2008). Treatment of co-occurring depression and substance dependence: using meta-analysis to guide clinical recommendations. *Psychiatric Annals, 38*(11) nihpa128505.

CHAPTER 3

1. **B.** Conditioned place aversion

Conditioned place preference and self-administration measure the reinforcing effect of a substance and are animal models relevant for the binge/

intoxication phase of the addiction cycle. Drug- and cue-induced reinstatement are relevant for the preoccupation/anticipation stage of the addiction cycle.

2. **B.** NPY

NPY is a neuromodulator shown to have anxio- lytic effects and is part of the brain's "anti-stress" system that functionally opposes CRF. Dynorphin is upregulated in withdrawal states and leads to increased dysphoria. Central noradrenergic sys- tems become activated in withdrawal and increase anxiety and agitation. The HPA axis becomes acti- vated in withdrawal and leads to elevated levels of CRF, ACTH, and glucocorticoids; ACTH does not counteract or modulate the effects of CRF.

3. **A.** Norepinephrine

Dopamine is ubiquitously important in directly or indirectly mediating the rewarding effect of all drugs of abuse. Alcohol directly affects GABA, serotonin, and opioid receptors in the binge/intox- ication stage. Norepinephrine is the least relevant neurotransmitter system in mediating the reward- ing effects of any substance of use. It is most rel- evant in the withdrawal/negative affect stage in which noradrenergic overactivity in the locus coe- ruleus is implicated in opioid withdrawal and can be effectively treated with central alpha-agonists such as clonidine or lofexidine.

4. **C.** Reinforcing drugs will lower the threshold for ICSS

The Olds and Milner classic experiment was an ICSS animal study showing that animals would perform a response (lever pressing) to self-admin- ister a stimulus delivered via implanted brain elec- trodes to brain reward circuits. ICSS provides a way to study substances' effects on brain reward thresholds. The addictiveness of substance is cor- related with its ability to lower ICSS threshold. Answer choice A describes conditioned place aver- sion, and answer choice B describes conditioned place preference.

5. **A.** Defensive burying

In defensive burying, the animal is placed in a box filled with woodchip bedding and an electrified probe protruding into the box. After touching the probe and receiving a shock, the animal generally buries the probe with the woodchips; observers will measure variables related to burying including the time to burying, the height of the woodchip mound, and the total time spent burying. These measures are sensitive for increased anxiety-like states. Choices B, C, D, and E do not measure anx- iety-like responses.

6. **B.** Negative reinforcement

In negative reinforcement, a negative stimulus is removed with a behavior, making it more likely that the behavior will be repeated. In this example, resumption of heroin use reduces opioid with- drawal symptoms. Removal of these highly aver- sive symptoms is a powerful negative reinforcer.

7. **D.** Operant conditioning

Operant conditioning refers to behavior modi- fication through use of punishing and rewarding consequences. Methadone maintenance programs use a contingency management approach through their allotment of take-home doses for patients who have demonstrated abstinence.

8. **A.** Glutamatergic projections from the PFC to dopamine neurons in the VTA

Incentive salience refers to cue-learning in which a stimulus becomes conditioned with a drug's rewarding effect, to the point in which the stimu- lus can induce motivation to drug-seek. Incentive salience is regulated through glutamatergic projec- tions from the PFC to dopamine neurons in the VTA.

9. **B.** Hallucinogens

According to data from large surveys of adult twins, hallucinogen use disorder has the low- est heritability among the common substances of abuse, whereas cocaine and opioids have among the highest (Ducci & Goldman, 2012).

10. **A.** GWAS

Answer choice B is an older method used to iden- tify chromosomal regions coinherited with the phenotype of interest (e.g., substance abuse) among related individuals. Linkage studies have largely been replaced by GWAS, which are performed by querying the genome with microarrays of thousands to millions of genetic markers to examine whether particular alleles are more common among individuals with the disease versus controls. Advantages of GWAS include the ability to identify multiple risk alleles with individual small effect sizes, although studies typically require very large sample sizes.

REFERENCE

Ducci, F., & Goldman, D. (2012). The genetic basis of addictive disorders. *Psychiatric Clinics of North America, 35*(2), 495–519. https://doi.org/10.1016/j.psc.2012.03.010.

CHAPTER 4

1. **A.** Her alcohol use is considered at-risk because she is drinking more than the accepted weekly amount for women.

   This question is testing your knowledge of the NIAAA standards of alcohol consumption for men and women. According to the NIAAA, women should drink no more than 7 standard drinks per week and no more than 3 standard drinks per occasion; men should drink no more than 14 standard drinks per week and no more than 4 drinks per occasion. Drinking more than these limits is considered to put individuals at risk for negative health and social outcomes.

2. **F.** Inpatient; he has no social supports involved in his treatment.

   This question is testing your application of the ASAM placement criteria to determine whether this patient can be managed as an outpatient. In general, patients who present with CIWA greater than 15 (indicating severe withdrawal), have unstable medical or psychiatric conditions that can complicate treatment of withdrawal, have high levels of recent alcohol consumption, have a history of withdrawal seizures or DTs, who do not have any social supports at home or cannot reliably present to an outpatient clinic daily should be managed in the inpatient setting.

3. **D.** Acamprosate did not outperform either placebo or naltrexone.

This question is testing your knowledge of the Project COMBINE research study. Disulfiram was not included as one of the study's three interventions, immediately ruling out answer choices B and E. Acamprosate was not associated with a significant reduction in drinking compared with placebo, either alone or in combination with naltrexone at the end of the 16-week treatment period. The treatment group that showed the best outcome received MM with naltrexone without the CBI.

4. **D.** Patients receiving medication management (naltrexone) + no behavioral intervention

   Of the nine treatment groups compared in the COMBINE study, the groups performing best at the end of the treatment period received medication management (with naltrexone) with and without behavioral intervention, and behavioral intervention with MM (with placebo).

5. **F.** No group showed statistically superior outcomes at 1-year follow-up.

   According to results from the COMBINE study, all between-group effects observed following the 16-week treatment period were no longer significant at 1-year follow-up.

6. **B.** Fomepizole prevents build-up of formaldehyde through inhibition of alcohol dehydrogenase.

   To answer this question, you need to know both methanol's metabolic pathway and fomepizole's mechanism of action. Methanol is metabolized to formaldehyde by alcohol dehydrogenase. Ethylene glycol is metabolized to glycolic acid, and ethanol is metabolized to acetaldehyde; neither of these byproducts are in the metabolic pathway of methanol. Fomepizole competitively inhibits ADH, not ALDH, and prevents metabolization of methanol to the highly toxic formaldehyde.

7. **A.** Production of calcium oxalate crystals, leading to renal injury

   Ethylene glycol is metabolized to glycolic acid, which is further broken down to calcium oxalate. Calcium oxalate crystals can then form in the kidneys, leading to renal injury. Answer choice B refers to the effects of methanol; answer choice C refers to the effects of ethanol; answer choice

D refers to the effects of isopropyl alcohol, which causes ketosis without metabolic acidosis.

8. **D.** EtG

Indirect biomarkers do not contain ethanol or its direct metabolites and include MCV, CDT, GGT, AST, and alanine aminotranferase. Direct measures include EtG, EtS, BAC, and breath alcohol concentrations.

9. **B.** Women have a lower expression of ADH in the gastric mucosa, reducing first-pass metabolism.

Gastric ADH is responsible for first-pass metabolism of alcohol. Women express less gastric ADH, which allows more alcohol to be absorbed into systemic circulation. Gastric ADH expression also declines with advancing age. There is no evidence for answer choice A. Answer choices C and D are true for individuals who express the ALDH*2 and ADH1B*2 isotype, common among those with East Asian heritage.

10. **B.** Elevated heart rate

Vital signs are not factored into overall scoring but are typically recorded each time the CIWA-Ar is administered. The decision not to include vital signs was based on data showing that pulse and blood pressure did not correlate as well with severity of alcohol withdrawal compared with the other signs and symptoms included in the CIWA-Ar.

11. **C.** ALDH; acetaldehyde

Alcohol flush reaction is common among individuals of East Asian descent because of a higher frequency of both the ADH1B*2 and ALDH2*2 alleles, both of which lead to accumulation of acetaldehyde. The ADH1B*2 allele metabolizes ethanol more rapidly to acetaldehyde, whereas the ALDH2*2 allele metabolizes acetaldehyde more slowly; the presence of one or both of these isotypes would lead to accumulation of acetaldehyde. Increased amounts of acetaldehyde lead to the release of histamines, which then causes vessel dilatation and skin redness.

12. **D.** Verbal learning

Some or all of the above cognitive domains have been found to become impaired in 50% to 70% of individuals with AUD. However, verbal learning impairments are most quick to reverse following cessation of use with some studies demonstrating recovery within the first 2 weeks of abstinence. As longer-term abstinence is reached, learning and memory issues are still present in some individuals.

13. **D.** Liver disease

In the United States, alcohol-related mortality has alarmingly doubled between 1999 and 2017. This has been the subject of extensive national discussion and was highlighted by recent publications by economists Anne Case and Angus Deaton. These deaths, also coined "deaths of despair," are primarily a result of liver disease (31%), followed by overdoses (18%) either with alcohol alone or in combination with other drugs, followed by cardiovascular disease (11%) based on mortality data from 2017. Globally, however, alcohol-related injuries (traffic accidents, self-harm, or violence) are the most common cause of alcohol-related mortality.

14. **B.** Naltrexone

Naltrexone is the only medication listed that primarily acts by reducing the euphoric and pleasant effects of alcohol by blocking opioid pathways projecting to the reward areas of the brain, thereby reducing alcohol-induced dopamine release and the positive reinforcing effects of alcohol. Disulfiram predominantly works by creating a highly aversive reaction (i.e., a punishment) in the presence of alcohol, thereby incentivizing the patient to avoid it completely. Acamprosate reduces symptoms of protracted withdrawal during abstinence and has no effect on the positive reinforcing effects of alcohol. Sertraline has little efficacy for use in AUD beyond treating a co-occurring psychiatric disorder. Gabapentin has no effects on the positive reinforcing properties of alcohol. Naltrexone is the best choice.

15. **C.** Acamprosate

Acamprosate should only be started when the patient has achieved abstinence; because of its GABAergic and antiglutamatergic activity, it is thought to attenuate the symptoms of protracted alcohol withdrawal that place patients at risk for relapse during early abstinence.

16. **A.** It is a positive allosteric modulator of GABA-A receptors.

Acamprosate is a positive allosteric modulator of the GABA-A receptor and an NMDA receptor antagonist; it reduces glutamatergic activity and increases GABAergic activity during early abstinence and can counteract the symptoms of protracted withdrawal. Answer choices B and D describe the mechanism of action for baclofen and gabapentin, respectively.

17. **D.** Alpha-2-receptor agonist

Gabapentin was designed to be a structural analog of GABA and closely resembles endogenous amino acids; despite this and despite its name, gabapentin does not directly agonize or antagonize the GABA-A or GABA-B receptor and does not modulate GABA activity. Gabapentin inhibits the alpha-2-delta-1 subunit of voltage-gated calcium channels.

18. **C.** ARND

This question is testing your knowledge of the diagnostic criteria for FASD. This patient meets criteria for ARND. Generally, the IQ of individuals with FASD is above the threshold for intellectual disability (IQ >70). If this same patient had two or more facial features of FAS, he would meet criteria for pFAS. The diagnosis of FAS requires four criteria: (1) two or more characteristic facial features (short palpebral fissures, thin vermillion border, or smooth philtrum), (2) growth retardation, (3) evidence of brain involvement, and (4) neurobehavioral impairments. Documented alcohol exposure is not required for the FAS diagnosis.

19. **C.** Coronary occlusion

Severe myocardial disease or coronary occlusion is an absolute contraindication to disulfiram use; the disulfiram–alcohol reaction can cause coronary vasospasm, chest pain, and in rare cases can cause cardiorespiratory death. Hepatic impairment is a relative but not absolute contraindication; disulfiram can cause a fatal drug-induced hepatitis in 1 in 30,000 patients, and increases risk for cholestatic and fulminant hepatitis. Physiological dependence on opioids is a contraindication for using naltrexone but not disulfiram. Depression (severe or otherwise) and migraines are not contraindications for using disulfiram.

20. **B.** High neuroticism

AUD is significantly associated with higher neuroticism and lower conscientiousness. It is not associated with differences in extraversion, openness to experience, or agreeableness.

21. **D.** Acamprosate

The FDA approved three medications to treat AUD: disulfiram, naltrexone, and acamprosate. Of these, acamprosate would be the preferred medication to use in patients with hepatic insufficiency. It is excreted in urine as an unmetabolized drug. As a result, it should not be used as a first-line agent for renal impairment patients. Naltrexone is metabolized hepatically via noncytochrome-mediated dehydrogenase and is subject to the extensive first-pass effect. Its use can be associated with increase serum transaminases, and it is contraindicated in patients with acute hepatitis or hepatic failure. Disulfiram is metabolized hepatically via glucuronidation. Its side effects include cholestatic hepatitis, fulminant hepatitis, and hepatic failure. It is relatively contraindicated in patients with hepatic cirrhosis. Gabapentin and ondansetron are used as second-line treatment options for AUD but are not FDA approved for this condition.

CHAPTER 5

1. **A.** Alpha-1 subunit of GABA receptor

Z-drugs have the greatest effect at the alpha-1 subunit which mediates sleep and amnestic effects, and weaker activity at alpha-2 and -3 subunits which mediates anxiolytic and anticonvulsant effects. Benzodiazepines exert their effects at alpha-1 through -3 and -5 subunits (answer choice C). Z-drugs do not interact with the NMDA or AMPA glutamate receptor.

2. **D.** Increase the duration of GABA channel opening

Barbiturates increase the duration of GABA channel opening (answer choice D), whereas benzodiazepines increase the frequency (answer choice E). Barbiturates are antagonists, not agonists, at the AMPA and kainate receptor, ruling out answer choices A and B. Barbiturates are indirect agonists and allosteric modulators of the GABA receptor, ruling out answer choice C.

3. **E.** There are no significant drug–drug interactions.

Most benzodiazepines are metabolized by CYP3A4 oxidation followed by glucuronide conjugation. The so-called "LOT" (lorazepam, oxazepam, and temazepam) benzodiazepines do not undergo oxidation and only undergo conjugation. Therefore, lorazepam does not have CYP-related drug–drug interactions, and answer choice E is correct. This characteristic of LOT benzodiazepines makes them the medication of choice in patients with hepatic impairment or where you wish to avoid drug–drug interactions.

4. **D.** Cleft palate

Although the absolute risk remains very low, benzodiazepines have been found to increase the risk of cleft palate from 6 in 10,000 to 11 in 10,000 based on retrospective case–control studies (Bellantuono et al., 2013). Neonatal abstinence syndrome (answer choice A) can occur following chronic maternal exposure to opioids. Placenta previa, stillbirth, and preeclampsia (answer choices B, C, and E) are not known risks of benzodiazepine exposure during pregnancy.

5. **B.** High lipophilicity

The three pharmacologic characteristics that can help predict all of the clinical effects of benzodiazepines are lipophilicity, elimination half-life, and potency. Alprazolam has a long elimination half-life (11–15 hours) but is highly lipophilic (answer choice B), which accounts for its rapid onset of action and short duration of clinical effect. While alprazolam does not have active metabolites, this does not explain why it has a short duration of effect. Alprazolam does not have activity at the GABA-B or NMDA receptor.

6. **B.** Lorazepam

Standard urine drug tests detect oxazepam, and all benzodiazepines that include oxazepam as one of their metabolic byproducts. This includes chlordiazepoxide, oxazepam, temazepam, and diazepam. However, some of the most commonly prescribed benzodiazepines (e.g., clonazepam, lorazepam, and alprazolam) do not share this metabolic pathway and are therefore not detected by routine urine drug tests.

7. **B.** Complex sleep-related behaviors

Following a number of reports serious injuries and deaths from sleep behaviors such as sleepwalking and sleep driving, the FDA placed a **black box warning** stating that use of zolpidem, zaleplon and eszopiclone is contraindicated in patients who have experienced an episode of a complex sleep behavior while taking one of these medications. Benzodiazepines, not Z-drugs, have a **black box warning** stating that taking benzodiazepines together with opioids can be fatal (choice A).

8. **C.** Memory impairment

Patients prescribed chronic benzodiazepines quickly build tolerance to their hypnotic, sedative, and anticonvulsant effects. Driving impairments and falls largely occur as a result of sedative side effects. However, individuals do not tend to build tolerance to the anxiolytic or amnesic effects of benzodiazepines (choice C) (Vinkers & Olivier, 2012).

9. **A.** Transition patient from lorazepam to clonazepam and perform a slow taper

For patients who have been on benzodiazepines longer term, it is generally recommended to perform a gradual taper after cross-tapering to a benzodiazepine with a longer duration of effect, such as clonazepam. Ancillary medications may be used to help with anxiety and sleep during the taper, for example, trazodone or hydroxyzine. Alprazolam has a short duration of effect and would not be a good choice for performing a taper (choice B). Starting an SSRI may be reasonable if clinically indicated, but answer choice A is still the next best step.

10. **C.** Naloxone

It is rare that a patient presenting to the emergency room with a solitary benzodiazepine overdose can reach a stuporous or comatose state; in these cases, benzodiazepines are typically co-ingested with other substances, such as alcohol or opioids. Recall that approximately 75% of benzodiazepine-related fatal overdoses involve co-ingestion with opioids. In this clinical scenario, the immediate next best step would be to administer naloxone (choice C). Flumazenil can be used in benzodiazepine over-dose, but it can precipitate withdrawal seizures in patients who are benzodiazepine dependent. Flu-mazenil is frequently used to reverse benzodiaze-pine-induced sedation for anesthesia or in cases of pediatric ingestion in which benzodiazepine dependence is less of an issue. Flurazepam is a lipophilic benzodiazepine with a long elimination half-life that has no role for treatment in this sce-nario (choice B). Activated charcoal is generally not recommended in cases of benzodiazepine overdose because of the risk of aspiration (choice D). Hemodialysis is not effective as a rapid elimi-nation technique (choice E).

REFERENCES

Bellantuono, C., Tofani, S., Di Sciascio, G., & Santone, G. (2013). Benzodiazepine exposure in pregnancy and risk of major malfor-mations: A critical overview. *General Hospital Psychiatry, 35*(1), 3–8. https://doi.org/10.1016/j.genhosppsych.2012.09.003.

Vinkers, C. H., & Olivier, B. (2012). Mechanisms underlying toler-ance after long-term benzodiazepine use: A future for subtype-selective GABA(A) receptor modulators? *Advances in Pharmaco-logical Sciences, 2012*, Article 416864.

CHAPTER 6

1. **C.** 60 to 80 mg

   Illicit opioid use was directly related to methadone dosage: in patients on doses above 70 mg per day, no heroin use was detected, whereas patients on doses below 50 mg per day were at higher risk of using heroin than those receiving higher doses. A meta-analysis of 21 studies concluded that metha-done dosages ranging from 60 to 100 mg per day were more effective than lower dosages in retain-ing patients and in reducing the use of heroin and cocaine use during treatment (Faggiano et al., 2003).

2. **C.** Fluconazole

   Methadone is metabolized by CYP3A4 and co-use of potent CYP3A inhibitors, such as certain HIV medications, antifungals, and antibiotics, can lead to increased serum levels of methadone.

3. **B.** 2.5 to 4 hours

   Methadone differs from other opioids in the drug's absorption, metabolism, and relative analgesic potency. Particular vigilance is necessary during treatment initiation and titration. Methadone can be detected in the blood 15 to 45 minutes after its oral administration and reaches its peak levels between 2 and 4 hours.

4. **D.** Dextromethorphan

   Many routinely prescribed medications are asso-ciated with false-positive urine toxicology results. If in doubt, such tests should be confirmed using gas chromatography-mass spectrometry. The "opi-ates" immunoassay used in standard urine drug screens uses antibodies specific for morphine metabolites and detects the presence of natural and some semisynthetic opioids, such as heroin, morphine, and codeine. Opiate false-positive results have been reported for dextromethorphan, quinolones, diphenhydramine, and rifampin. Dextromethorphan has a chemical structure that is similar to morphine and can lead to a urine drug screen that is false-positive for opiates or phencyclidine.

5. **B.** Meperidine

   Meperidine is known to induce seizures because of the accumulation of meperidine's metabolite, normeperidine, norpethidine. The use of meperi-dine in the elderly and patients with underlying hepatic or renal disease should be avoided. The use of meperidine, in combination with serotonergic medications or herbs, has also been linked with the development of serotonin syndrome.

6. **C.** The requirement for 7 days of abstinence from opioids before naltrexone initiation

   Extended-release naltrexone is an FDA-approved treatment for OUD. Initiation requires detoxifi-cation from opioids first because it precipitates withdrawal symptoms in individuals dependent on opioids. It is recommended for patients to abstain from opioids for 7 to 10 days before ini-tiation. This can be a significant barrier for many patients, particularly those being induced in the outpatient setting, but naltrexone is still a practical treatment approach for many individuals with OUD.

7. **D.** OUD, moderate

In the *Diagnostic and Statistical Manual of Mental Disorders*, Fifth Edition, a patient must meet at least two diagnostic criteria to qualify for an OUD. Severity is characterized as "mild" if two or three criteria are met, "moderate" if four or five criteria are met, and "severe" if six or more criteria are met. The patient above meets at least four criteria, which qualifies him for a moderate OUD. He demonstrates tolerance to opioids, is using more and for longer than intended, has increased time spent obtaining opioids, and has failed to fulfill work obligations.

REFERENCE

Faggiano, F., Vigna-Taglianti, F., Versino, E., & Lemma, P. (2003). Methadone maintenance at different dosages for opioid dependence. *Cochrane Database Syst Rev*(3), Article CD002208.

CHAPTER 7

1. **B.** Varenicline

Among the available pharmacotherapies, which include NRT, bupropion, and varenicline, varenicline has the highest efficacy in achieving abstinence. These findings have been demonstrated in several large studies and were one of the main findings of the Evaluating Adverse Events in a Global Smoking Cessation Study (EAGLES) trial (Anthenelli et al., 2016).

2. **D.** Decreased heart rate

Nicotine withdrawal symptoms usually reach their peak 2 to 3 days after discontinuation. Smoking cessation may lead to decreased heart rate, tremors, irritability, insomnia, and increased appetite.

3. **C.** 14 mg every 24 hours

Dosing is determined by the number of cigarettes a person smokes daily when the patch is started. If the person smokes more than 10 cigarettes per day, it is recommended to begin with a 21 mg/day patch for the first 6 weeks, then 14 mg/day for 2 weeks, and then 7 mg/day for 2 weeks. If the person is smoking less than 10 cigarettes per day, it is recommended to start with the 14 mg/day patch for 6 weeks, followed by 7 mg/day for 2 weeks.

4. **A.** Not wearing the patch during nighttime

Leaving the patch on overnight can cause side effects such as insomnia and vivid dreams. If patients experience this, they can remove the patch before bedtime and replace it in the morning. Smoking cessation rates are similar whether the patch is left on for 24 hours or taken off at night. It is not recommended to wear a patch for more than 24 hours as it can cause an adverse reaction to the skin. It is also not recommended for people to wear more than one patch at a time.

5. **B.** Nasal spray

Nicotine nasal spray tends to be used for a longer time and has been linked with a higher potential abuse than other forms of nicotine replacement.

6. **C.** Nortriptyline

A Cochrane systematic review found multiple controlled trials of nortriptyline as smoking cessation. The data shows that nortriptyline can double the odds of quitting smoking (Hughes et al., 2005).

REFERENCES

Anthenelli, R. M., Benowitz, N. L., West, R., St Aubin, L., McRae, T., Lawrence, D., Ascher, J., Russ, C., Krishen, A., & Evins, A. E. (2016). Neuropsychiatric safety and efficacy of varenicline, bupropion, and nicotine patch in smokers with and without psychiatric disorders (EAGLES): A double-blind, randomised, placebo-controlled clinical trial. *Lancet (London, England), 387*(10037), 2507–2520.
Hughes, J. R., Stead, L. F., & Lancaster, T. (2005). Antidepressants for smoking cessation. *Cochrane Syst Rev.*

CHAPTER 8

1. **B.** Short-term memory impairment

Of the answer choices provided, answer choices B and D are well-known effects of cannabis intoxication. Cannabis intoxication does not cause long-term memory impairments, respiratory depression, or dementia (answer choices A, C, and E). Answer choice B is the correct answer; short-term memory impairments can lead to difficulties with learning and academic performance which is most relevant to his presenting problem.

2. **B.** Higher affinity for the CB1 receptor

Synthetic cannabinoids are full agonists at the CB1 receptor and have a much higher receptor affinity (approximately 100 ×) for CB1 compared to plant-based THC. Unlike plant-based cannabis, synthetic cannabinoids do not contain CBD which would modulate the psychotomimetic effects of CB1 agonism.

3. **A.** The perceived risk of marijuana use has declined among this age group

There has been a sea change in public policy and opinion regarding the safety and efficacy of cannabis; this has accompanied the widespread legalization and decriminalization of cannabis use in many U.S. states. There is an inverse relationship between perceived risk and substance use; as the perceived risk of cannabis has been declining among high schoolers, cannabis use has increased. Over the past several decades, the average proportion of THC has increased while CBD has decreased, ruling out answer choices C and D. Despite being legalized in a number of states, marijuana remains a Schedule I drug, ruling out answer choice E.

4. **A.** Tachypnea

Because of the co-localization of CB1 receptors with beta-adrenergic receptors, cannabis intoxication can lead to adrenergic-like effects including tachycardia, tachypnea (answer choice A), and blood pressure variability, ruling out answer choice B. Cannabis typically causes dry mouth, not hypersalivation (answer choice D). Piloerection commonly occurs with opioid withdrawal, not cannabis intoxication (answer choice C). Cannabis intoxication typically causes time dilatation or a sense of time slowing down, ruling out answer choice E.

5. **B.** CM

This is an example of CM, which is based on the principle of operant conditioning. In contingency management, a patient with a substance use disorder would perform a toxicology test, and if negative, the patient would get to draw from a bucket of tickets with prizes of variable monetary value. The most effective evidence-based psychosocial intervention for cannabis use disorder is abstinence-based voucher CM + CBT; this combination is more effective than either intervention alone.

6. **D.** The majority of individuals who try cannabis once will not develop a cannabis use disorder

Although there is a positive association between cannabis use and schizophrenia, the direction of causality has not been established, ruling out answer choices A, B, and C. Among individuals who have tried cannabis once, approximately 9% will eventually develop a cannabis use disorder, which rules out answer choice E.

7. **C.** Butane hash oil

The boards may ask about the relative THC potency of different products derived from the cannabis plant. In general: *cannabis leaves and stems* (0.5%–5%); *sinsemilla*, or the cannabis flowering tops of unpollinated female plants (7%–14%); *hashish oil* (15%–50%); *"dab"* or *butane hash oil* (up to 90%). *Hashish* is dried cannabis resin with compressed flowers and variable THC potency (2–8%).

8. **B.** Dronabinol

Dronabinol is synthetically produced delta-9-THC and will cause a positive UDS for THC because it is structurally identical. Sativex is 1:1 delta-9-THC:CBD and will also cause a positive toxicology test. Of the two, this patient is most likely being prescribed dronabinol, which is commonly used for cancer-induced nausea; Sativex is approved for the treatment of spasticity in multiple sclerosis. Nabilone is a synthetic analog of THC with distinct metabolites and will not cause a positive test on a standard urine drug screen. CBD is not detected on standard urine drug screens, ruling out answer choices D and E.

9. **C.** Increased risk of preterm birth

Cannabis use during pregnancy is associated with an increased risk of preterm birth and infants who are small for gestational age or require transfer to the NICU. It is not associated with increased risk of preeclampsia, neonatal abstinence syndrome, or stillbirth (Corsi et al., 2019).

10. **C.** CB1 antagonism; suicidality

Rimonabant is a CB1 receptor antagonist and a weight-loss drug whose use was limited due to the adverse effect of suicidality. Rimonabant is no longer available in the United States.

11. **C.** Cannabis use has no effect on the risk of driving accidents.

Cannabis intoxication increases the risk of car accidents by a factor of 2; for comparison, alcohol with a BAL greater than 0.08% increases risk of car accidents by a factor of 5 (Sewell et al., 2009). Cannabis intoxication leads to delayed reaction time, poorer hand–eye coordination, and impairs automatic motor behaviors that are important in driving. States that have legalized recreational marijuana have seen a significant increase in cannabis-related car accidents.

REFERENCES

Corsi, D. J., Walsh, L., Weiss, D., Hsu, H., El-Chaar, D., Hawken, S., Fell, D. B., & Walker, M. (2019). Association between self-reported prenatal cannabis use and maternal, perinatal, and neonatal outcomes. *JAMA, 322*(2), 145–152.

Sewell, R. A., Poling, J., & Sofuoglu, M. (2009). The effect of cannabis compared with alcohol on driving. *The American Journal on Addictions, 18*(3), 185–193.

CHAPTER 9

1. **D.** Bupropion

Combined with CM, bupropion has been proven to reduce cocaine use more effectively than either treatment alone or placebo (Poling et al., 2006).

2. **E.** Rivastigmine

Medications enhancing cholinergic transmission, especially cholinesterase inhibitors, have shown promise for the treatment of stimulant use disorder. Rivastigmine has reduced methamphetamine-associated increases in diastolic blood pressure and self-reported feelings of anxiety as well as the desire for the use of methamphetamine (De La Garza et al., 2012).

3. **A.** CM

Several behavioral treatments have been used for cocaine use disorder treatment, including CBT and CM. The goal of CBT is to teach strategies and enhance coping abilities to prevent drug use behavior. The efficacy of CBT for cocaine use disorder has been demonstrated in multiple studies. CM can be combined with other forms of psychotherapy or medications, and from the available options is the only treatment that is based on the principles of operant conditioning

4. **A.** It induces intracellular dopamine-containing vesicles to release dopamine into the synaptic cleft and blocks the reuptake of dopamine.

Cocaine acts primarily by blocking the reuptake of released dopamine in the synaptic clefts of the mesolimbic dopamine neurons. Caffeine competitively binds to adenosine receptors affecting the release of catecholamines and other neuropeptides. Methamphetamine blocks the dopamine transporter from pumping dopamine back into the transmitting neuron and causes the intracellular release of neurotransmitters to the synaptic cleft. From the options, methamphetamine is the only one that is commonly manufactured in illegal hidden laboratories by mixing various chemicals and over-the-counter medications.

5. **D.** Mirtazapine

Mirtazapine is a medication currently used to treat depression, which antagonizes noradrenergic alpha-2 receptors and the serotonin 5-HT2A/C and 5-HT3 receptors. It has demonstrated efficacy in reducing the rewarding effect of cocaine.

6. **C.** Amphetamine

Stimulant intoxication presents with hypertension, chest pain, anxiety, and diaphoresis. Tobacco intoxication would involve some gastrointestinal symptoms. Alcohol intoxication would present with disinhibition and slurred speech. Opioid use would present with decreased respiration, lethargy, and constricted pupils.

7. **D.** CAMK4

The CAMK4 and the presence of CHRNB3-A6 are linked with a higher susceptibility for cocaine use disorder. VNTRs in the *DAT1* gene are also associated with cocaine and methamphetamine-induced psychosis.

8. **D.** Bruxism

Bruxism is frequently seen in MDMA intoxication. The grinding of teeth usually goes away within 24 to 48 hours after ingestion of the drug.

REFERENCES

De La Garza, R., 2nd, Newton, T. F., Haile, C. N., Yoon, J. H., Nerumalla, C. S., Mahoney, J. J., 3rd, & Aziziyeh, A (2012). Rivastigmine reduces "Likely to use methamphetamine" in methamphetamine-dependent volunteers. *Progress in Neuro-psychopharmacology & Biological Psychiatry, 37*(1), 141–146.

Poling, J., Oliveto, A., Petry, N., Sofuoglu, M., Gonsai, K., Gonzalez, G., Martell, B., & Kosten, T. R. (2006). Six-month trial of bupropion with contingency management for cocaine dependence in a methadone-maintained population. *Archives of General Psychiatry, 63*(2), 219–228.

CHAPTER 10

1. **C.** Decrease the amount of coffee as tolerated

   Caffeine is a stimulant to the CNS and chronic use can cause physical dependence. If the person in this case stops taking caffeine abruptly, he may experience withdrawal symptoms. Some of the symptoms of caffeine withdrawal include anxiety, irritability, low mood, and difficulty concentrating. The recommendation is to decrease the amount as tolerated.

2. **B.** Adenosine

   Caffeine is an adenosine-receptor antagonist and is also a nonspecific phosphodiesterase inhibitor; the adenosine-2a receptor forms a heteromer with D2 receptors, which is believed to indirectly mediate the dopaminergic effects of caffeine. Caffeine does not directly affect dopamine, serotonin, or glycine receptors.

3. **C.** Toluene

   Exposure to toluene vapors found in paint thinners and other industrial products severely impacts the CNS. The patient in this case presents with mild brain atrophy, a prominent abnormality in toluene leukoencephalopathy cases. Other common findings in toluene intoxication include hypokalemia, metabolic acidosis, renal tubular acidosis, and muscle paralysis.

4. **A.** DXM

   DXM is commonly abused by teenagers and young adults for their dissociative and euphoric effects. At low doses, DXM has opioid-like effects (which account for its efficacy as a cough suppressant); at higher doses, it acts as a dissociative and hallucinogen through its NMDA receptor antagonism, popularly referred to as "robotripping."

5. **E.** Naloxone

   Naloxone is effective in antagonizing the effects of opioids. DXM is a synthetic analog of levorphanol, which is an opioid that is structurally similar to morphine. Based on case reports, naloxone can work to reverse coma and respiratory depression in cases of severe DXM overdoses. N-acetylcysteine is an important therapeutic consideration in DXM overdoses, as many cough syrup preparations contain acetaminophen.

6. **B.** PCP intoxication

   The hallmark clinical findings of PCP intoxication are nystagmus, hypertension, and an altered mental status.

7. **D.** Ayahuasca

   Almost all hallucinogens carry the potential risk of serotonin syndrome owing to their primary serotonergic effects through the 5-HT2 receptor, and that risk increases when combined with any other serotonergic agent. However, ayahuasca is unique in that it contains both DMT and naturally occurring MAOIs. The combination of fluoxetine and an MAOI leads to a higher risk of serotonin syndrome.

CHAPTER 11

1. **A.** A decrease in renal function

   Ibuprofen, an NSAID agent, reduces prostaglandin synthesis via cyclooxygenase inhibition. NSAIDs can induce sodium retention and antagonize diuretics, impairing free-water clearance and causing hyponatremia, creating lower-leg edema resulting in weight gain in the patient.

2. **C.** Psychiatric evaluation

   The patient in this case appears to meet the criteria for a mood disorder. Symptoms of a mood disorder are common in patients suffering from chronic pain. It has been reported that at least one-third of patients presenting to chronic pain clinics have an active major depression disorder. This patient would benefit from a psychiatric evaluation to diagnose and treat current symptoms.

3. **B.** Nociceptive pain

Nociceptive pain is acute pain that usually consists of acute tissue damage and not a direct nerve injury. It presents as dull aching pain at the site of the injury. Neuropathic pain includes a direct nerve tissue injury.

CHAPTER 12

1. **C.** SUD prevalence rates among emergency physicians and anesthesiologists are higher than the general population.

SUD is as commonly prevalent among physicians as the general population (around 10% lifetime prevalence). Emergency physicians and anesthesiologists are more likely to have an SUD than other physicians, whereas pediatricians and surgeons are less likely to have an SUD. Psychiatrists are most likely to use benzodiazepines, whereas anesthesiologists are most likely to use opioids. The prognosis for physicians with an SUD is better than the general population, likely due to the fear of losing one's license acting as an alternate reinforcer. Physician health programs are typically separate from the state medical boards and offer supervision that further improves physicians' prognosis for recovery.

2. **D.** A positive drug test indicates recent drug use.

Drug testing demonstrates recent drug use. Using substances does not necessarily mean that the individual has a diagnosable SUD. Such a positive drug test gives us no information about whether the individual needs diagnostic criteria for an SUD. Drug test requests are categorized as *random* or *for-cause*. *For-cause* testing refers to situations when a drug test is ordered when there is reasonable suspicion that the person had used the drug.

In contrast, *random* testing refers to a situation when a drug test is ordered without reasonable suspicion that the person had used the drug. *Random* tests are most effective in identifying frequent users rather than occasional users. Hair testing for biomarkers of excessive alcohol use is not recommended as a monitoring strategy to ensure abstinence for someone who is recently charged with a DUI. Doing it provides retrospective information about excessive alcohol use over the past 2 to 3 months, but not about recent alcohol use. As such, breath alcohol monitoring combined might be more appropriate in such situations.

3. **C.** A 19-year-old man with schizophrenia and phencyclidine intoxication

The relationship between substance use and violence and criminal behavior has been studied extensively. Major epidemiological studies, including the MacArthur Violence Risk Assessment Study, found that persons with nonaddictive psychiatric disorders are more likely to be the victims of violent encounters than the perpetrators. In contrast, those with substance use disorders, particularly if intoxicated, carry an increased risk of violence or criminal behaviors. Furthermore, co-occurring addictive and nonaddictive psychiatric disorders have an even greater risk. Younger age, male gender, and psychosis are also associated with an increased risk of violence in persons who use drugs or alcohol.

CHAPTER 13

1. **A.** Precontemplation

This patient's disinterest in treatment and minimization of the adverse consequences of his substance use suggests that he is in the precontemplation stage of change. He did not demonstrate any ambivalence about wanting to address his substance use. Patients in this stage are not considering change and present with active resistance. The main clinical risk during this stage is dropout from treatment. The other stages of change are:

- Contemplation: Patients in this stage are ambivalent about changing their behaviors.
- Preparation: Patients in this stage are taking steps toward changing their behaviors and present with increasing confidence in their decision to change.
- Action: Patients in this stage are overtly modifying their behaviors and factors in the environment that support continued substance use. The main clinical risk during this stage is relapse.

- Maintenance: The goals for this stage include sustaining changes, consolidating gains, learning alternative coping strategies, and recognizing triggers.
- Relapse and recycling: This stage is not inevitable. During this stage, patients' main clinical risk is to feel stuck in their old ways. As such, the primary goal of treatment is avoiding becoming stuck and redefining the relapse as an opportunity for further self-improvement.
- Termination: Patients in this stage have reached their ultimate goals and can exit the cycle of change without fear of relapse.

2. **C.** It sounds like you are interested in quitting but are worried about how quitting may affect your performance.

Reflections are likely the most important aspect of MI. Different types of reflections include simple reflections (for example: "So you are saying that alcohol is causing a drift in your relationship."), double reflections (e.g., "So on the one hand, alcohol helps you cope with stress caused by work, and on the other hand, it is causing a drift in your relationship."), or amplified reflections (for example, after a patient tells you that they enjoy drinking alcohol, you overshoot and respond: "I see, drinking alcohol has been a very positive experience in your life and you have no interest in cutting down."). In this clinical vignette, the patient is expressing a desire to address her cocaine use but is identifying potential barriers. Reflecting her statements will allow her to expand on her motivating factors and will lead to her using more change talk.

3. **D.** Using point-of-care testing at home three times a week and rewarding her with random gift certificates occasionally when she tests negative.

CM is based on the principles of introducing alternative reinforcers that are valued more than using drugs or alcohol (such as monetary rewards). CM as therapy involves positive reinforcement by rewarding patients with incentives for achieving their treatment goals such as abstinence. CM is most effective when the rewards are given immediately following a negative test (rather than days later if the drug screen is performed at a laboratory) and delivered with a variable frequency (rather than following every negative test).

4. **B.** Commitment to participating in 12-step–based mutual-support groups and to abstinence.

Multiple studies investigating the effectiveness of 12-step–based mutual-support groups have consistently found that group participants who are committed to the group process and to the goal of achieving abstinence tend to fare better and have better long-term abstinence outcomes. Twelve-step-based mutual-support groups meetings involve group members sharing their experiences and are encouraged to "work through" the 12 steps. Twelve-step-based mutual-support group principles include taking responsibility, finding humility, and using honesty. The process uses tools based on psychological principles, including stimulus control and cue reactivity, reconditioning, and positive reinforcement.

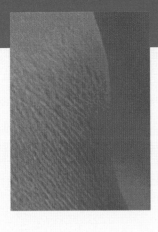

PRACTICE TESTS ANSWER KEY (CHAPTER 14)

BLOCK 1

1. **C.** Precontemplation

   According to Prochaska and DiClemente's Stages of Change, precontemplation is characterized by either denial of the problem or an unwillingness to change (DiClemente et al., 2004).

2. **B.** Nabilone

   Both dronabinol and nabilone are FDA-approved to treat cancer-related nausea and vomiting. Dronabinol is a synthetic delta-9-tetrahydrocannabinol (THC), and nabilone is a THC analog with minimal euphoric effects. For this patient, nabilone would be the best choice. Rimonabant is a cannabinoid 1 (CB1)-receptor antagonist studied to treat cannabis use disorder but was pulled from the worldwide market due to serious psychiatric side effects, including suicidal ideation (answer choice C). Although cancer is a qualifying condition in many states for medical marijuana, medical marijuana does not have FDA approval for any situation. It has varying amounts of CBD and delta-9-THC, the latter of which produces psychoactive effects (answer choice D). Cannabidiol alone would not be the most effective cannabinoid to treat his condition (answer choice E).

3. **E.** Assess the severity of her opioid withdrawal and begin buprenorphine.

   This patient is coming to your clinic seeking treatment using medications for OUD. Buprenorphine might be a better option than naltrexone, given her history of chronic pain and continued pain despite treating an opioid agonist. Given that she is currently in withdrawal, you might be able to begin office-based buprenorphine induction on the same day, maximizing the chances for her recovery once she starts having mild to moderate symptoms of opioid withdrawal. In contrast, prescribing her clonidine and other medications for opioid withdrawal and discharging her with a follow-up appointment in 1 week will increase the likelihood that she will continue using illicit opioids after leaving your office to relieve the withdrawal symptoms. Further, while having a history of suicide attempts and substance use disorder (SUD) are major risk factors for suicide, the patient is not currently suicidal or depressed. There is no indication to send her to the psychiatric emergency room.

4. **B.** Send him to the emergency room.

   This patient should be evaluated urgently in an emergency room setting. His history of intravenous drug use, sharing needles, chest pain, fever, and tachycardia elevate his risk for infective myocarditis and endocarditis. Injecting drugs increases the likelihood of bacterial injections from nonsterile injection procedures. Drug and alcohol use are associated with behavioral disinhibition, which could further increase the risk of bacterial infections. Bacteria, most commonly *Staphylococcus*, can travel with blood and deposit as vegetations on cardiac valves (most commonly the tricuspid valve). Bacterial endocarditis is lethal if untreated. Treatment involves a long course of intravenous antibiotics and, at times, valve replacement.

5. **E.** Aripiprazole

   A variety of neuropharmacological strategies are being researched to find an effective treatment for methamphetamine use disorder. Aripiprazole did not have an effect on cue-induced methamphetamine craving but was associated with an increase in some of the rewarding and stimulatory effects produced by methamphetamine use (Newton et al., 2008).

6. **C.** Nitrous oxide

Nitrous oxide is an odorless, colorless gas and effective sedative with a rapid onset and recovery. However, if it is misused and abused it can lead to the irreversible inactivation of vitamin B_{12}. A neurological examination can reveal sensory ataxia and pseudoathetosis in the upper limbs with reduced vibration sensation bilaterally. Laboratory studies can show low serum vitamin B_{12} concentration, mild macrocytosis, and raised serum homocysteine concentration.

7. **D.** Serotonin

3,4-Methylenedioxymethamphetamine (MDMA) use is associated with deficits in sleep, sexual dysfunction, reduced immune-competence, and increased oxidative stress. Serotonin plays an essential role in mood, sleep, and appetite regulation. The excess release of serotonin by MDMA can cause a depletion of serotonin causing a dysregulation of emotions, impulsiveness, and aggression.

8. **C.** Twelve-step facilitation (TSF)

Project MATCH compared three psychosocial interventions for treatment of alcohol use disorder: CBT, MET, and TSF. Its main finding was that all three interventions produced roughly equivalent clinical improvement. Subgroup analysis found that MET was better for angrier patients with lower initial motivation. CBT was superior for patients with less severe alcohol use disorder, and TSF was superior for patients with little social support for abstinence (Matching alcoholism treatments to client heterogeneity, 1998).

9. **B.** Naltrexone

The COMBINE study was a multicenter, randomized placebo-controlled trial that compared different combinations of three interventions for alcohol use disorder; two of the interventions were medication management with naltrexone and/or

acamprosate, and the third was a combined behavioral intervention (CBI). One of the striking findings of this study was that acamprosate did not outperform placebo in reducing drinking when given alone or in combination with CBI. At the end of the 16-week treatment period, among the best treatment outcomes were observed in patients receiving naltrexone with or without CBI (Anton et al., 2006). Only naltrexone and acamprosate were studied in this trial, ruling out answer choices C, D, and E.

10. **E.** Inhibition of dopamine-beta-hydroxylase

Disulfiram inhibits dopamine-beta-hydroxylase (DBH), which metabolizes dopamine to norepinephrine. Inhibiting DBH increases dopamine levels, which is believed to reduce the positive, rewarding effect of cocaine. Disulfiram inhibits aldehyde dehydrogenase, its relevant mechanism of action for treating alcohol use disorder (answer choice A); it does not inhibit alcohol dehydrogenase (answer choice B). Ditiocarb is a metabolite of disulfiram, which has been found to have antineoplastic effects through its interference with the ubiquitin-proteasome system (answer choice C). Disulfiram is not a monoamine oxidase inhibitor (answer choice D) (Kosten et al., 2013).

11. **C.** CBT conceptualizes the interconnections between thought processes, emotional responses, and behaviors reactions in drug and alcohol use.

As adapted for SUD, CBT is based on the Relapse Prevention (RP) model by Marlatt (and Gordon), which is based on social learning theory and operant conditioning principles. The model posits that relapse follows immediate determinants of substance use (such as triggering people, places, and things; coping strategies; or outcome expectancies) and covert antecedents to substance use, including lifestyle factors and craving. Answer A describes psychodynamic therapies. Answer B describes motivational interviewing. Answer D describes contingency management. Answer E describes mindfulness-based interventions.

12. **C.** Naloxone

Naloxone is a mu-opioid receptor antagonist that is used in opioid overdoses to counteract life-threatening effects on the central nervous system and respiratory system. Naloxone has no potential for abuse. Naloxone wears off in 20 to 90 minutes, and a person may require administration of more than one dose.

13. **A.** Precontemplation

The transtheoretical model of change (TTM) is a useful model to determine a given patient's readiness to change their behaviors as it applies to substance use. It includes the following stages:

- Precontemplation: Patients in this stage are not considering change and present with active resistance. The patient in this vignette appears to be in the precontemplation stage. The main clinical risk during this stage is dropout from treatment.
- Contemplation: Patients in this stage are ambivalent about changing their behaviors.
- Preparation: Patients in this stage are taking steps toward changing their behaviors and present with increasing confidence in their decision to change.
- Action: Patients in this stage are overtly modifying their behaviors and factors in the environment that support continued substance use. The main clinical risk during this stage is relapse.
- Maintenance: The goals for this stage include sustaining changes, consolidating gains, learning alternative coping strategies, and recognizing triggers.
- Relapse and recycling: This stage is not inevitable. The main clinical risk during the stage is for patients to feel stuck in their old ways and as such, the primary goal of treatment is avoiding becoming stuck and redefining the relapse as an opportunity for further self-improvement.
- Termination: Patients in this stage have reached their ultimate goals and are able to exit the cycle of change without fear of relapse.

14. **B.** CBT

CBT is a combination of two therapeutic approaches, cognitive therapy and behavioral therapy. CBT helps a person remove self-sabotaging thoughts and high-risk situations while working on avoidance skills by focusing on how a person's

ideas influence mood, thoughts, physical reactions, and behaviors. Dialectical behavior therapy is based on CBT, focusing on emotional and social aspects, and was developed to help people cope with extreme or unstable emotions, sense of emptiness, and harmful behaviors. MET is a counseling approach that helps resolve ambivalence about engaging in treatment, evoking rapid and internally motivated change, reducing substance use, and stopping drug use.

15. **C.** Bupropion

There are no FDA-approved medications for treating cocaine or methamphetamine use disorders. Bupropion is a norepinephrine–dopamine reuptake inhibitor with a structure similar to amphetamine. Some studies have found it helpful during the initial treatment of cocaine and methamphetamine use disorder. It has been found to significantly reduce cravings and treat depressive symptoms, which are common during withdrawal of methamphetamines and other stimulants.

16. **B.** Flumazenil binds to the benzodiazepine-binding site on the GABA-A receptor.

Flumazenil competitively antagonizes the GABA-A receptor at the benzodiazepine binding site, where both benzodiazepines and Z-drugs bind. Given its mechanism of action, flumazenil can reverse benzodiazepines and Z-drug overdoses, but not barbiturate or alcohol poisoning.

17. **B.**

Delta-9-tetrahydrocannabinol can be easily identified by its long aliphatic chain which renders it highly lipophilic and hydrophobic. Answer choice A is the chemical structure for phencyclidine. Answer choice C is the chemical structure of 3,4,-methylenedioxymethamphetamine (MDMA). Answer choice D is the chemical structure for amphetamine. For both MDMA and amphetamine, you can observe the phenethylamine structure, which is common to many psychoactive compounds. Answer choice E is the chemical structure for heroin.

18. **E.** CBD

Prescription CBD (marketed as Epidiolex) was recently FDA-approved for the treatment of seizures in Dravet and Lennox-Gastaut syndrome for patients aged 2 years and older. Dronabinol is synthetic delta-9-THC that is FDA-approved for the treatment of chemotherapy-related nausea and vomiting, as well as weight loss in AIDS (answer choice A). Nabilone is a THC analogue with minimal euphoric effects that is FDA-approved for cancer chemotherapy-related nausea and vomiting (answer choice B). Rimonabant is a CB1 receptor antagonist that was studied for the treatment of cannabis use disorder and was pulled from the global market due to serious psychiatric side effects (answer choice C). Medical marijuana is not FDA-approved for any condition (answer choice D).

19. **E.** The onset of action of edibles is longer and harder to predict.

Cannabis edibles have exploded in popularity over the past decade, as have cannabis-related visits to the emergency room from their consumption. The primary reason is that patients, frequently younger and more inexperienced users, will consume more edibles to pursue a psychoactive effect not realizing that the onset of action of edibles is longer and more variable, ranging from 1 to 3 hours. Compared with patients who consume cannabis via the smoked route, patients presenting with cannabis intoxication from edibles present with more severe intoxication and psychiatric symptoms. Although edible cannabis does in fact have lower bioavailability, this does not explain the phenomenon described in the vignette (answer choice D) (Monte et al., 2019).

20. **D.** Levamisole

Levamisole is an anthelmintic agent used illicitly as a cocaine adulterant. It looks like cocaine and acts as a bulking agent, increasing the total weight of the sample, so the selling street price increases. Levamisole can cause neutropenia, agranulocytosis, and skin necrosis.

21. **D.** Topiramate

Topiramate is believed to decrease the dopamine release in the corticomesolimbic system involved in reward and reinforcement mechanisms of using cocaine; however, clinical trials' conflicting results do not definitively provide topiramate's efficacy in managing cocaine use disorder (Shinn & Greenfield, 2010).

22. **E.** Naltrexone

Naltrexone is approved by the FDA to treat alcohol and opioid use disorders. Naltrexone inhibits dopamine release in the nucleus accumbens and ventral pallidum, reducing gambling urges. Other medications, such as the selective serotonin reuptake inhibitors (SSRIs), have been tested based on the hypothesis that serotonin dysfunction could be a potential mediator of gambling addiction.

23. **A.** Cannabis is categorized as Schedule I, but the judicial branch of the federal government issued a memorandum indicating the states would not be prosecuted for having a state-legal cannabis enterprise.

Under U.S. federal law, cannabis is a Schedule I controlled substance with no currently accepted medical use; however, individual states can have medical and recreational cannabis programs because of a memorandum released by the U.S. Department of Justice in 2013 called the Cole Memorandum, indicating that state-legal cannabis enterprises would not be prosecuted.

24. **E.** Passive inhalation of cannabis smoke is unlikely to result in a positive test.

In the vast majority of cases, passive inhalation of cannabis smoke will not produce positive urine tests at commonly utilized cutoff concentrations used for UDS testing of cannabis (answer choice A). Extreme cannabis smoke exposure (e.g., sitting in a nonventilated room for an hour or longer next to individuals smoking high-potency cannabis) may rarely result in a positive test, but this is likely limited to the hours following cannabis exposure. Both ibuprofen and pantoprazole can rarely test false positives for THC, but confirmation with GC-MS rules out these possibilities (answer choices B and C). Bupropion can test false positive for amphetamines, not for THC (answer choice D). In this vignette, it is not plausible that his reported exposure would result in a positive UDS test (Cone et al., 2015).

25. **A.** CB1 receptors are expressed in very low density in the brainstem.

Many drug overdose deaths are primarily caused by respiratory failure. However, cannabis does not have significant respiratory effects because of the low density of CB1 receptors in the brainstem, regulating respiratory drive. The highest concentration of CB1 receptors is found in the hippocampus and basal ganglia, but this is not directly relevant to the question (answer choice B). CB2 receptors are mostly expressed in immune cells, although they can be found in the central nervous system (answer choice D). Endocannabinoids regulate several critical physiological functions, but the respiratory drive is not one of them (answer choice E).

26. **B.** Assess the severity of the patient's depression and current suicidal thoughts.

The most critical risk factor for suicide is having a history of past suicide attempts. SUD is a significant risk factor for attempted and completed suicide. Additionally, acute and severe psychosocial stressors further increase the risk. As a result, this patient presents with a very high risk for suicide and should be evaluated for current suicidal thinking. Ensuring patient safety if he is suicidal might require inpatient hospitalization. This patient is undoubtedly at risk of contracting HIV and HCV. However, laboratory testing for these infections should be offered after acute stabilization and assessment of imminent threats (answer choice A). Having a history of suicide attempts or obtaining buprenorphine from illicit sources is not a contraindication for buprenorphine treatment (answer choices C and D). This patient might benefit from treatment with an SSRI. However, it is preferable to wait until he completes medically assisted opioid detoxification and reassess his depressive symptoms before prescribing an antidepressant medication (answer choice E).

27. **D.** Perform a psychiatric evaluation for co-occurring psychiatric disorders.

The prevalence of co-occurring psychiatric disorders among patients with an SUD is approximately 50%. This patient should receive a full psychiatric evaluation for co-occurring psychiatric disorders and be longitudinally reassessed. Naltrexone would not be an appropriate treatment for prolonged alcohol withdrawal symptoms (answer choice A). Acamprosate may be the right choice but still does not preclude a full psychiatric evaluation (answer choice B). There is no evidence that this patient requires readmission for detoxification after 1 month of inpatient rehabilitation (answer choice C). Symptoms secondary to substance intoxication or withdrawal will generally resolve without psychotropic medication, but this is unlikely given the time course of his symptomatology (answer choice E).

28. **C.** The patient's current dose of lorazepam may be too low to adequately treat his anxiety disorder.

This question is testing your assessment of "pseudoaddiction," which is the notion that certain patients may be receiving inadequate doses of medication for their condition. They may repeatedly request increases in dosages and may be incorrectly seen as being "drug-seeking" owing to ostensibly having an SUD. In the context of benzodiazepine use and the treatment of anxiety, approaches to these patients include increasing the dose or frequency of dosing, or considering a longer-acting agent.

29. **B.** Operant conditioning

The primary influence on human behavior is learning from the environment. Positive reinforcement strengthens an action by providing a reward. In this case, he has known the rewarding feeling of sitting at the table and gambling. Sitting at the table ensures that he would repeat the action again and again. The removal of an unpleasant reinforcer can also strengthen behavior. This is known as negative reinforcement. Classical conditioning is a condition discovered by Pavlov, a physiologist (answer choice C). A stimulus is paired with and precedes the unconditioned stimulus (until the conditioned stimulus alone is sufficient to elicit a response). Classical conditioning is a reductionist explanation of behavior by breaking it down into smaller stimulus-response units of action (answer choice E).

30. **B.** Women with alcohol use disorder have a higher risk of negative medical sequelae.

Women have a lower prevalence of alcohol use disorder, including binge drinking, begin drinking at a later age, and are more likely to have a co-occurring psychiatric disorder than men. However, women have a shorter time from initiation of alcohol use to the onset of alcohol-related problems, commonly referred to as "telescoping." Women appear to be more vulnerable to the neurotoxic effects of alcohol use and the development of medical sequelae (e.g., cirrhosis and alcoholic cardiomyopathy) than men. Variations may be due to differences in alcohol metabolism, as women have a slower rate of alcohol metabolism, a lower percentage of total body water, and lower first-pass metabolism (Ceylan-Isik et al., 2010).

31. **A.** Ventral tegmental area (VTA), nucleus accumbens (NAc)

This question is testing your knowledge of basic brain reward circuitry. The reward pathway is the mesolimbic dopamine pathway. It includes dopaminergic cell bodies in the VTA in the midbrain that project to the NAc in the ventral striatum. All drugs directly or indirectly exert their main reinforcing effects through the VTA–NAc pathway. Opioids inhibit GABAergic interneurons in the VTA, disinhibiting VTA dopaminergic neurons and increasing dopaminergic neurotransmission to the NAc. Opioids also act directly on opioid receptors present in the NAc (Nestler, 2005).

32. **C.** Neuropeptide Y

Neuropeptide Y is a neuromodulator with anxiolytic effects. It is part of the brain's "antistress" system; it functionally opposes corticotropin-releasing factor. Alcohol withdrawal decreases neuropeptide Y expression in the amygdala, increasing vulnerability to negative emotional states. Dynorphin is an opioid peptide that is upregulated in withdrawal states and leads to increased dysphoria (answer choice A). Noradrenergic systems are upregulated during withdrawal, leading to anxiety and agitation (answer choice B). CRF mediates the physiological stress response and regulates the hypothalamic–pituitary–adrenal axis (answer choice D). CREB is a transcription factor that is upregulated by substance use and leads to increased dynorphin (answer choice E).

33. **A.** Activation of CRF and norepinephrine in the amygdala and VTA

In this vignette, the patient undergoes stress-induced reinstatement following the death of his wife. Stress-induced reinstatement depends on the activation of CRF and norepinephrine in the amygdala and the VTA (Koob & Volkow, 2016). Answer choice B describes the neurocircuitry relevant for drug-induced reinstatement. Answer choice C describes the neurocircuitry relevant for cue-induced reinstatement. Answer choice D describes the basic neurocircuitry of the reward pathway. Answer choice E describes the biological effects of opioids on reward circuitry.

34. **E.** It sounds like you are worried that your anxiety will worsen if you stop drinking while at the same time recognizing the need to address your alcohol use.

In motivational interviewing, patients are encouraged to explore both the positive (such as disinhibition, socialization, and pleasure, or in this case, self-medicating) and the negative and harmful aspects of using drugs or alcohol. Reflections are likely the most critical aspect of motivational interviewing, includes simple considerations (e.g., "So you are saying that alcohol is causing a drift in your relationship."), double reflections (e.g., "So on the one hand, alcohol helps you cope with stress caused by work, but on the other hand, it is causing a drift in your relationship."), or amplified reflections (.e.g, after a patient tells you that they enjoy drinking alcohol, you overshoot and respond: "I see, drinking alcohol has been a very positive experience in your life, and you have no interest in cutting down."). The statement in option E is an example of a double reflection.

35. **E.** Weekly drug testing at home and rewarding her with money any time she tests negative for marijuana.

CM is based on the introduction of alternative reinforcers that are valued more than using drugs or alcohol (such as monetary rewards) that tip the balance in favor of abstinence and help promote recovery. CM as a therapy involves positive reinforcement by rewarding patients with incentives for achieving their treatment goals such as abstinence (hence answer C is incorrect). The immediate reward of negative tests serves an important reinforcement purpose. As a result, utilizing point-of-care testing at home would be more effective than drug testing at a laboratory in which results can take several days to be reported (hence answer D is incorrect).

36. **D.** Oxytocin

Oxytocin is a hormone secreted by the posterior lobe of the pituitary gland. It has been shown to modulate substance use-related reward and seeking behaviors in the subthalamic nucleus of people abusing methamphetamine.

37. **B.** Norpethidine

Meperidine is known to induce seizures from the accumulation of meperidine's metabolite, norpethidine. It would be best to avoid meperidine in the elderly and patients with underlying hepatic or renal disease. The medication increases the risk of normeperidine accumulation and increased risk for seizures. The use of meperidine in combination with other agents known to increase serotonin has been linked with serotonin syndrome development.

38. **C.** CREB

Opioid, cocaine, and alcohol use can lead to the upregulation of CREB in the NAc. This creates an upregulation of dynorphin, binds to kappa-opioid receptors, and produces a dysphoria-like response. These adaptations are believed to lead to drug tolerance and a dysphoric state in the absence of the drug. Delta-FosB is another key transcription factor relevant in addiction; in contrast to CREB, its levels rise more slowly with repeated substance use and remain high for months following abstinence. Higher levels of delta-FosB lead to increases in the positive, rewarding effect of the substance (answer choice A). Neuropeptide Y is not a transcription factor (answer choice B). Myocyte-enhancing factor-2 and nuclear factor κB are both transcription factors under study for addiction, but neither upregulates dynorphin (answer choices D and E) (Robison & Nestler, 2011).

39. **B.** Persons with SUD learn to utilize the social activities and chores to model change and rely on their new community to practice cognitive and behavioral changes conducive to change and recovery.

The effectiveness of TC is thought to result from the community serving as a model context for prosocial relationships and activities. TC staff are described as "rational authorities" and are often peers in recovery rather than SUD experts. Programs focus on accountability, responsibility, and structuring a socially productive life. The TC model has been adapted to correctional settings. When combined with community-based TC on release from incarceration, such models are associated with improved substance use and criminal outcomes. The therapeutic focus on "resocialization" is that isolation and dysfunctional social and interpersonal coping mechanisms precede the long-term facility presentation for many patients.

40. **A.** Women show higher dropout rates and more use during treatment than men.

There are significant gender differences in the use of methamphetamines. Women initiate methamphetamine use at an earlier age, have more severe use, higher attrition rates from treatment, yet they respond better to treatment than men. Women have a lower incidence of emergency department-related deaths involving methamphetamine (Dluzen & Liu, 2008).

41. **A.** Alcohol withdrawal

Symptoms of alcohol withdrawal can start as early as 5 to 6 hours after the last drink. After the first 48 hours, alcohol withdrawal symptoms can include seizures; high blood pressure; and tactile, auditory, and visual hallucinations. Particularly in patients who are unable to provide a reliable clinical history, it is important to always keep other intoxication or withdrawal syndromes on the differential.

42. **C.** Hyperthermia

Methamphetamine use can lead to cardiovascular, gastrointestinal, and renal complications. Tachycardia and hypertension are frequently observed in methamphetamine intoxication. The patient is presenting with methamphetamine intoxication with hyperthermia. In hyperthermia, early diagnosis and treatment are crucial. Administration of 100% oxygen via a nonrebreather mask, ensuring the patient has intravenous access to administer fluids, removing sheets and blankets, and lowering the room temperature are a few of the measures recommended to reduce core body temperature.

43. **A.** Benzodiazepines increase the odds of a future suicide attempt.

According to a recent meta-analysis, benzodiazepines increase the odds of attempting or completing suicide by three to five times (Dodds, 2017). Given her increased baseline risk of suicide, this is an essential consideration in prescribing this medication. Possible mechanisms for increasing suicide risk include increased impulsivity, withdrawal symptoms, or overdose toxicity. For patients presenting with acute anxiety or agitation where you may wish to avoid benzodiazepines, antihypertensives (clonidine, beta-blockers), and second-generation antipsychotics can be considered. As for the other answer choices, tobacco use disorder is not a contraindication for benzodiazepine use, although caution should be taken for any patient with a past or current substance use disorder (answer choice B). SSRIs and tricyclic antidepressants are as effective for generalized anxiety disorder as benzodiazepines (answer choice C). Lorazepam is not metabolized through CYP liver enzymes and has minimal drug–drug interactions (answer choice D). Patients who come requesting specific medications are frequently assumed to be drug-seeking but should not be refused an indicated medication on this basis (answer choice E).

44. **E.** The patient was started on higher than the recommended dose of zolpidem.

In 2013, the FDA informed the manufacturers of zolpidem that the recommended dose for women should be lowered from 10 mg to 5 mg given evidence from clinical trials that women eliminate zolpidem more slowly than men, leading to residual effects that could impair women in tasks requiring alertness, such as driving (Farkas et al., 2013).

Prescription of a long-acting zolpidem may potentially worsen these side effects if the dosage is not appropriately adjusted.

45. **C.** Opioids are involved in the majority of benzodiazepine overdose deaths.

Benzodiazepine-related overdose deaths have increased dramatically over the past two decades; they have jumped fivefold between 1996 and 2013. However, benzodiazepines alone can rarely lead to an overdose death; opioids were involved in approximately 75% of benzodiazepine-related overdose deaths. Conversely, benzodiazepines are estimated to be involved in approximately 30% of opioid overdose deaths (Bachhuber et al., 2016).

46. **B.** Perform a taper with clonazepam over the course of months.

For patients who have been on benzodiazepines longer term, it is generally recommended to perform a gradual taper after cross-tapering to a benzodiazepine with a longer duration of effect. In this case, the patient is already on a long-acting benzodiazepine and would not require a cross-taper. In cases where you do not want to prescribe a benzodiazepine or where you need to discontinue the benzodiazepine quickly, you can manage the withdrawal syndrome with antiepileptics such as valproic acid or carbamazepine, although this is not clinically indicated in this case. His previous failure appears to be due to the fact that he abruptly discontinued clonazepam; detoxification would not be the next best step.

47. **A.** Increased cardiac workload and systemic vascular resistance

Cocaine use is associated with significant cardiovascular pathologies, which could potentially cause angina and myocardial ischemia. Cocaine causes hypertension, increased systemic vascular resistance, and vasoconstriction. In addition to the standard protocols used for non-cocaine-related cardiac events, the medical treatment of cocaine-related angina and myocardial infarction should include benzodiazepines. Benzodiazepines might be necessary to manage hypertension and tachycardia. They help to decrease the central stimulatory effects of cocaine.

Other causes of cocaine-induced coronary artery disease involve vasculopathy and vasoconstriction. Cocaine use can also cause left ventricular hypertrophy, hyperthrombotic states, aortic dissection and rupture, and arrhythmias. Cocaine's vascular and cardiotoxic effects are not dose related.

48. **D.** Start nicotine replacement therapy

Hospitalized smokers benefit from NRT because it has a rapid onset of action. Varenicline and bupropion are slower to reduce symptoms of irritability and craving.

49. **B.** AA has no dogma, theology, or creed.

Even though AA utilizes spiritual concepts, it is not a religion and has no dogmas or creeds. It is best described as a spiritually driven program and a way of life. Techniques used to promote change rely on experiential learning, building structure, learning coping strategies, and strengthening social networks. The goals of such a group include promoting self-efficacy and a new identity. Although AA is an abstinence-based and community support group program, it does not posit that persons with alcohol use disorder can learn to drink in moderation once in recovery. In large-scale studies, commitment to abstinence was demonstrated to be the most important predictor of prognosis and sustained recovery.

50. **A.** A 43-year-old banker who has been drinking a bottle of wine daily for the past 6 months in the context of increased stress at work.

SBIRT refers to an evidence-based practice to identify, reduce, and prevent maladaptive substance use in primary care or other non-SUD-focused settings. SBIRT serves as a public health initiative to identify persons at risk for developing an SUD or with an undetected SUD at the primary care level. It offers those with less severe substance use simple interventions to address simple substance use problems and refer those with more complex substance use treatment needs to specialized services. Evidence supporting brief interventions (BIs) efficacy is strongest for maladaptive alcohol use. BI is particularly effective for patients with less severe alcohol use problems where the intervention goal is typically a reduction of alcohol consumption rather

than complete abstinence. BI for alcohol is associated with an overall decrease in alcohol use, drinking days, binge drinking, and alcohol-related deaths.

BONUS ANSWER

51. **D.** Clozapine

Cigarette smoking and daily dose have positive correlations with the plasma concentration of medications metabolized by the CYP450 enzyme CYP1A2. Because clozapine is a substrate of the enzyme being induced by smoking, the medication concentration of the medication and its efficacy in most cases might be affected. Remember that smoking and not nicotine induces the isoenzyme CYP1A2. CYP1A2 activity is higher in heavy smokers than in nonsmokers, and quitting can normalize the CYP1A2 activity.

BLOCK 2

1. **A.** As applied to SUD, CBT aims to establish a functional analysis framework identifying high risk antecedents and consequences of their use.

The CBT model in SUD treatment relies on the same fundamental principle that thought processes, emotional responses, and behavioral reactions are interconnected. As adapted for SUD, CBT is based on the Relapse Prevention (RP) model by Marlatt based on social learning theory and operant conditioning principles. The model posits that relapse follows immediate determinants of substance use (such as triggering people, places and things, coping strategies, or outcome expectancies) and covert antecedents to substance use, including lifestyle factors and craving. During the treatment course, the therapist and patient develop a functional analysis framework identifying high-risk antecedents and consequences of their use. Patients practice identifying and avoiding high-risk situations and learn specific coping strategies (including stimulus control and urge-management techniques and relapse road maps) to enhance the patient's self-efficacy in maintaining sobriety. Network therapy, not mentalization-based therapy, uses family and peers to support patients with SUD in their recovery process.

The mentalization-based therapy approach is founded on psychoanalytic and social attachment theory. Deficits and impairments in mentalization contribute to maladaptive cognitive patterns associated with substance use. TSF is not a 12-step mutual support group; it is a manualized and structured 12-session approach that aims to promote the patient's engagement in 12-step mutual support groups.

2. **C.** ALDH; acetaldehyde

Alcohol flush reaction is common among individuals of East Asian descent owning to a higher frequency of both the ADH1B*2 and ALDH2*2 alleles, both of which lead to accumulation of acetaldehyde. The ADH1B*2 allele metabolizes ethanol more rapidly to acetaldehyde, whereas the ALDH2*2 allele metabolizes acetaldehyde more slowly; the presence of one or both of these isotypes would lead to accumulation of acetaldehyde. Increased amounts of acetaldehyde lead to the release of histamines, which then causes vessel dilatation and skin redness.

3. **C.** Less than 0.5%

Approximately 0.4% of the population had a methamphetamine use disorder in 2017 with clinically significant impairment, including disability and failure to meet responsibilities at work, school, or home.

4. **D.** Capsaicin can provide effective symptomatic relief.

This question is testing your knowledge of cannabinoid hyperemesis syndrome, a syndrome of cyclic vomiting associated with cannabis use. Patients typically present to their providers or the emergency room with intractable vomiting and nausea, and are predominantly young males who have been using cannabis regularly for at least a year. Patients will frequently report taking hot showers compulsively with symptom relief. Symptomatic treatments include topical capsaicin or dopamine antagonists such as haloperidol. Cessation of cannabis use is the only known effective treatment (Sorensen et al., 2017).

5. **D.** Anandamide

The two endogenous ligands of the CB1 receptor that you should know are anandamide and 2-arachidonoylglycerol (2-AG). Anandamide is released postsynaptically but acts in a retrograde manner on presynaptic CB1 cannabinoid receptors; it also has some activity at CB2 receptors. Dynorphin and enkephalin are endogenous ligands of the opioid receptor (answer choices A and B); dynorphin is particularly important in stress response and mediates the negative affective experience of withdrawal states. Cannabidiol binds CB1 but is not an endogenous ligand (answer choice C). Neuropeptide Y is also important for stress regulation but is not an endogenous cannabinoid (answer choice E).

6. **A.** AKT1

Marijuana is associated with psychosis, particularly among individuals with a genetic vulnerability. Individuals with the AKT1 C/C genotype have sevenfold odds of experiencing psychotic symptoms with daily cannabis use compared to lower-risk T/T carriers. AKT1 encodes a protein kinase that is important for cellular signaling and dopamine transmission. ADH2 encodes alcohol dehydrogenase, which is relevant for alcohol use disorder, not cannabis use, and psychosis (answer choice B). CNR1 encodes the cannabinoid type I receptor, and individuals with increased AAT repeats have a higher risk of a cannabis use disorder, however, there is no known association with psychosis risk (answer choice C). FAAH encodes fatty acid amide hydrolase, the enzyme that metabolizes anandamide and is associated with the severity of cannabis withdrawal. However, it has no relevance to psychosis risk (answer choice D). OPRM1 encodes the mu-opioid receptor and is relevant for OUD (answer choice E) (Di Forti et al., 2012).

7. **C.** *C. indica* has a higher ratio of CBD to THC.

C. indica and *C. sativa* are the two main subspecies of the cannabis family that are most relevant for the medical and nonmedical use of cannabis, although there are over 700 different types of plants within the cannabis family. *C. indica* and *C. sativa* have distinct appearances, but the main difference is that *C. indica* has a higher ratio of CBD to THC compared to *C. sativa*. The female plants of both subspecies produce higher concentrations of cannabinoids compared to male plants (answer choice A). *C. indica* does not have a negligible amount of THC (answer choice B). *C. indica* may be legal to grow in some states with legalized marijuana; however, cannabis remains Schedule I and federally illegal (answer choice D). For both *C. indica* and *C. sativa*, the highest cannabis potency is in the flowering tops of the female plant, not the leaves and stems (answer choice E).

8. **C.** Vitamin E acetate (VEA) in THC cartridges

This question is testing your knowledge of e-cigarette or vaping associated lung injury (EVALI). Vitamin E acetate (VEA) in black-market THC cartridges has been identified as the likely cause of EVALI; VEA is frequently added as a diluent or filler in THC products. According to a recent study of 160 patients with EVALI in California, VEA was detected in 84% of the THC products and none of the nicotine products. Several states have now banned VEA as an additive in any vaping product. Carbon monoxide is present in cannabis and tobacco smoke but is minimal in cannabis and nicotine vapor; neither are believed to cause EVALI (answer choice A and B). Propylene glycol is a common additive in vaping pens but is generally recognized as safe (answer choice E) (Heinzerling et al., 2020).

9. **E.** Immediately

Guidelines recommend starting HAART as soon as possible. There is no recommended CD4 count cutoff at which to initiate therapy. Evidence suggests that starting HAART when CD4 counts are high is associated with improved long-term outcomes. HAART use is related to improved CD4 count, virologic suppressionn and preserved immune function. Earlier HAART initiation may result in better immunologic responses and clinical outcomes, reductions in AIDS and non-AIDS-associated morbidity and mortality, and a significant reduction in HIV transmission risk. Although it is certainly preferable that patients with HIV abstain from drug and alcohol use, HAART is not contraindicated in actively using patients.

10. **D.** Fentanyl

An overdose of fentanyl is the most likely cause of her symptoms. The patient is showing the signs and symptoms of an acute opioid overdose including a decreased level of consciousness, pupillary constriction, respiratory depression, and hypothermia. Initial treatment involves supporting the patient's airway and breathing by providing oxygen and intubating where needed. Naloxone, a short-acting opioid receptor antagonist, is the treatment of choice to reverse opioid poisoning. Fentanyl is among the most potent opioids, and frequently requires higher than the typically administered doses of naloxone to reverse the signs of an opioid overdose. Doxepin is a tricyclic antidepressant that can cause tachycardia, drowsiness, dry mouth, nausea, hypotension, seizures, and cardiac dysrhythmias in overdose. Acetaminophen poisoning may include nausea, vomiting, abdominal pain, seizures, and liver failure.

11. **C.** Standard deviation

Standard deviation is a measure of the amount of variation that shows how closely the data are clustered around the mean value. Most methadone doses will be close to the mean value. If the bell curve is flattened, fewer of the methadone doses will be clustered around the mean, and the standard deviation will be higher. If the bell curve is steep, more of the data is clustered around the mean, and the standard deviation will be lower.

12. **B.** Mood disorders are the most common psychiatric disorder seen in this group.

Mood disorders are the most diagnosed psychiatric disorders co-occurring in pregnant women with an OUD. Older pregnant women with an OUD exhibit higher rates of comorbid mood disorders than younger pregnant women with OUD. Pregnant women with OUD frequently suffer from more than one psychiatric disorder.

13. **C.** Specificity

Confirmation of presumptive positive UDS tests, necessary to minimize the reporting of false-positive results, can be costly and time-consuming. In this vignette, specificity is the proportion of the methadone patients not using illicit opioids who have a negative result on UDS tests. Sensitivity is defined as the proportion of individuals with illicit opioid use who have a positive result on a diagnostic test. A test that has higher specificity will have fewer false positives, whereas a test with higher sensitivity will have fewer false negatives. Positive predictive value is the probability that patients who have a positive screening test result have the disease. In contrast, the negative predictive value is the probability that a negative test result means that the patient does not have a disease.

14. **A.** Formation of cocaethylene

Concomitant alcohol and cocaine use can form a third active compound, ethylbenzoylecgonine, commonly known as cocaethylene. The plasma half-life of cocaethylene is longer and can cause behavioral and physiological effects similar to cocaine.

15. **D.** Mirtazapine

Mirtazapine is currently used to treat depression. It antagonizes noradrenergic alpha-2 receptor and the serotonin 5-HT2A/C and 5-HT3 receptors. It has demonstrated efficacy in reducing the rewarding effect of cocaine and methamphetamine.

16. **B.** Tobacco use disorder

Tobacco use disorder is the most common SUD in the United States. Approximately 60% to 80% of current smokers meet criteria for tobacco use disorder. Nicotine is the primary addictive substance in tobacco. Among those who experiment with cigarettes, 20% to 30% will meet tobacco use disorder criteria in their lifetime.

17. **C.** OPRM1

The *OPRM1* gene encodes the mu-opioid receptor. Patients treated with naltrexone who have the G allele of the A118G SNP of the *OPRM1* gene have been found to have a lower rate of relapse compared to patients homozygous for the A allele; this genetic polymorphism may help identify patients who are more likely to respond to naltrexone. AUTS2 is associated with alcohol use disorder in genome-wide association studies (answer choice A). SLC6A4 encodes the serotonin transporter protein studied as a potential moderator of treatment

response in alcohol use disorder, though this does not include naltrexone (answer choice B). CYP2A6 encodes the cytochrome P450 2A6 enzyme, which metabolizes nicotine; specific polymorphisms are associated with heavier smoking (answer choice D). Specific polymorphisms of the *AKT1* gene increase the risk for psychosis in cannabis users (answer choice E) (Anton et al., 2008).

18. **B.** Naltrexone

The timeframe and description of symptoms are most consistent with precipitated opioid withdrawal from methadone because of oral naltrexone administration. This vignette demonstrates why it is essential to educate patients on the importance of letting all their health care providers know that when they are taking methadone, especially given that methadone is not listed on state prescription monitoring programs when prescribed from an opioid treatment program. In this case, the patient likely did not disclose that he was on methadone and was prescribed naltrexone for his alcohol use disorder, leading to precipitated withdrawal. Disulfiram reaction is another possibility, but it is less likely given that he was not drinking or intoxicated at the time this occurred; disulfiram reactions occur minutes after alcohol consumption and include cutaneous flushing, head throbbing, tachycardia, nausea, vomiting, and respiratory difficulties. Gabapentin, baclofen, and acamprosate are not known to cause this reaction (answer choices C, D, and E).

19. **C.** CBT

CBT is a short-term, goal-oriented psychotherapy treatment that focuses on developing skills to manage factors that influence relapse. Its goal is to change patterns of thinking or behavior.

20. **B.** Crack

Crack cocaine is the free-base form of cocaine that can be smoked. Benzoylecgonine is the active compound tested in UDS tests for cocaine.

21. **C.** Opioids have a significant impact on reinforcement mechanisms in the VTA.

The VTA is the most sensitive site for the brain's self-administration of opioids. When animals self-administer heroin, they respond to a decrease in dose by increasing the frequency of injections. The administration of opioids into the VTA increases opioid self-administration, whereas injection of opioid receptor antagonists in this region does not affect heroin self-administration.

22. **C.** She should start breastfeeding immediately; the benefits outweigh the risks.

Methadone is the treatment of choice for pregnant women with OUD. Its long half-life prevents the fetus from undergoing withdrawal. There is no contraindication to breastfeeding for patients with hepatitis C or those using methadone. However, women who are HIV positive should not breastfeed, as they can pass HIV on to the infant through maternal milk.

23. **D.** Cannabis-induced anxiety

Cocaine use should be suspected, but a negative urine toxicology screen ruled that out. Because of the symptoms' chronology, it is unlikely that the patient is experiencing alcohol withdrawal syndrome. The symptoms described here are consistent with a panic attack induced by cannabis use. Anxiety caused by cannabis often occurs in inexperienced users. The higher the dose, the more likely anxiety is to appear. Paranoid thoughts are also frequent in marijuana intoxication, precipitating fear, and anxiety. Synthetic marijuana usually does not show up in ordinary urine drug assays, and dilated pupils will not accompany the withdrawal syndrome.

24. **B.** Ammonium chloride

Amphetamines are weak bases that get trapped in acidic environments, making them neutral and lipid soluble. If an acid like ammonium chloride is added, the amphetamine is ionized and is excreted in the urine. Bicarbonate is used to treat overdoses with weak acid drugs, such as barbiturates and aspirin. Flumazenil is used to treat overdoses of benzodiazepines, and naloxone is used to treat opioid overdoses. Naltrexone is used to prevent relapse in patients with OUD.

25. **B.** Recommend varenicline and behavioral modification.

The patient is unable to quit despite his best intentions. Varenicline has demonstrated superior efficacy in clinical trials when compared with placebo and bupropion. Smoking cessation is best managed with a combination of pharmacotherapy and behavioral modification.

26. **D.** Sertraline

In the case in Question 26, pornography use is adversely affecting the patient's life. It has resulted in a damaged relationship with his wife, financial instability, and difficulties at work. The use of SSRIs in treating sexual addiction is based on the proposed mechanism of serotonergic dysfunction of sexual behavior. Naltrexone was not found to be more effective than a placebo in one study but is effective in treating gambling disorder. Stimulants, dopamine agonists, and tricyclic antidepressants have not been found to have efficacy in treating sexual addiction.

27. **D.** Brain imaging studies revealed a loss of brain tissue and cognitive impairments are noted on neuropsychological testing.

Persons with alcohol use disorder or chronic history of excessive alcohol use may present with neurocognitive impairment. These impairments can be detected on neuropsychological testing and brain imaging. Magnetic resonance imaging studies and diffusion tensor imaging reveal a loss of brain tissue with accelerating gray matter loss. In more than half of persons with alcohol use disorder, abnormalities can be seen on CT imaging even in the absence of cognitive deficits. Some of these changes may be reversible with abstinence, suggesting that the abnormalities might be at least in part evidence of brain tissue dehydration.

28. **E.** Antisocial personality disorder

SUDs are often comorbid with personality disorders, most commonly antisocial personality disorder, borderline personality disorder, and schizotypal personality disorder. Of these, an antisocial personality disorder is the most common.

29. **D.** There are off-label medications that can be prescribed to alleviate cannabis withdrawal symptoms.

Currently, there are no FDA-approved treatments for cannabis use disorder, although a number of commonly used psychiatric medications have been studied, are currently under study, or are used off-label. Some medications that are used off-label to alleviate cannabis withdrawal include quetiapine, mirtazapine, and gabapentin. Rimonabant is a CB1 receptor antagonist and an antiobesity medication that showed efficacy for treatment of cannabis use disorder in preliminary clinical trials, but its serious psychiatric side effects led to discontinuation of its study (answer choice A). Given the time course of the patient's symptoms, cannabis withdrawal is more likely than the development of a depressive episode (answer choice B). There is no evidence that genetic testing can help determine the correct medication approach for cannabis use disorder (answer choice E) (Brezing & Levin, 2018).

30. **E.** None of the above

The FDA has approved three medications to treat OUD: buprenorphine, methadone, and naltrexone. But no medication is approved specifically for comorbid OUD and PTSD. No medications are explicitly approved for any SUD comorbid with any other psychiatric disorder, for that matter.

31. **E.** PCP

PCP is an N-methyl-D-aspartate (NMDA) receptor antagonist and D2 partial agonist causing paranoia and depersonalization. Psychosis, agitation, and dysphoria can occur as well as occasional unprovoked aggressive behavior such as in this case. The management of PCP intoxication mainly consists of supportive care.

32. **B.** Bradycardia

GHB overdose is among the most dangerous because of its steep dose-response curve; its LD50 is only five times greater than the typical recreational dose. Common signs and symptoms in GHB intoxication include vomiting (more common with ethanol co-ingestion), seizures, respiratory distress, hypothermia, hypotension and bradycardia. Death from GHB overdose most commonly occurs because of respiratory arrest. According to a case series of patients presenting to the emergency room with GHB intoxication, 38% presented with bradycardia (Liechti et al., 2006).

33. **B.** Sedative withdrawal

One of the key differences between benzodiazepine and alcohol withdrawal is that the timing, severity, and range of symptoms is more variable in benzodiazepine withdrawal; the withdrawal syndrome depends on the dose, duration, and half-life of the ingested benzodiazepine and their metabolites. Recall that standard urine drug screens do not detect some of the most commonly used and abused benzodiazepines (e.g. clonazepam, alprazolam, and lorazepam). In this vignette, the patient may have ingested a longer-acting benzodiazepine (e.g., clonazepam) that is missed by standard UDS tests. The timing and nature of the patient's symptoms are not consistent with alcohol, cocaine, or opioid withdrawal, nor with a psychotic episode.

34. **D.** Gabapentin

Despite its name and the fact that it is structurally similar to GABA, gabapentin does not exert its effects through the GABA-A or GABA-B receptor. Gabapentin binds to a voltage-gated calcium channel containing the alpha-2-delta-1 subunit that is distributed throughout the central nervous system. Baclofen and GHB are both GABA-B receptor agonists. Propofol is a GABA-A agonist and has NMDA antagonist activity as well. Phenobarbital is a barbiturate and is a positive allosteric modulator of the GABA-A receptor.

35. **A.** Open-label clinical trial

An open-labeled clinical trial is a clinical trial type in which information on the study is not withheld from the researchers and participants, which is in contrast with a blinded experiment, in which data are withheld to reduce bias.

36. **B.** Larger doses of opioids are needed for analgesia.

Opioids are a mainstay of acute pain management. However, long-term use of opioids can create tolerance and induced hyperalgesia, a paradoxical increase in pain with opioid administration. The mechanism of opioid tolerance is complex. The mechanisms can include those mediated by opioid receptor desensitization and internalization, glutamate receptors, and the cAMP-protein kinase A pathway. Glutamate receptors have long proved a a key component in the synaptic networks responsible for behavioral tolerance.

37. **D.** Contingency management

Contingency management provides rewards for the desired behaviors, such as negative urine toxicology screen tests. It is effective for various issues and conditions, including impulsive behaviors, defiance, and substance use disorders.

38. **A.** Heroin

Some signs and symptoms of heroin intoxication include flushing of the skin, dry mouth, pupillary constriction, sedation, and reduced respiratory rate. Heroin withdrawal symptoms include pupillary dilation, muscle spasms, lacrimation, yawning, restlessness, pain, gastrointestinal upset, and increased heart rate and blood pressure. The Clinical Opiate Withdrawal Scale (COWS) is a great tool to quantify the severity of opiate withdrawal symptoms.

39. **D.** Nucleus accumbens

The nucleus accumbens is a crucial site in mediating reward behavior, and it is directly involved in reinforcing addictive behavior for both SUD and behavioral addictions.

40. **C.** He should be screened for depression upon admission and reassessed frequently thereafter.

It is not uncommon for patients with substance use disorders to present with various co-occurring psychiatric symptoms, particularly mood and neurovegetative symptoms. It is important to assess any such symptoms seriously on an ongoing basis to determine whether the patient requires active treatments, including with medications and specialized psychotherapies, and to prevent serious complications of untreated psychiatric illnesses, including profound functional decline and/or suicidal behaviors. Many patients with substance-induced mood disorders would be expected to improve after being abstinent for a few weeks. Others might suffer from independent or secondary psychiatric disorders.

41. **C.** Alcohol withdrawal

This patient presents with a history of anxiety symptoms and panic attacks that occurs mostly in the mornings after abstaining from any alcohol use overnight. Consuming alcohol leads to a resolution of his symptoms. This is consistent with alcohol withdrawal–related panic attacks and anxiety. Panic attacks related to substance use are seen most commonly with marijuana and lysergic acid diethylamide (LSD) intoxication and alcohol withdrawal. The vignette does not provide enough information to support the diagnosis of generalized anxiety disorder or panic disorder. Further, alcohol use would not be expected to prevent panic attacks or treat anxiety in patients with a generalized anxiety disorder or panic disorder.

42. **C.** Diagnosis of depression made at least 1 week after the patient discontinues drinking

A meta-analysis of placebo-controlled trials of antidepressant medications among patients with SUD and depressive disorders by Nunes and Levin (2008) found that diagnosing depression after at least 1 week of abstinence was associated with a greater effect of antidepressant medication treatment. A depressive disorder that persists after 1 week or more of abstinence is likely independent of substance use and should be treated. For patients who cannot achieve any amount of abstinence, the meta-analysis recommended using clinical judgment in making decisions to treat depressive disorder based on the patient's history, past episodes of independent depression, and severity of the depressive disorder. Further, most positive studies included tricyclic antidepressants or antidepressants with noradrenergic or mixed mechanisms, such as serotonin and norepinephrine reuptake inhibitors. Most studies using SSRI were negative.

43. **E.** Start an antidepressant medication after this patient completes the medically supervised alcohol detoxification if he remains symptomatic.

In this clinical situation, it is unclear whether this patient's depressive symptoms are substance induced and likely to resolve spontaneously or represent an independent depressive disorder. Given that there are no acute safety concerns reported in the vignette, it is not unreasonable to hold off on starting antidepressant medications until he completes alcohol detoxification and withdrawal symptoms subside. When thinking about the psychiatric manifestations of SUD, one must differentiate between:

- The expected effects of the substance: Drugs and alcohol intoxication or withdrawal cause psychiatric signs and symptoms that are part of the normal toxidrome of a given substance. For example, feeling euphoric after using cocaine or anxious when going through alcohol withdrawal are expected effects of cocaine intoxication or alcohol withdrawal and should not be labeled as a manic or anxiety syndrome.
- Substance induced disorders: This category refers to the presence of psychiatric symptoms that:
    - Vastly exceed the expected effects of being intoxicated with or withdrawing from a substance
    - Meet diagnostic criteria for a psychiatric disorder (psychotic, bipolar, depressive, anxiety, obsessive compulsive, sleep, sexual, or neurocognitive disorder)
    - Develop during or soon after substance intoxication or withdrawal
    - Improve after a period of abstinence
- Co-occurring primary psychiatric disorders: This category refers to psychiatric disorders that either preceded or followed the onset of an SUD, but neither condition played a causative role in the onset of the other. For example, tobacco use disorder and schizophrenia often co-occur, but schizophrenia does not cause the onset of tobacco use disorder, and tobacco use disorder does not cause the onset of schizophrenia.
- Secondary psychiatric disorders: This category refers to psychiatric disorders that follow the onset of an SUD, with the SUD playing a causative role in the onset of the co-occurring psychiatric disorder. Unlike substance-induced disorders, with secondary psychiatric disorders, the symptoms do not improve after a period of abstinence.

44. **C.** Oxazepam

Traditional immunoassay tests for benzodiazepines detect both oxazepam and nordiazepam. Diazepam is metabolized to nordiazepam and temazepam, and those compounds are further metabolized to oxazepam. Chlordiazepoxide and clorazepate are both metabolized to nordiazepam. Clonazepam, alprazolam, and lorazepam are not metabolized to oxazepam. Their metabolites have limited cross-reactivity with traditional immunoassay, resulting in false negatives.

45. **A.** OUD

OUD is defined as a problematic pattern of opioid use leading to clinically significant impairment or distress. The patient in this case has been isolating more, and his drug use has been affecting his social functioning and school responsibilities. He is using opioids in increasing amounts and for longer than 12 months, and has continued using opioids despite the negative consequences of their use. The patient meets criteria for an OUD.

46. **A.** Rifampicin

When reading a drug testing report, it is crucial to understand the specific compounds tested in a given immunoassay. For example, in the SAMHSA-5 assays, the "opiates" immunoassay uses antibodies specific for morphine metabolites and detects the presence of natural and some semisynthetic opioids such as heroin, morphine, and codeine. Detecting synthetic opioids, such as tramadol, hydrocodone, oxycodone, buprenorphine, or fentanyl, requires an extended opioid panel. The following substances are reported to cause false-positive UDS results:

Drug tested	Substance used causing false-positive UDS result
Amphetamines	Labetolol, ranitidine, buproprion, pseudoephedrine, ephedrine, amantadine, desipramine, selegeline, trazodone, methylphenidate, Vicks inhalers
Benzodiazepines	Sertraline
Barbiturates	Phenytoin, nonsteroidal antiinflammatory drug
Marijuana	Proton pump inhibitors, dronabinol, nonsteroidal antiinflammatory drug
Opiates	Ofloxacin, rifampicin, poppy seeds (papaverine), fluoroquinolone
PCP	Venlafaxine, dextromethorphan, ketamine

47. **C.** Cannabis

Cannabis remains an illegal substance federally in the United States. Caffeine is the most commonly used psychogenic substance, alcohol is the most widely used addictive substance, marijuana is the most commonly used illicit substance, and opioid pain medications are the most commonly abused prescription drug (except in high school students who most commonly abuse prescribed amphetamines). This question is tricky because it is not asking about which SUD is most prevalent, that would be alcohol use disorder (or cannabis use disorder in adolescents). This question is not asking about the most widely used substance with psychotropic effects; that would be caffeine (caffeine and alcohol, not illicit substances). This question is not asking about the substance whose use increased the most over the past 2 decades, which would be opioids.

48. **A.** Glaucoma

Excessive alcohol use can cause significant problems in cardiovascular, pulmonary, and liver function, but not glaucoma. Some complications include dilated cardiomyopathy marked by hypercontractility, reduced cardiac output with increased systemic vascular resistance caused by both the toxic effects of alcohol and acetaldehyde accumulation, portal venous diseases, and portal hypertension marked by hyperdynamic cardiovascular function with increased cardiac output and decreased systemic vascular resistance. Excessive alcohol use can also cause arrhythmias including atrial fibrillation (holiday heart). Osteonecrosis of the hip is almost always due to excessive alcohol or steroid use. It presents with dull groin pain.

49. **E.** Distortion of senses

Hallucinogens such as the lysergic acid diethylamide (LSD) and other centrally acting agents can affect body temperature. People who use LSD can experience visual hallucinations, an artificial sense of euphoria, and a distortion of one's sense of time and identity.

50. **B.** Naltrexone

Naltrexone is the only medication listed that primarily acts by reducing the euphoric and pleasant effects of alcohol by blocking opioid pathways projecting to the reward areas of the brain, thereby reducing alcohol-induced dopamine release and the positive reinforcing effects of alcohol. Disulfiram predominantly works by creating a highly aversive reaction (i.e., a punishment) in the presence of alcohol, thereby incentivizing the patient to avoid it completely. Acamprosate reduces symptoms of protracted withdrawal during abstinence and has no effect on the positive reinforcing effects of alcohol. Sertraline has little efficacy for use in AUD beyond treating a co-occurring psychiatric disorder. Gabapentin has no effects on the positive reinforcing properties of alcohol. Naltrexone is the best choice.

BLOCK 3

1. **D.** Alcohol intoxication at the time of the commission of the crime does not negate specific intent or mens rea.

A security guard at a bar told Mr. Saille that he could no longer drink because he appeared intoxicated and asked him to leave. Mr. Saille went home, grabbed a gun, and returned to shoot the guard but accidentally shot another patron. In court, he contended that voluntary intoxication should negate malice and mens rea (evil intent). The California Supreme Court ruled that voluntary intoxication did not reduce criminal responsibility. The court reasoned that evidence of mental illness should not be admitted showing or negating the capacity to form any mental state.

2. **E.** (1): Beneficence and (2): autonomy

Autonomy, beneficence, nonmaleficence, and justice are the four principles of medical ethics.

Autonomy principle requires that patients are free to make their own choices as long as they are competent and have autonomy in their thought process, intentions and actions when making medical decisions. As such, the medical decision-making process must be free of coercion or undue influence.

- Beneficence principle requires that any medical decision offered, or any clinical intervention performed, serve to promote the health and welfare of patients. It requires that clinical providers acquire the necessary knowledge and skills.
- Nonmaleficence principles require that any medical decision offered, or any clinical intervention performed, does not harm the patient.
- Justice principle requires that health care providers make medical decisions that treat patients equally and that the burden and benefits of new or experimental interventions are distributed fairly across all patients.

In this case, the physician's actions suggest a paternalistic approach. The physician valued promoting the health and welfare of the patient (seeking to improve the burden of the patient's depression) over the patient's autonomy and professed choice to continue smoking marijuana.

3. **B.** Deontological theory

In medical practice, it is not uncommon to face situations where there is discordance in applying the autonomy, beneficence, nonmaleficence, and justice ethical principles. Different ethical theories can help guide clinical decision making in such situations:

- Dialectical principlism theory is based on the major moral principles and requires the balancing of competing principles in order to find a rich and ethically acceptable solution.

- Deontological theory deals with the clinician's duty and moral obligation to "do the right thing."
- Utilitarianism theory aims to achieve the greatest good for the greatest number of people.
- Liberal individualism theory places paramount importance on the patient's rights and autonomy.
- Virtue theory examines whether the clinical provider intended to do good by the patient, showing good character and moral values while placing less emphasis on strictly following the rules and consequences.
- Consequentialism theory determines the moral worth of an action based on whether its outcomes or consequences are good or bad.

In this case, the psychiatrist determined that protecting the beneficence principle would violate the patient's autonomy and vice versa. The psychiatrist used a paternalistic approach, prioritizing the health and welfare of the patient (beneficence) over the patient's autonomy. This is consistent with the deontological theory.

4. **C.** A 27-year-old athlete prescribed codeine after a meniscal injury surgical repair.

In a standard UDS test commonly referred to as an SAMHSA-5 assay, the "opiates" immunoassay uses antibodies specific for morphine metabolites. It detects the presence of natural and some semisynthetic opioids such as heroin, morphine, and codeine. Detecting synthetic opioids such as meperidine, methadone, hydrocodone, oxycodone, buprenorphine, or fentanyl requires an extended opioid panel.

5. **C.** Acamprosate

Acamprosate should only be started when the patient has achieved abstinence; because of its GABAergic and antiglutamatergic activity, it is believed to attenuate the symptoms of protracted alcohol withdrawal that place patients at risk for relapse during early abstinence.

6. **A.** It is a positive allosteric modulator of GABA-A receptors.

Acamprosate is a positive allosteric modulator of the GABA-A receptor and an NMDA receptor antagonist. It reduces glutamatergic activity and increases GABAergic activity during early abstinence and can counteract protracted withdrawal symptoms. Answer choices B and D describe the mechanism of action for baclofen and gabapentin, respectively. Answer choice E describes the mechanism of action for naltrexone.

7. **D.** Alpha-2-delta-1 subunit of voltage-gated calcium channels antagonist

Gabapentin was designed to be a structural analog of GABA and closely resembles endogenous amino acids. Gabapentin does not directly agonize or antagonize the GABA-A or GABA-B receptor and does not modulate GABA activity. Gabapentin inhibits the alpha-2-delta-1 subunit of voltage-gated calcium channels.

8. **E.** Confirmation by GC-MS can help identify false positives from true positives.

Standard UDS tests utilize immunoassays to detect the presence of specific compounds. Any positive test on a UDS should be sent to GC-MS confirmation testing. Poppy seeds may cause a false-positive opiate test on UDS. GC-MS confirmation or hair drug testing would not result in a false-positive result. Ofloxacin, rifampicin, and fluoroquinolone can also result in false-positive opiate tests on UDS.

9. **B.** Hair drug testing is often accurate and should not be used in clinical situations.

Drug testing utilizing a blood matrix has the shortest window of detection. Most drugs are cleared from circulating blood within hours. As a result, blood has a concise window of detection, making it an impractical matrix for drug testing. In contrast, hair has the most extended window of detection, up to 3 months. Urine drug testing tests utilize immunoassays to detect the presence of specific compounds.

10. **B.** pH: 6; temperature: 98°F; urine creatinine: 18 mg/dL; specific gravity: 1.007; nitrites: 4 mg/dL

A normal urine sample is valid for testing if:

- No gross adulterants are identified on visual examination

- Temperature between 90°F and100°F
- pH between 4.5 and 8.5
- Nitrites less than 5 mg/dL
- Urine creatinine between 2 and 20 mg/dL
- Specific gravity between 1.0030 and 1.0200

Upon review by the medical review officer, UDS results are reported as:

- Negative: No drug metabolites found, and all validity testing parameters listed above within normal range
- Negative—dilute: No drug metabolites found, creatinine concentration between 2 and 20 mg/dL AND the specific gravity between 1.0010 and 1.0030, but all other validity testing parameters within normal range
- Positive with drug metabolites noted: Drug metabolites found, and all validity testing parameters within normal range
- Positive with drug metabolites noted—dilute: Drug metabolites found, creatinine concentration between 2 and 20 mg/dL, AND the specific gravity between 1.0010 and 1.0030, but all other validity testing parameters within normal range
- Adulterated: Nitrite concentration greater than 500 mg/dL, urine pH less than 4 or greater or equal than 11, or if the presence of chromium, halogens, glutaraldehyde, pyridine, surfactants or any other adulterant is verified
- Substituted: Creatinine concentration less than 2.0 mg/dL AND the specific gravity less than 1.0010 or greater than 1.0200
- Invalid: Inconsistent creatinine and specific gravity values or if urine pH is between 4 and 4.5 or between 9 and 11

11. **C.** Alcohol-related neurodevelopmental disorder

This question is testing your knowledge of the diagnostic criteria for fetal alcohol spectrum disorders (FASD). This patient meets the criteria for the alcohol-related neurodevelopmental disorder. Generally, individuals with FASD are above the threshold for intellectual disability (IQ > 70). If this same patient had two or more FAS facial features, he would meet partial FAS criteria. The diagnosis of FAS requires four criteria: (1) two or more characteristic facial features (short palpebral fissures, thin vermillion border, or smooth philtrum), (2) growth retardation, (3) evidence of brain involvement, and (4) neurobehavioral impairments. Documented alcohol exposure is not required for the FAS diagnosis.

12. **C.** Coronary occlusion

Severe myocardial disease or coronary occlusion is an absolute contraindication to disulfiram use. The disulfiram–alcohol reaction can cause coronary vasospasm, chest pain, and, in rare cases, cardiorespiratory death. Hepatic impairment is a relative but not absolute contraindication to its use. Disulfiram can cause fatal drug-induced hepatitis in 1/30,000 patients and increase cholestatic and fulminant hepatitis. Physiological dependence on opioids is a contraindication for using naltrexone, but not disulfiram. Depression (severe or otherwise) and migraines are not contraindications for using disulfiram.

13. **B.** High neuroticism

Alcohol use disorder is significantly associated with higher neuroticism, lower conscientiousness, and lower agreeableness. It is not associated with differences in extraversion or openness to experience (Malouff et al., 2007).

14. **C.** Operant conditioning

Methadone maintenance programs provide incentives for abstinence by reducing required days of attendance based on the duration of abstinence; conversely, active substance use is punished by the removal of take-home medication privileges. Contingency management is an evidence-based treatment approach that systematically reinforces desired behaviors by using rewarding and punishing reinforcements and is an example of operant conditioning. Classical conditioning describes how a neutral (unconditioned) stimulus elicits a response after being paired with a biological potent (conditioned) stimulus (answer choice A). Incentive salience refers to the desire or motivation to use a substance after being exposed to substance-related cues (answer choice B). Contingency management in MMTP utilizes both positive and negative reinforcements (answer choices D and E),

and the use of these reinforcements to promote behavior change is an example of operant conditioning (Stitzer & Petry, 2006).

15. **D.** Negative reinforcement

Drug courts have a strong behavioral orientation and generally utilize negative reinforcements more often than positive support to maintain the desired behavior. In negative reinforcement, a negative stimulus (in this case, required program attendance) is reduced with a behavior (continued abstinence). In positive reinforcement, a reward is provided for the desired behavior (e.g., praise or a small monetary reward).

16. **C.** Family-based treatment

Studies have consistently demonstrated the efficacy of family-based therapy for adolescents with cannabis use disorder, with some studies showing superiority compared with other individual and group-based treatments. Family-based treatment addresses a wider scope of issues, including family communication, peer networks, work, and school attendance. Answer choices A, B, and E do not have a strong evidence based for treatment of adolescent cannabis use disorder. Relapse prevention (answer choice D) would not be appropriate for an individual who is actively using substances and ambivalent about stopping (Hogue & Liddle, 2009).

17. **B.** The prevalence of SUDs among physicians is similar to that in the general population. Physicians with SUDs have a good prognosis, as the potential to lose one's license serves as an alternative reinforcer for sobriety.

Physicians, in general, are as likely as the general population to be diagnosed with an SUD. Among physicians, anesthesiologists and emergency physicians have the highest rates of SUDs. Once the SUD is identified and the physician submits to treatment and monitoring for SUD, prognosis for treatment is good as nearly four in five physicians achieve and sustain recovery. The fear of losing one's license combined with the highly structured treatment programs offered through the physician's health programs contribute to these high recovery rates. SUD in physicians should be suspected when they exhibit signs or symptoms (albeit often non-specific) such as the deterioration in their physical appearance, irritability, behavioral changes, significant weight changes, changes in sleeping patterns, or smelling of alcohol.

18. **B.** A 27-year-old man who assaulted another patron at a bar after someone "roofied" him by surreptitiously putting flunitrazepam (Rohypnol) in his drink

Engaging in a criminal act does not necessarily mean that the person is criminally responsible or that they would be adjudicated guilty of the crime. Legal incompetence, insanity, and involuntary intoxication represent three exceptions whereby a person may commit unlawful behavior without being adjudicated guilty. Involuntary intoxication refers to situations in which a person is tricked, forced under duress or undue influence to consume an intoxicating substance, or experience an atypical reaction to a substance or an intoxicating medication side effect.

19. **E.** Alcohol Use Disorders Identification Test (AUDIT)

The Alcohol Use Disorders Identification Test (AUDIT) is a validated questionnaire identifying excessive or otherwise maladaptive patterns of alcohol use. Its short version, the AUDIT-C consists of three questions:

- How often do you have alcohol?
- How many standard drink units (SDUs) do you drink on a typical day?
- How often do you have six or more drinks on one occasion?

A score of four or more for men or three or more for women is considered positive. Of the options listed, the AUDIT is the only tool that was validated in multiple controlled studies.
The MAST screens for alcohol use in the elderly; the TWEAK (tolerance, worry, eye-opener, amnesia, K-cutting down) questionnaire screens for alcohol use in pregnant women; the CAGE questionnaire is not a validated instrument with wide applicability in SBIRT; ASI assesses SUD severity in seven potential problem areas (medical status, employment and support, drug use, alcohol use, legal status, family and social status, and psychiatric status) but is not widely utilized in SBIRT.

20. **C.** He has developed tolerance to alcohol and can withstand higher alcohol levels

Patients without alcohol tolerance who present with a blood alcohol level between 300 and 400 mg/dL are at risk for coma, respiratory depression, and death. In this case, the patient very likely is a heavy chronic alcohol user and has developed a high tolerance to its intoxicant effects. Neither cocaine nor a concurrent manic episode would explain this patient's functional status at this serum alcohol level (answer choices A and B). Even if the patient had a genetic polymorphism that allowed him to rapidly metabolize alcohol, it would not explain his functional status at this alcohol level (answer choice E).

21. **C.** GABAergic underactivity and glutamatergic overactivity

Alcohol enhances inhibitory GABA-A receptor function and inhibits excitatory glutamatergic NMDA receptors. Cessation of alcohol use in an individual who is alcohol dependent results in the pathophysiology of alcohol withdrawal: loss of GABAergic inhibition, glutamatergic overactivity, and a severe hyperadrenergic state.

22. **E.** Ability to abstain from alcohol temporarily

Cloninger's typology is frequently referred to in clinical practice and is a validated approach to categorizing alcohol use disorder. Type I patients typically develop alcohol use disorder later in life, are more likely to suffer from other psychiatric disorders, affect men and women equally, and typically respond better to treatment. In contrast, type II patients are defined as having earlier onset of alcohol use disorder (<25 years of age), a prominent family history of alcohol use disorder, higher prevalence of antisocial behaviors, are predominantly men, and are often unable to abstain from alcohol even temporarily (Leggio et al., 2009).

23. **D.** Courage

AA meetings involve an opening ritual that includes the serenity prayer, group members sharing their experiences, and closing rituals. AA principles include taking responsibility, finding humility, and using honesty. AA uses tools based on psychological principles, including stimulus control and cue reactivity (surrounding oneself with sober social connections and avoiding people, places, and things associated with alcohol use), reconditioning (or counterconditioning: learning healthier behaviors for managing urges and substituting addictive behaviors such as seeking support from a sponsor, desensitization, assertion, and cognitive counters to irrational assertions), and positive reinforcement (offering "chips" to celebrate the duration a member has been sober).

The Serenity Prayer is: "God, grant me the serenity to accept the things I cannot change, the courage to change the things I can, and the wisdom to know the difference."

24. **D.** Step 9

Twelve-step-based programs rely on active rather than passive participation. The model views SUD as a chronic disease rather than a temporary state of excessive substance use. The principles focus on acceptance, surrendering, and actively participating in meetings and activities related to recovery. Members are encouraged to "work through" the 12 steps of AA, surrender to a higher power, and select a sponsor who can provide mentorship, guidance, and support to help the member work through the steps. The 12 steps of AA are:

- I can't (We are powerless over alcohol and our lives have become unmanageable.)
- God can (Power greater than ourselves can restore us to sanity.)
- Let God (Turn our will and our lives over to the care of God as we understood Him.)
- Look within (Made a searching and fearless moral inventory of ourselves.)
- Admit wrongs (Admitted to God, to ourselves, and to another human being the exact nature of our wrongs.)

- Ready self for change (Were entirely ready to have God remove all these defects of character.)
- Seek God's help (Humbly asked Him to remove our shortcomings.)
- Become willing (Made a list of all persons we had harmed and became willing to make amends to them all.)
- Make amends (Made direct amends to such people wherever possible, except when to do so would injure them or others.)
- Daily inventory (Continued to take personal inventory and when we were wrong promptly admit it.)
- Pray and meditate (Sought through prayer and meditation to improve our conscious contact with God as we understood Him, praying only for knowledge of His will for us and power to carry that out.)
- Give it away (Having had a spiritual awakening as the result of these steps, we tried to carry this message to alcoholics and to practice these principles in all our affairs.)

25. **C.** ADHD treatment, including the use of stimulants, does not increase the risk of SUD.

Persons with ADHD are more likely to develop SUD and do so at an earlier age. Treating ADHD, including the use of stimulants as treatment, does not increase the risk of SUD, and the data suggest that it might reduce the risk of having an SUD. The misuse of prescription stimulants for treating ADHD is seen most commonly among friends of persons with ADHD rather than among individuals with ADHD.

26. **C.** An essential aspect of treating patients with comorbid borderline personality disorder and alcohol use disorder involves setting and maintaining strict therapeutic limits and boundaries.

Patients with personality disorders, particularly borderline and antisocial personality disorders, may present with personality traits that are easily confused with substance-induced characterological traits and behaviors. A careful history and longitudinal assessment can help identify the true etiology of such traits. When treating patients with comorbid personality disorders and SUD, an emphasis on structure and limit-setting is required. Effective treatment often involves acceptance of vulnerability and of being ordinary. Personality disorders are highly comorbid with SUD, and among men with SUD, antisocial personality disorder is particularly prevalent. Overall, two-thirds of persons with cannabis or stimulant use conditions and one-third of those with nicotine or alcohol use disorder will have a comorbid mood, anxiety, or personality disorder.

27. **C.** Her medication regimen caused a recurrence of psychotic symptoms.

Disulfiram blocks dopamine beta-hydroxylase, the enzyme responsible for metabolizing dopamine, which results in increased dopamine levels in the central nervous system. Such newly elevated dopamine levels may trigger a recurrence of psychotic symptoms, as was seen in this case. Disulfiram is not contraindicated in patients with schizophrenia. However, ample psychoeducation should be provided to patients and their families to recognize early signs of a possible psychotic decompensation.

28. **E.** All of the above are possible

The relationship between substance use, SUDs, and psychiatric symptoms is complex. When thinking about the psychiatric manifestations of SUD, one must differentiate between:

- The expected effects of the substance: Drugs and alcohol intoxication or withdrawal cause psychiatric signs and symptoms that are part of the normal toxidrome of a given substance.
- Substance induced disorders: This category refers to the presence of psychiatric symptoms that:
  - Vastly exceed the expected effects of being intoxicated with or withdrawing from a substance
  - Meet diagnostic criteria for a psychiatric disorder (psychotic, bipolar, depressive, anxiety, obsessive compulsive, sleep, sexual, or neurocognitive disorder)
  - Develop during or soon after substance intoxication or withdrawal
  - Improve after a period of abstinence
- Co-occurring primary psychiatric disorders: This category refers to psychiatric disorders that either preceded or followed the onset of an SUD, but neither condition played a causative role in the onset of the other.
- Secondary psychiatric disorders: This category refers to psychiatric disorders that follow the onset of an SUD, with the SUD playing a causative role in the onset of the co-occurring psychiatric disorder. Unlike substance-induced disorders, with secondary psychiatric disorders, the symptoms do not improve after a period of abstinence

29. **D.** Intellectual disability

Suicide risk assessments involve examining specific factors, precipitants, and features that may generally increase or decrease the risk for suicide and that may serve as modifiable targets for both acute and ongoing interventions and address the patient's immediate safety and determine the most appropriate treatment setting. Once factors are identified, the psychiatrist can determine if they are modifiable. Risk factors can be categorized as being either dynamic and modifiable or static and unmodifiable. Modifiable risk factors are those that are amenable to change. This is an important point, as the identification of modifiable risk factors should be used to direct decision-making regarding intervention and support planning. Static risk factors cannot be changed, such as history (including a history of suicide attempts, comorbid psychiatric diagnoses including SUD), family history, and demographic characteristics. While static factors are essential to identify baseline risk, they cannot be the focus of intervention. Instead, mental health experts can decrease a patient's suicide risk by recognizing and mitigating dynamic suicide risk factors (such as current intoxication, access to means for suicide), and promoting or strengthening protective factors. All of the above answer choices are risk factors for suicide, with the exception of intellectual disability, which is associated with a lower odds of suicide (Harris & Barraclough, 1997).

30. **A.** Chlordiazepoxide

Chlordiazepoxide is metabolized hepatically. It has a longer half-life of active metabolites compared to the other options. The other benzodiazepines listed above are metabolized by glucuronide conjugation. This enzyme is more rapid and produces inactive metabolites, making it safer for liver disease patients. Gabapentin metabolism is not primarily hepatic.

31. **D.** Liver transplant

This patient presentation is consistent with liver cirrhosis caused by chronic untreated HCV. Up to 60% to 80% of injection drug users are HCV positive. Untreated, it can lead to progressive hepatic disease, cirrhosis, and hepatocellular carcinoma. It can cause hepatorenal syndrome, a renal failure in patients with acute and severe liver failure from decompensated cirrhosis or acute fulminant hepatitis, causing jaundice, coagulopathy, and hepatic death and renal failure or variceal bleeding. Hepatic cirrhosis manifests with signs and symptoms of hepatitis in addition to portal venous disease, portal hypertension, ascites, bacterial peritonitis, hepatocellular carcinoma, varices, and hepatic failure. This condition is irreversible even with discontinuation of alcohol use. Liver transplants are the only effective therapeutic intervention for cirrhosis. Hepatic cirrhosis is associated with a 50% 2-year mortality rate and is the second most common cause of liver transplants. To be eligible for a transplant, one must abstain from alcohol use for at least 6 months. Transplants are indicated with ascites, encephalopathy, jaundice, or portal hypertension.

32. **B.** TSF aims to encourage attendance and meaningful utilization of 12-step meetings.

TSF is not a 12-step mutual support group. It is a manualized and structured 12-session approach that promotes the patient's engagement in 12-step mutual support groups. In TSF, the therapist encourages the patient to participate in 12-step mutual support groups and guides them through the first four steps. Participation in TSF increases the likelihood that SUD patients will affiliate with a mutual support group and reduce their substance use (data supporting its effectiveness in alcohol is strongest).

33. **C.** HCV is most prevalent among those born between 1945 and 1965.

HCV is the most common chronic bloodborne infectious agent, four times more prevalent than HIV. Its prevalence is highest among those born between 1945 and 1965 (between 3% and 4%), the group known as the Baby Boomer generation. Up to 60% to 80% of injection drug users are HCV positive. Untreated, it can lead to progressive hepatic disease, cirrhosis, and hepatocellular carcinoma. Risk factors for worse prognosis include alcohol use, HCV genotype 1, older age at the time of infection, male gender, co-occurring HBV, and higher viral load at the time of treatment initiation. The medical management of HCV includes ensuring that the person is vaccinated against HAV/HBV and limiting alcohol consumption. Historically, HCV treatment consisted of interferon and ribavirin. Newer interferon-free HCV antivirals have been developed and are becoming more easily accessible. These include sofosbuvir, simeprevir, and ledipasvir.

34. **D.** Efavirenz

Antiretroviral medications used to treat patients with HIV include nucleoside reverse transcriptase inhibitors (NRTI), nonnucleoside reverse transcriptase inhibitors (NNRTI), protease inhibitors (PI), or integrase inhibitors (II). Highly active antiretroviral therapy (HAART) refers to a customizable combination of antiretroviral medications to help patients with HIV achieve an undetectable viral load. Standard HAART protocols typically include two NRTIs combined with one NNRTI, or one PI or one II. Efavirenz, an NNRTI, is the antiretroviral medication most associated with psychiatric adverse effects, including anxiety, depression, suicidal ideation, confusion, and hallucinations.

35. **E.** Performing multiple longitudinal psychiatric assessments

When thinking about the psychiatric manifestations of substance use, one has to differentiate between:

■ The expected effects of the substance: Drugs and alcohol intoxication or withdrawal cause psychiatric signs and symptoms that are part of the normal toxidrome of a given substance. For example, feeling euphoric after using cocaine or anxious when going through alcohol withdrawal are expected effects of cocaine intoxication or alcohol withdrawal and should not be labeled as a manic or anxiety syndrome.

■ Substance-induced disorders: This category refers to the presence of psychiatric symptoms that:

  ■ Vastly exceed the expected effects of being intoxicated with or withdrawing from a substance

  ■ Meet diagnostic criteria for a psychiatric disorder (psychotic, bipolar, depressive, anxiety, obsessive compulsive, sleep, sexual or neurocognitive disorder)

  ■ Develop during or soon after substance intoxication or withdrawal

  ■ The symptoms improve after a period of abstinence

■ Co-occurring primary psychiatric disorders: This category refers to psychiatric disorders that either preceded or followed the onset of a SUD, but neither condition played a causative role in the onset of the other. For example, tobacco use disorder and schizophrenia often co-occur, but schizophrenia does not cause the onset of tobacco use disorder and tobacco use disorder does not cause the onset of schizophrenia.

■ Secondary psychiatric disorders: This category refers to psychiatric disorders that follow the onset of an SUD, with the SUD playing a causative role in the onset of the co-occurring psychiatric disorder. Unlike substance-induced disorders, with secondary psychiatric disorders, the symptoms do not improve after a period of abstinence

A comprehensive clinical evaluation that is performed multiple times longitudinally will assist the prudent psychiatrist in making the correct diagnostic determination.

36. **D.** How many times did you have five or more drinks in a single day for men or four or more drinks for women over the past year?

The NIAAA single-question alcohol screen has been validated as a single-item screen for detecting alcohol use disorder with a sensitivity and specificity equivalent to longer screening instruments like the AUDIT. Persons who screen positive should then receive an in-depth assessment to determine the risk level. Brief intervention and advice follow (per the SBIRT model).

37. **B.** Naloxone

Naloxone is used in opioid overdoses to counteract life-threatening effects on the central nervous system and respiratory system.

38. **C.** Screening and brief intervention

SBIRT serves as a public health initiative to identify persons at risk for developing a SUD or with an undetected SUD at the primary care level. It offers less severe substance use simple interventions to address simple substance use problems and refer those with more complex substance use treatment needs to specialized services. There's no information in the vignette suggesting that this patient requires a referral to specialized SUD treatment services, and as a result, screening and a brief intervention would suffice. Motivational interviewing (MI) is an evidence-based psychotherapeutic intervention aiming to resolve ambivalence and increase motivation to change maladaptive behaviors. Brief interventions are often modeled on the MI approach.

39. **D.** A 34-year-old man who drinks 5 alcoholic beverages 6 days a week seen at his primary care clinic for his annual physical exam.

SBI refers to an evidence-based practice to identify, reduce, and prevent maladaptive substance use used in primary care or other non-SUD-focused settings. Evidence supporting BI efficacy is strongest for maladaptive alcohol use. BI is particularly useful with patients with less severe alcohol use problems. BI for alcohol is associated with an overall reduction in alcohol use, drinking days, binge drinking, and alcohol-related deaths. Studies examining BI for illicit drug use found BI to be ineffective and costly, and as such, BI is not recommended to address the needs of patients with illicit drug use.

40. **A.** The perceived risk of marijuana use has declined among this age group.

For over the past decade, the perceived risk of cannabis use has been declining, accompanied by an increase in cannabis use among teenagers and young adults. The inverse relationship between perceived risk and use also applies to cigarette smoking, which has declined among this age group, as its perceived risk has been increasing. The THC content in cannabis has steadily been increasing due to selective breeding for higher THC: CBD plants (answer choice C and D). Marijuana is classified as an illegal Schedule I drug by the federal government (answer choice E).

41. **D.** Liver disease

In the United States, alcohol-related mortality has alarmingly doubled between 1999 and 2017. This has been the subject of extensive national discussion and was highlighted by the economists Anne Case and Angus Deaton. These deaths, also coined "deaths of despair," are primarily due to liver disease (31%), followed by overdoses (18%), either with alcohol alone or in combination with other drugs, followed by cardiovascular disease (11%) based on mortality data from 2017. However, globally, alcohol-related injuries (traffic accidents, self-harm, or violence) are the most common cause of alcohol-related mortality.

42. **B.** Placental abruption

The increased level of catecholamines caused by cocaine use during pregnancy can cause vasospasm in the uterine blood vessels, increasing the risk of experiencing placental separation and abruption.

43. **B.** Phencyclidine

Both ketamine and phencyclidine are NMDA receptor antagonists. They mainly affect the central nervous system causing hallucinations, lightheadedness, headache, nightmares, and sensory changes.

44. **A.** Low birth weight

Exposing the fetus to heroin and other illicit substances can cause central nervous system hyperirritability, autonomic nervous system dysfunction, and gastrointestinal disturbances. Low birth weight, oligohydramnios, and a decreased head circumference are common findings.

45. **D.** State-dependent learning

State-dependent learning occurs when behavior acquired in the presence of a particular drug is performed better on subsequent occasions when that drug is present than when it is absent. Tolerance can be created by the constant and chronic use of a substance, and a higher amount is needed to have the same desire wanted, while the suddenly reduced dose might cause withdrawal. These symptoms can be mild (e.g., nausea or vomiting) or more serious (e.g., psychosis or seizures).

46. **D.** Discontinue zolpidem

Zolpidem, zaleplon, and eszopiclone are all known to rarely induce complex behaviors while asleep, including sleepwalking, driving, eating, preparing food, and having sex. The patient generally has no recollection of these actions. Because of case reports of serious injuries and fatalities, the FDA added a contraindication to prescribing these medications for any patient with a history of complex sleep behaviors while on these medications. It is also contraindicated to continue prescribing these medications if patients experience complex sleep behavior after taking any medications (Dyer, 2019).

47. **B.** The requirement for at least 7 days of abstinence before beginning treatment

It is recommended not to start naltrexone until 7 to 14 days of opioid abstinence to decrease the likelihood of precipitating withdrawal symptoms. During this period, patients may drop out of care or lose interest, making this a potential disadvantage of naltrexone.

48. **C.** Naltrexone

Naltrexone effectively reduces the frequency and intensity of gambling urges and should be considered a first-line treatment for pathologic gambling. No significant difference has been shown between bupropion, mood stabilizers, and placebo in reducing the frequency and intensity of gambling urges in recent studies (Yau & Potenza, 2015).

49. **D.** Acamprosate

The FDA approved three medications for the treatment of alcohol use disorder: disulfiram, naltrexone, and acamprosate. Of these, acamprosate would be the preferred medication to use in patients with hepatic insufficiency. It is excreted in urine as an unmetabolized drug. As a result, it should not be used as a first-line agent for patients with renal impairment. Naltrexone is metabolized hepatically via non-cytochrome–mediated dehydrogenase. It is subject to an extensive first-pass effect and can be associated with an increase in serum transaminases. It is contraindicated in patients with acute hepatitis or hepatic failure. Disulfiram is metabolized hepatically via glucuronidation and possible side effects include cholestatic hepatitis, fulminant hepatitis, and hepatic failure. It is relatively contraindicated in patients with hepatic cirrhosis. Gabapentin and ondansetron are used as second-line treatment options for alcohol use disorder but are not FDA approved for this condition.

50. **D.** Verbal learning

Some or all of the above cognitive domains have been found to become impaired in 50% to 70% of individuals with alcohol use disorder; however, verbal learning impairments are most quick to reverse following cessation of use with some studies demonstrating recovery within the first 2 weeks of abstinence. As longer-term abstinence is reached, learning and memory issues are still present in some individuals.

REFERENCES

Anton, R. F., O'Malley, S. S., Ciraulo, D. A., Cisler, R. A., Couper, D., Donovan, D. M., et al. COMBINE Study Research Group. (2006). Combined pharmacotherapies and behavioral interventions for alcohol dependence: The COMBINE study: A randomized controlled trial. *Journal of the American Medical Association, 295*(17), 2003–2017.

Anton, R. F., Oroszi, G., O'Malley, S., Couper, D., Swift, R., Pettinati, H., et al. (2008). An evaluation of mu-opioid receptor (OPRM1) as a predictor of naltrexone response in the treatment of alcohol dependence: Results from the Combined Pharmacotherapies and Behavioral Interventions for Alcohol Dependence (COMBINE) study. *Archives of General Psychiatry, 65*(2), 135–144.

Bachhuber, M. A., Hennessy, S., Cunningham, C. O., & Starrels, J. L. (2016). Increasing benzodiazepine prescriptions and overdose mortality in the United States, 1996-2013. *American Journal of Public Health, 106*(4), 686–688.

Brezing, C. A., & Levin, F. R. (2018). The current state of pharmacological treatments for cannabis use disorder and withdrawal. *Neuropsychopharmacology, 43*(1), 173–194.

Ceylan-Isik, A. F., McBride, S. M., & Ren, J. (2010). Sex difference in alcoholism: who is at a greater risk for development of alcoholic complication? *Life Sciences, 87*(5-6), 133–138.

Cone, E. J., Bigelow, G. E., Herrmann, E. S., Mitchell, J. M., LoDico, C., Flegel, R., et al. (2015). Non-smoker exposure to secondhand cannabis smoke. I. Urine screening and confirmation results. *Journal of Analytical Toxicology, 39*(1), 1–12.

DiClemente, C. C., Schlundt, D., & Gemmell, L. (2004). Readiness, and stages of change in addiction treatment. *American Journal of Addiction, 13*(2), 103–119.

Di Forti, M., Iyegbe, C., Sallis, H., Kolliakou, A., Falcone, M. A., Paparelli, A., et al. (2012). Confirmation that the AKT1 (rs2494732) genotype influences the risk of psychosis in cannabis users. *Biological Psychiatry, 72*(10), 811–816.

Dluzen, D. E., & Liu, B. (2008). Gender differences in methamphetamine use and responses: A review. *Gender Medicine, 5*(1), 24–35.

Dodds, T. J. (2017). Prescribed benzodiazepines and suicide risk: A review of the literature. *The Primary Care Companion for CNS Disorders, 19*(2), 16r02037.

Dyer, O. (2019). FDA issues black box warnings on common insomnia drugs. *British Medical Journal, 365*, l2165.

Farkas, R. H., Unger, E. F., & Temple, R. (2013). Zolpidem and driving impairment-identifying persons at risk. *The New England Journal of Medicine, 369*(8), 689–691.

Harris, E. C., & Barraclough, B. (1997). Suicide as an outcome for mental disorders. A meta-analysis. *British Journal of Psychiatry: The Journal of Mental Science, 170*, 205–228.

Heinzerling, A., Armatas, C., Karmarkar, E., Attfield, K., Guo, W., Wang, Y., et al. (2020). Severe lung injury associated with use of e-cigarette, or vaping, products—California, 2019. *JAMA Internal Medicine, 180*(6), 861–869.

Hogue, A., & Liddle, H. A. (2009). Family-based treatment for adolescent substance abuse: Controlled trials and new horizons in services research. *Journal of Family Therapy, 31*(2), 126–154.

Koob, G. F., & Volkow, N. D. (2016). Neurobiology of addiction: A neurocircuitry analysis. *The Lancet Psychiatry, 3*(8), 760–773.

Kosten, T. R., Wu, G., Huang, W., Harding, M. J., Hamon, S. C., Lappalainen, J., et al. (2013). Pharmacogenetic randomized trial for cocaine abuse: Disulfiram and dopamine β-hydroxylase. *Biological Psychiatry, 73*(3), 219–224.

Leggio, L., Kenna, G. A., Fenton, M., Bonenfant, E., & Swift, R. M. (2009). Typologies of alcohol dependence. From Jellinek to genetics and beyond. *Neuropsychology Review, 19*(1), 115–129.

Liechti, M. E., Kunz, I., Greminger, P., Speich, R., & Kupferschmidt, H. (2006). Clinical features of gamma-hydroxybutyrate and gamma-butyrolactone toxicity and concomitant drug and alcohol use. *Drug and Alcohol Dependence, 81*(3), 323–326.

Malouff, J. M., Thorsteinsson, E. B., Rooke, S. E., & Schutte, N. S. (2007). Alcohol involvement and the Five-Factor model of personality: A meta-analysis. *Journal of Drug Education, 37*(3), 277–294.

Matching alcoholism treatments to client heterogeneity: Project MATCH three-year drinking outcomes. (1998). *Alcoholism: Clinical and Experimental Research, 22*(6), 1300–1311.

Monte, A. A., Shelton, S. K., Mills, E., Saben, J., Hopkinson, A., Sonn, B., et al. (2019). Acute illness associated with cannabis use, by route of exposure: An observational study. *Annals of Internal Medicine, 170*(8), 531–537.

Nestler, E. J. (2005). Is there a common molecular pathway for addiction? *Nature Neuroscience, 8*(11), 1445–1449.

Newton, T. F., Reid, M. S., De La Garza, R., Mahoney, J. J., Abad, A., Condos, R., et al. (2008). Evaluation of subjective effects of aripiprazole and methamphetamine in methamphetamine-dependent volunteers. *International Journal of Neuropsychopharmacology, 11*(8), 1037–1045.

Nunes, E. V., & Levin, F. R. (2008). Treatment of co-occurring depression and substance dependence: Using meta-analysis to guide clinical recommendations. *Psychiatric Annals, 38*(11), nihpa128505.

Robison, A. J., & Nestler, E. J. (2011). Transcriptional and epigenetic mechanisms of addiction. *Nature Reviews. Neuroscience, 12*(11), 623–637.

Shinn, A. K., & Greenfield, S. F. (2010). Topiramate in the treatment of substance-related disorders: A critical review of the literature. *Journal of Clinical Psychiatry, 71*(5), 634–648.

Sorensen, C. J., DeSanto, K., Borgelt, L., Phillips, K. T., & Monte, A. A. (2017). Cannabinoid hyperemesis syndrome: Diagnosis, pathophysiology, and treatment—A systematic review. *Journal of Medical Toxicology, 13*(1), 71–87.

Stitzer, M., & Petry, N. (2006). Contingency management for treatment of substance abuse. *Annual Review of Clinical Psychology, 2*, 411–434.

Yau, Y. H., & Potenza, M. N. (2015). Gambling disorder and other behavioral addictions: Recognition and treatment. *Harvard Review of Psychiatry, 23*(2), 134–146.

INDEX

Page numbers followed by '*f*' indicate figures, '*t*' indicate tables, '*b*' indicate boxes.